Nutritional Influences on Bone Health

Peter Burckhardt · Bess Dawson-Hughes
Connie Weaver
Editors

Nutritional Influences on Bone Health

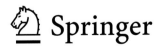 Springer

Peter Burckhardt, MD
Internal Medicine Department
Clinique Bois-Cerf/Hirslanden
Lausanne
Switzerland

Bess Dawson-Hughes, MD
USDA Human Nutrition
Research Centre on Aging
Tufts University Boston
Boston, MA
USA

Connie Weaver, PhD
Foods and Nutrition Department
Purdue University
West Lafayette, IN
USA

ISBN: 978-1-84882-977-0 e-ISBN: 978-1-84882-978-7

DOI: 10.1007/978-1-84882-978-7

Springer Dordrecht Heidelberg London New York

A catalogue record for this book is available from the British Library

Library of Congress Control Number: 2010925795

Springer Science+Business Media (www.springer.com)

Preface

The seventh symposium on "Nutritional Aspects of Osteoporosis" continues to be the primary forum for scientists to focus on the impact of nutrition on bone health in general. Since 1991, the year of the first symposium, research in this field has increased impressively and has become an established part of research and science in osteology. This symposium in particular featured many global comparisons in diet and the effect on bone. As Western diet permeates more of the globe and the population continues to grow, it is meaningful to study the impact of these changes on bone health as diet is one of the few major modifiable factors which in turn affects health care costs. Calcium, vitamin D, and acid-base balance continued to dominate the discussion. The symposium offered an opportunity to learn about theories and data in nutritional research concerning bone as well as methodological approaches to classify diets. The proceedings allow the reader to capture the new messages, to analyze the new scientific data presented, and to use the book as a source of references in this field.

Peter Burckhardt
Bess Dawson-Hughes
Connie Weaver

Acknowledgments

This work comprises papers from the 7th International Symposium on Nutritional Aspects of Osteoporosis in 2009 in Lausanne, Switzerland. The sponsors of this event are listed below:

Main Sponsors
Nestlé
Nycomed
Sandoz

Sponsors
Amgen
Coca-Cola Beverage Institute
Dairy Australia
DSM Nutritional Products (Roche)
Lallemand US
Pharmative US
Procter&Gamble
Servier
Wyeth

Contributors
Glaxo SmithKline
Eli Lilly
International Osteoporosis Foundation
Merck Sharp Dome
National Dairy Council US
Opfermann
Swiss Dairy Producers

Endorsement
International Osteoporosis Foundation

Contents

Contributors

Laura K. Bachrach, MD Clinical Research Center and Columbia University, Helen Hayes Hospital, West Haverstraw, NY, USA

C.W. Binns, MPH, PhD School of Public Health, Curtin University of Technology, Perth, Australia

Heike Bischoff-Ferrari, MD DrPH Centre on Aging and Mobility, Department of Rheumatology and Institute of Physical Medicine, University Hospital Zurich, Zurich, Switzerland

Jean-Philippe Bonjour, MD Division of Bone Sciences, Department of Rehabilitation and Genetics, Geneva University Hospitals and Faculty of Medicine, Geneva, Switzerland

Peter Burckhardt, MD Internal Medicine Department, Clinique Bois-Cerf/Hirslanden, Lausanne, Switzerland

David A. Bushinsky, MD Department of Medicine, University of Rochester School of Medicine, Rochester, NY, USA

Kevin D. Cashman, BSc PhD Department of Food and Nutritional Sciences, University College Cork, Cork, Ireland

Thierry Chevalley, MD Division of Bone Sciences, Department of Rehabilitation and Genetics, Geneva University Hospitals and Faculty of Medicine, Geneva, Switzerland

Kristin L. Cobb, PhD Clinical Research Center and Columbia University, Helen Hayes Hospital, West Haverstraw, NY, USA

Meredith Curtis Clinical Research Center and Columbia University, Helen Hayes Hospital, West Haverstraw, NY, USA

Robin M. Daly, PhD Department of Medicine (RMH/WH), The University of Melbourne, Western Hospital, Melbourne, Australia

Andrea L. Darling, BSc (Hons) Division of Nutritional Sciences, Faculty of Health and Medical Sciences, University of Surrey, Guildford, UK

Bess Dawson-Hughes, MD USDA Human Nutrition Research Centre on Aging, Tufts University Boston, Boston, MA, USA

A. Devine, PhD School of Exercise, Biomedical and Health Science,
Edith Cowan University, Australia

Weijing Du, PhD National Institute for Nutrition and Food Safety,
Chinese Center for Disease Control and Prevention, Beijing, China

Regina Ebert, PhD Orthopedic Center for Musculoskeletal Research,
Orthopedic Department, University of Wuerzburg, Wuerzburg, Germany

Lynda A. Frassetto, MD Clinical Research Center, University of California
San Francisco, San Francisco, CA, USA

G.R. Goldberg, PhD MRC Human Nutrition Research, Elsie Widdowson
Laboratory, Cambridge, UK

Gail Greendale, MD Clinical Research Center and Columbia University,
Helen Hayes Hospital, West Haverstraw, NY, USA

Yian Gu, PhD Clinical Research Center and Columbia University,
Helen Hayes Hospital, West Haverstraw, NY, USA

Véronique Habauzit Human Nutrition Unit, UMR1019, INRA Clermont/Theix,
St-Genès Champanelle, France

Christine Hamann, MD Department of Orthopedics, Technical University,
University of Dresden Medical Center, Dresden, Germany

Antonia C. Hardcastle, PhD MSc BSc Department of Applied Medicine,
University of Aberdeen, Foresterhill, Aberdeen, UK

Kathleen M. Hill Foods and Nutrition Department, Purdue University,
West Lafayette, IN, USA

Kenji Hirota, MD Department of Obstetrics and Gynecology,
Nissay Hospital, Osaka, Japan

Takako Hirota, PhD RD Department of Health and Nutrition,
Kyoto Koka Women's University, Kyoto, Japan

Lorenz C. Hofbauer, MD Division of Endocrinology, Diabetes,
and Metabolic Bone Diseases, Department of Medicine III (LCH),
and Department of Orthopedics (CH), Technical University, Dresden, Germany

Marie-Noëlle Horcajada, PhD Nutrition and Health, Nestle Research Center,
Lausanne, Switzerland

Xiaoqi Hu, MD National Institute for Nutrition and Food Safety,
Chinese Center for Disease Control and, revention, Beijing, China

Franz Jakob, MD Orthopedic Center for Musculoskeletal Research,
Orthopedic Department, University of Wuerzburg, Wuerzburg, Germany

Heini Karp, MSc Calcium Research Unit, Department of Applied Chemistry
and Microbiology, University of Helsinki, Helsinki, Finland

Izumi Kawasaki, PhD Research Laboratory, Tsuji Academy of Nutrition,
Osaka, Japan

Jennifer L. Kelsey, PhD Clinical Research Center and Columbia University, Helen Hayes Hospital, West Haverstraw, NY, USA

Virpi Kemi, MSc Calcium Research Unit, Department of Applied Chemistry and Microbiology, University of Helsinki, Helsinki, Finland

D.A. Kerr, PhD School of Public Health, Curtin University of Technology, Perth, Australia

Christa Kitz, MD DTMH Department of Tropical Medicine, Medical Mission Hospital, Wuerzburg, Germany

Sonja Kukuljan, PhD Deakin University, School of Exercise and Nutrition Sciences, Burwood, Melbourne, Australia

Christel Lamberg-Allardt, PhD Calcium Research Unit, Department of Applied Chemistry and Microbiology, University of Helsinki, Helsinki, Finland

Susan A. Lanham-New, BA MSc PhD Division of Nutritional Sciences, Faculty of Health and Medical Sciences, University of Surrey, Guildford, UK

Joan M. Lappe, PhD RN Department of Nursing and Medicine, Creighton University, Omaha, NE, USA

Warren T.K. Lee, PhD RD Division of Nutritional Sciences, Faculty of Health and Medical Sciences, University of Surrey, Guildford, UK

Lars Libuda, MSc Department of Nutrition and Health, Research Institute of Child Nutrition, Dortmund, Germany

Paul Lips, MD PhD Internal Medicine Division, Section of Endocrinology, University Medical Center, Amsterdam, The Netherlands

Ailing Liu, PhD National Institute for Nutrition and Food Safety, Chinese Center for Disease Control and Prevention, Beijing, China

Jose Luchsinger, MD Clinical Research Center and Columbia University, Helen Hayes Hospital, West Haverstraw, NY, USA

Guansheng Ma, PhD National Institute for Nutrition and Food Safety, Chinese Center for Disease Control and, revention, Beijing, China

Helen M. Macdonald, PhD MSc BSc Department of Applied Medicine, University of Aberdeen, Foresterhill, Aberdeen, UK

Kathryn Melsop, MS Clinical Research Center and Columbia University, Helen Hayes Hospital, West Haverstraw, NY, USA

X. Meng, MD School of Medicine and Pharmacology, University of Western Australia, Perth, Australia

School of Public Health, Curtin University of Technology, Perth, Australia

Jeri W. Nieves, PhD Clinical Research Center and Columbia University, Helen Hayes Hospital, West Haverstraw, NY, USA

Elizabeth Offord, MD Nutrition and Health, Nestle Research Center, Lausanne, Switzerland

A. Prentice, PhD MRC Human Nutrition Research, Elsie Widdowson Laboratory, Cambridge, UK

Richard L. Prince, MD School of Medicine and Pharmacology, University of Western Australia, Perth, Australia

Sir Charles Gairdner Hospital, Perth, Australia

Peter Raab, MD Orthopedic Center for Musculoskeletal Research, Orthopedic Department, University of Wuerzburg, Wuerzburg, Germany

Thomas Remer, PhD Department of Nutrition and Health, Research Institute of Child Nutrition, Dortmund, Germany

René Rizzoli, MD Division of Bone Sciences, Department of Rehabilitation and Genetics, Geneva University Hospitals and Faculty of Medicine, Geneva, Switzerland

Nikolaos Scarmeas, MD Clinical Research Center and Columbia University, Helen Hayes Hospital, West Haverstraw, NY, USA

Olga Schmidlin, MD Department of Medicine, University of California San Francisco, San Francisco, CA, USA

I. Schoenmakers, PhD MRC Human Nutrition Research, Elsie Widdowson Laboratory, Cambridge , UK

Anthony Sebastian, MD Department of Medicine, University of California San Francisco, San Francisco, CA, USA

Lothar Seefried, MD Orthopedic Center for Musculoskeletal Research, Orthopedic Department, University of Wuerzburg, Wuerzburg, Germany

Sue A. Shapses, PhD Nutritional Sciences, Rutgers University, NJ, USA

V. Solah, PhD School of Public Health, Curtin University of Technology, Perth, Australia

MaryFran Sowers, PhD Clinical Research Center and Columbia University, Helen Hayes Hospital, West Haverstraw, NY, USA

Barbara Sponholz, PhD Institute for Geography, University of Wuerzburg, Wuerzburg, Germany

Yaakov Stern, PhD Clinical Research Center and Columbia University, Helen Hayes Hospital, West Haverstraw, NY, USA

August Stich, MD Department of Tropical Medicine, Medical Mission Hospital, Wuerzburg, Germany

Deeptha Sukumar, MS Nutritional Sciences, Rutgers University, NJ, USA

Elizabeth Vasquez Clinical Research Center and Columbia University, Helen Hayes Hospital, West Haverstraw, NY, USA

X. Wang, PhD Department of Preventative Medicine, Shenyang Medical College, Shenyang, China

Xiaoyan Wang, PhD National Institute for Nutrition and Food Safety, Chinese Center for Disease Control and Prevention, Beijing, China

Connie M. Weaver, PhD Foods and Nutrition Department, Purdue University, West Lafayette, IN, USA

Lu Wu, PhD Foods and Nutrition Department, Perdue University, West Lafayette, IN, USA

L. Yan, PhD MRC Human Nutrition Research, Elsie Widdowson Laboratory, Cambridge, UK

Jing Yin, PhD National Institute for Nutrition and Food Safety, Chinese Center for Disease Control and Prevention, Beijing, China

Qian Zhang, PhD National Institute for Nutrition and Food Safety, Chinese Center for Disease Control and Prevention, Beijing, China

B. Zhou, PhD Department of Preventative Medicine, Shenyang Medical College, Shenyang, China

K. Zhu, PhD School of Public Health, Curtin University of Technology, Perth, Australia

Kun Zhu, PhD Department of Endocrinology and Diabetes, Sir Charles Gairdner Hospital, Nedlands, Australia

Dietary Protein and Bone Mass Accrual

René Rizzoli, Jean-Philippe Bonjour, and Thierry Chevalley

1.1 Introduction

For most parts of the skeleton, peak bone mass is achieved by the end of the second decade of life. Puberty is the period during which the sex difference in bone mass observed in adult subjects becomes expressed. More than 60% of the variance of peak bone mass, the amount of bone present in the skeleton at the end of its maturation process, is genetically determined. The remainder is influenced by factors amenable to intervention, such as adequate dietary intake of calcium and proteins or dairy products as a source of these nutrients. A significant positive association can be found between long-term protein intakes, and periosteal circumferences, cortical area, bone mineral content, and with a calculated strength strain index.

In a recent study, we found that BMD/BMC in prepubertal boys were positively associated with spontaneous protein intake. But in this study, increased physical activity was associated with greater BMC at both axial and appendicular sites under high, but not low, protein intake. Thus to optimize bone mass accrual through dietary and physical exercise measures, these interactions as a valuable primary measure for the prevention of fractures later in life should be taken into account.

1.2 Bone Mass Acquisition

Childhood and adolescence are periods characterized by growth, development, and maturation of the various body systems, including the skeletal tissue.[1] Bone modeling begins with the development of the skeleton during fetal life and continues until the end of the second decade, when the epiphyseal growth plates are closed and longitudinal growth of the skeleton is completed. During childhood and adolescence, bones are modeled by bone formation and resorption occurring in distinct locations, leading to the various bone shapes in adults. Although bone remodeling also starts during fetal life, the highest level of remodeling is achieved during adolescence. Remodeling replaces an old bone with a new one without changing the shape of the bone. This process allows for the preservation of skeletal mechanical integrity (e.g., through (micro-)fracture repair) and the control of calcium homeostasis by releasing calcium into the circulation when necessary. Peak bone mass, which is defined as the amount of bone present in the skeleton at the end of its maturation process, is considered to be achieved by the end of the second decade of life.[1] Indeed, prospective observational studies suggest that more than 95% of the adult skeleton is formed by the end of adolescence.[2] Some consolidation, particularly in the cortical bone of male individuals and representing a few percents, can take place during the third decade of life.

An estimate of bone strength derived from the size and the cortical thickness of the distal radius indicates a marked increase of resistance to bending throughout puberty.[3,4] In adolescents, the peak of high longitudinal growth precedes by 1–2 years the peak in bone mineral mass accrual during pubertal spurt, highlighting a dissociation between longitudinal growth and bone mass accumulation.[5] For the midfemoral shaft, this dissociation in time is detectable in males, but less in females.

R. Rizzoli (✉)
Division of Bone Diseases, Department of Rehabilitation and Geriatrics, Geneva University Hospitals and Faculty of Medicine, 1211 Geneva 14, Switzerland
e-mail: rene.rizzoli@unige.ch

P. Burckhardt et al. (eds.), *Nutritional Influences on Bone Health*,
DOI: 10.1007/978-1-84882-978-7_1, © Springer-Verlag London Limited 2010

1.2.1 Factors Influencing Bone Mineral Mass Gain and Peak Bone Mass Acquisition

Bone mineral mass gain during childhood and adolescence is influenced by many factors including heredity and ethnicity, gender, diet (calcium and protein intakes), physical activity, endocrine status (such as sex hormones, vitamin D, growth hormone, and insulin-like growth factor (IGF)-I) (Fig. 1.1),[1,6] as well as exposure to risk factors such as cigarette smoking and alcohol intake. Sixty to eighty percent of the variance in peak bone mass is explained by genetic factors suggesting that the remainder may be amenable to interventions aimed at maximizing peak bone mass within its genetically predefined variance.[7] As a 10% increase in peak bone mass corresponds to a gain of 1 standard deviation in bone mineral density in adulthood, osteoporotic fracture risk may be reduced by up to 50% by interventions aimed at maximizing peak bone mass in a sustainable manner. According to a computer simulation of the bone remodeling process, a 10% higher than the mean young adult areal BMD (aBMD) corresponds to menopause being delayed by 13 years.[8]

1.2.1.1 Dietary Intakes and Bone growth

Dietary proteins provide the body with the necessary amino acids for building the bone matrix.[9] Dietary proteins influence bone growth, as they modify the secretion and action of the osteotropic hormone IGF-I.[10] As such, dietary proteins may modulate the genetic potential of peak bone mass attainment.[11] Low protein intake was shown to have deleterious effects on bone mineral mass acquisition by impairing the production and effects of IGF-I.[10,12,13] IGF-I promotes bone growth by stimulating the proliferation and differentiation of chondrocytes in the epiphyseal growth plate and directly affects the osteoblasts, the bone-forming cells.[14] In addition, IGF-I increases the renal conversion of 25 hydroxy-vitamin D_3 into the active hormone 1,25 dihydroxy-vitamin D_3 and thereby contributes to increased calcium and phosphorus absorption in the gut.[15] Furthermore, IGF-I directly increases the renal tubular reabsorption of phosphorus.[15]

1.2.2 Evidence from Association Studies

Prospective observational studies suggest that both calcium and protein intakes are independent variables

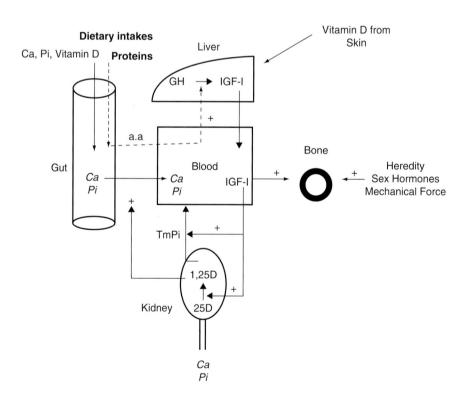

Fig. 1.1 Dietary intakes and bone/calcium–phosphorus homeostasis

Fig. 1.2 Influence of protein intake on the impact of physical activity on bone mineral content, bone scanned projected area, and areal bone mineral density of the femoral neck (FN) in prepubertal boys. From Chevalley et al.[20] With permission from the American Society for Bone and Mineral Research

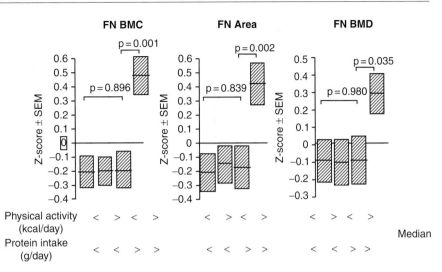

of bone mineral mass acquisition, particularly before the onset of pubertal maturation.[2,11,16–18] Therefore, it is possible that both protein and calcium play a role in the greater gain of total body aBMD/BMC, which has been observed in milk-supplemented adolescent girls.[19] In a recent study, we found that BMD/BMC changes in prepubertal boys were positively associated with spontaneous protein intake.[20] In addition, this study has also shown that protein intake modulates the effect of calcium supplementation on bone mineral mass gain in prepubertal boys.[21] Hence, in prepubertal boys, the favorable effects of calcium supplements were mostly detectable in those with a lower protein intake. At higher protein intake, the effect of calcium was not significant, suggesting possibly that calcium requirements for optimal bone growth could be lower at high levels of dietary protein. In the same study, increased physical activity was associated with greater BMC at both axial and appendicular sites under high, but not low, protein intake[20] (Fig. 1.2).

Furthermore, nutritional environmental factors seem to affect bone accumulation at specific periods during infancy and adolescence. In a prospective survey carried out in a cohort of female and male subjects aged 9–19 years, food intake was assessed twice, at a 1-year interval, using a 5-day dietary diary method with weighing of all consumed foods.[2] In this cohort of adolescents, we found a positive correlation between yearly spine or midshaft femur bone mass gain and calcium or protein intake. This correlation appeared to be significant mainly in prepubertal children, but not in those having reached a peri- or postpubertal stage.

It remained statistically significant after adjustment for spontaneous calcium intake.

In a prospective longitudinal study performed in healthy German children and adolescents of both genders between the age of 6 and 18, dietary intakes were recorded over 4 years, using an yearly administered 3-day diary.[22] Bone mass and size were measured at the radius diaphysis by peripheral quantitative computerized tomography. A significant positive association was found between long-term protein intakes, on the one hand, and periosteal circumferences, cortical area, bone mineral content, and with a calculated strength strain index, on the other hand (Fig. 1.3). The relatively high mean protein intakes in this cohort with a Western style diet should be highlighted. Indeed, protein intakes were around 2 g/kg body weight × day in prepubertal children, whereas they were around 1.5 g/kg × day in pubertal individuals. Note that the minimal requirements for protein intakes in the corresponding age groups are 0.99 and 0.95 g/kg × day, respectively. There was no association between bone variables and intakes of nutrients with high sulfur-containing amino acids or intake of calcium. Overall, protein intakes accounted for 3–4% of the bone parameters variance. However, even when they are prospective and longitudinal, observational studies do not allow one to draw conclusion on a causal relationship. Indeed, it is quite possible that protein intake could be, to a large extent, related to growth requirement during childhood and adolescence. Only intervention studies could reliably address this question. A recent study suggests that the effects of protein intake on bone may depend on the

Fig. 1.3 Relationship between radius bone variables, as assessed by peripheral quantitative tomography, and long-term dietary protein intakes in 229 healthy subjects aged 6–18 years. From Alexy et al.[22] With permission from the publisher

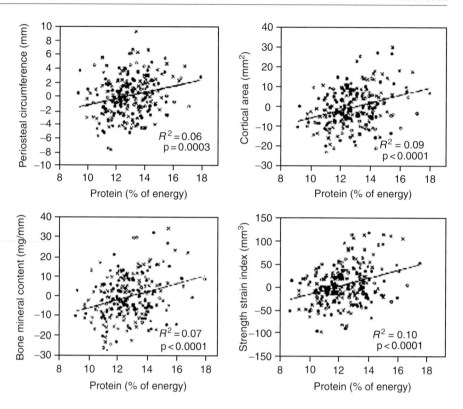

type of proteins. Increased intakes of aromatic amino acids, as found in soy, cereals, and dairy products, were shown to lead to higher serum IGF-I levels than were found with increased intake of branched chain amino acids.[23] We may thus hypothesize that the dietary intake of particular proteins might play a greater role in bone modeling and in the acquisition of PBM than others.

In addition to calcium, phosphorus, calories, and vitamins, one liter of milk provides 32–35 g of protein, mostly casein, but also whey proteins which contain numerous growth-promoting elements. Casein may enhance calcium absorption and mineral retention. In a balanced diet, about 70% of dietary calcium come from milk and dairy products, 16% from the few vegetables and dried fruits that are considered as good sources of calcium, and the remainder from minerals and drinking water or other discrete sources.

The correlation between dairy products intake and bone health has been investigated in cross-sectional and longitudinal observational studies, and in intervention trials (Table 1.1).[24] In growing children, long-term milk avoidance is associated with smaller stature and lower bone mineral mass, either at specific sites or at the whole body levels.[25–27] Low milk intake during

childhood and/or adolescence increases the risk of fracture before puberty mainly of the distal radius, generally occuring after a low energy trauma such as a fall from standing height (+2.6-fold), and possibly later in life.[28,29] In a 7-year observational study, there was a positive influence of dairy products consumption on a BMD at the spine, hip, and forearm in adolescents, leading thereby to a higher peak bone mass.[30] In contrast to widespread preconception, milk consumption was not associated with excessive weight gain or increased body fat, but was associated with increased body height. Of interest, calcium supplements did not affect spine aBMD in this study. In addition, higher dairy products intakes were associated with greater total and cortical proximal radius cross-sectional area. Regular intake of dairy products throughout adolescence increased aBMD at the hip and the spine, while calcium supplements had no effect at the spine. These observations may suggest that calcium supplementation essentially affects bone remodeling, while dairy products are likely to exert an additional effect on bone modeling, resulting in increased bone growth and periosteal bone apposition. These observations are consistent with earlier reports indicating that children who did not consume any dairy products had smaller stature

Table 1.1 Positive influence of dairy products on bone mass accrual

	Bone variable measured
Observational studies	
Alexy et al[22]	Radius
Black et al[25]	Whole body, spine, radius, proximal femur
Budek et al[17]	Whole body, spine
Esterle et al[18]	Spine
Hoppe et al[11]	Height
Matkovic et al[46]	Metacarpal
Matkovic et al[30]	Spine, neck, radius
Moore et al[47]	Whole body
Teegarden et al[19]	Whole body, spine, radius
Wiley[31]	Height
Intervention trials	
Baker et al[48]	Height
Budek et al[35]	Turnover
Cadogan et al[36]	Whole body
Cheng et al[37]	Spine
Du et al[38]	Whole body
Lau et al[49]	Whole body, spine, neck
Leighton and Clark[34]	Height
Merrilees et al[50]	Spine, proximal femur
Orr[51]	Height
Zhang et al[43]	Whole body
Zhu et al[40]	Metacarpal
Zhu et al[42]	Whole body
Zhu et al[41]	Metacarpal
Zhu et al[52]	Whole body

Study duration, populations investigated and outcome were different, but all the data support a favorable influence of dairy products on bone growth[11,17–19,22,25,30,31,34–43,46–52]

due to short bones. In agreement with this observation, milk consumption frequency and milk intake at age 5–12 and 13–17 years were significant predictors of the height of 12–18-year-old adolescents, studied in the NHANES 1999–2002.[31,32] After menarche, girls with milk intakes below 55 mL/day had significantly lower aBMD, BMC, and IGF-I as well as higher PTH compared to girls consuming over 260 mL/day of milk alongside other dairy products. Finally, consuming less than a glass of milk per week during childhood and/or adolescence was associated with a 3% reduction in hip BMC and aBMD and with a twofold increase in fracture risk during adulthood.[33]

1.2.3 Evidence from Randomized Controlled Intervention Trials

The earliest controlled intervention trials were published more than 80 years ago by Orr[51], and by Leighton and Clark.[34] They reported that a daily intake of 400–600 mL of milk, in addition to a normal diet, had a positive effect on height gain in Scottish school children over a 7-month observation period. In one randomized study with 8-year-old boys, high milk intake (1.5 L/day), but not high meat intake (250 g/day), and identical protein included in the normal diet for 7 days reduced bone turnover as assessed by biochemical markers of bone resorption (C-terminal telopeptides of type I collagen, CTx) and formation (serum osteocalcin, OC and bone-specific alkaline phosphatase, BSAP) vs. baseline.[35] After 7 days, the average daily protein intake increased in both groups by 47.5 g, yet the milk group had higher ($p < 0.0001$) calcium intake, suggesting that calcium and/or some milk-derived compounds, rather than the total protein intake, accounted for the decrease in bone turnover.

Three more recent intervention trials confirmed the beneficial effect of milk/dairy products on bone mineral mass during growth. In the first study, the effect of milk supplementation on total body bone mineral acquisition in adolescent girls, with a mean age 12.2 years, was evaluated in an open randomized intervention trial.[36] The intervention group received 568 mL (one pint) of whole or reduced fat milk per day for 18 months, the control group did not. With this milk supplement, the differences between the treated and control groups in calcium and protein intakes at the end of the study were around 420 mg/day and 14 g/day, respectively, taking into consideration the spontaneous consumption. Compared to the control group, the intervention group had greater increases of whole body bone mineral density and bone mineral content. Among the various skeletal sites, pelvis and legs showed the highest response to milk supplements. Serum levels of IGF-I were significantly higher than in the control group (+17%). In another open randomized controlled study with healthy 10–12-year-old girls with low dietary calcium intakes at inclusion, increasing calcium intake by consuming cheese (1,000 mg calcium daily) appeared to be more beneficial for cortical bone mineral mass accrual than was tablet form supplementation of the same amount of calcium.[37] The largest randomized controlled intervention trial with dairy products was conducted in 10-year-old Chinese girls in nine primary schools. In the first and the second group, the subjects received 330 mL milk fortified with calcium, with or without vitamin D supplementation, on school days for 2 years.[38,39] A third group served as control. Significantly higher gains in height, body weight, BMC and aBMD were observed in the groups receiving milk, with or without vitamin D, indicating that school-milk programs during childhood may improve bone growth. In addition, greater increases in cortical thickness measured in metacarpal bone and higher IGF-I concentrations at 24 months were observed in both groups receiving milk.[40–43]

1.2.4 Consequences of Milk Displacement from Diet

Overall, increased dietary intake of dairy products enhances bone mineral acquisition in children and adolescents and could contribute to maximize PBM. In addition, milk intake at a younger age may instigate similar habits of milk intake later in life. Calcium intakes do not currently meet recommended dietary intakes (RDI) in many countries. In France, for example, where the RDI for calcium is 1,200 mg/day for adolescents, 41–48% of the boys and 63–73% of the girls consume less than two thirds of the RDI between 11 and 17 years of age. One of the proposed explanations is that in western diet milk has been displaced by soft drinks and that the displacers are beverages containing caffeine and phosphoric acid, such as cola, which may have additional and direct deleterious effects on bone due to the relative metabolic acidosis and high levels of phosphate they induce. This hypothesis was tested in a short-term 10-day study that showed that high intake of cola along with a low-calcium diet induced increased bone turnover compared to a high intake of milk with a low-calcium diet, suggesting that the current trend toward a replacement of milk with cola and other soft drinks may negatively affect bone health.[44] In 2004, the American Academy of Pediatrics Committee on School Health issued a preventive statement indicating that the displacement of milk consumption by soft drinks resulted in calcium deficiency with an increased risk of osteoporosis and fractures.[45]

1.3 Conclusions

Athough more than 60% of the variance of peak bone mass, the amount of bone present in the skeleton at the end of its maturation process, is genetically determined, other factors amenable to positive intervention, such as adequate dietary intake of calcium and proteins, or dairy products as a source of these nutrients, can influence bone mass accrual. Indeed, a significant positive association can be found between long-term protein intakes, and bone mineral mass or bone size. In prepubertal boys, the positive association between spontaneous bone growth spontaneous and protein intake modulates the effects of increased physical activity. Indeed, greater BMC at both axial and appendicular sites in boys with increased physical exercise was found under high but not low protein intake. Thus to optimize bone mass accrual through dietary and physical exercise measures, these interactions as a valuable primary measure for the prevention of fractures later in life should be taken into account.

References

1. Bonjour JP, Rizzoli R (2001) Bone acquisition in adolescence. Academic Press, San Diego.
2. Theintz G, Buchs B, Rizzoli R et al (1992) Longitudinal monitoring of bone mass accumulation in healthy adolescents: evidence for a marked reduction after 16 years of age at the levels of lumbar spine and femoral neck in female subjects. J Clin Endocrinol Metab 75:1060-1065.
3. Schoenau E, Neu CM, Rauch F, Manz F (2001) The development of bone strength at the proximal radius during childhood and adolescence. J Clin Endocrinol Metab 86: 613-618.
4. Seeman E (2003) The structural and biomechanical basis of the gain and loss of bone strength in women and men. Endocrinol Metab Clin North Am 32:25-38.
5. Fournier PE, Rizzoli R, Slosman DO, Theintz G, Bonjour JP (1997) Asynchrony between the rates of standing height

gain and bone mass accumulation during puberty. Osteoporos Int 7:525-532.

6. Rizzoli R, Bonjour JP, Ferrari SL (2001) Osteoporosis, genetics and hormones. J Mol Endocrinol 26:79-94.

7. Ferrari S, Rizzoli R, Slosman D, Bonjour JP (1998) Familial resemblance for bone mineral mass is expressed before puberty. J Clin Endocrinol Metab 83:358-361.

8. Hernandez CJ, Beaupre GS, Carter DR (2003) A theoretical analysis of the relative influences of peak BMD, age-related bone loss and menopause on the development of osteoporosis. Osteoporos Int 14:843-847.

9. Rizzoli R, Bonjour JP (2004) Dietary protein and bone health. J Bone Miner Res 19:527-531.

10. Thissen JP, Ketelslegers JM, Underwood LE (1994) Nutritional regulation of the insulin-like growth factors. Endocr Rev 15:80-101.

11. Hoppe C, Molgaard C, Thomsen BL, Juul A, Michaelsen KF (2004) Protein intake at 9 mo of age is associated with body size but not with body fat in 10-y-old Danish children. Am J Clin Nutr 79:494-501.

12. Bonjour JP, Ammann P, Chevalley T, Rizzoli R. Protein intake and bone growth. *Can J Appl Physiol*. 2001;26(suppl): S153-S166.

13. Bonjour JP, Schurch MA, Chevalley T, Ammann P, Rizzoli R (1997) Protein intake, IGF-1 and osteoporosis. Osteoporos Int 7(suppl 3):S36-S42.

14. Ohlsson C, Mohan S, Sjogren K et al (2009) The role of liver-derived insulin-like growth factor-I. Endocr Rev 30:494-535.

15. Caverzasio J, Montessuit C, Bonjour JP (1990) Stimulatory effect of insulin-like growth factor-1 on renal Pi transport and plasma 1, 25-dihydroxyvitamin D3. Endocrinology 127:453-459.

16. Bonjour JP, Rizzoli R (2001) Bone acquisition in adolescence. In: Marcus R, Feldman D, Kelsey J (eds) Osteoporosis. Academic Press, San Diego, pp 621-638.

17. Budek AZ, Hoppe C, Ingstrup H, Michaelsen KF, Bugel S, Molgaard C (2007) Dietary protein intake and bone mineral content in adolescents-The Copenhagen Cohort Study. Osteoporos Int 18:1661-1667.

18. Esterle L, Sabatier JP, Guillon-Metz F et al (2009) Milk, rather than other foods, is associated with vertebral bone mass and circulating IGF-1 in female adolescents. Osteoporos Int 20:567-575.

19. Teegarden D, Lyle RM, Proulx WR, Johnston CC, Weaver CM (1999) Previous milk consumption is associated with greater bone density in young women. Am J Clin Nutr 69:1014-1017.

20. Chevalley T, Bonjour JP, Ferrari S, Rizzoli R (2008) High-protein intake enhances the positive impact of physical activity on BMC in prepubertal boys. J Bone Miner Res 23:131-142.

21. Chevalley T, Ferrari S, Hans D, et al. Protein intake modulates the effet of calcium supplementation on bone mass gain in prepubertal boys. *J Bone Miner Res*. 2002;17(suppl 1): S172.

22. Alexy U, Remer T, Manz F, Neu CM, Schoenau E (2005) Long-term protein intake and dietary potential renal acid load are associated with bone modeling and remodeling at the proximal radius in healthy children. Am J Clin Nutr 82:1107-1114.

23. Dawson-Hughes B, Harris SS, Rasmussen HM, Dallal GE (2007) Comparative effects of oral aromatic and branched-chain amino acids on urine calcium excretion in humans. Osteoporos Int 18:955-961.

24. Huncharek M, Muscat J, Kupelnick B (2008) Impact of dairy products and dietary calcium on bone-mineral content in children: results of a meta-analysis. Bone 43:312-321.

25. Black RE, Williams SM, Jones IE, Goulding A (2002) Children who avoid drinking cow milk have low dietary calcium intakes and poor bone health. Am J Clin Nutr 76: 675-680.

26. Hidvegi E, Arato A, Cserhati E, Horvath C, Szabo A (2003) Slight decrease in bone mineralization in cow milk-sensitive children. J Pediatr Gastroenterol Nutr 36:44-49.

27. Henderson RC, Hayes PR (1994) Bone mineralization in children and adolescents with a milk allergy. Bone Miner 27:1-12.

28. Goulding A, Rockell JE, Black RE, Grant AM, Jones IE, Williams SM (2004) Children who avoid drinking cow's milk are at increased risk for prepubertal bone fractures. J Am Diet Assoc 104:250-253.

29. Konstantynowicz J, Nguyen TV, Kaczmarski M, Jamiolkowski J, Piotrowska-Jastrzebska J, Seeman E (2007) Fractures during growth: potential role of a milk-free diet. Osteoporos Int 18: 1601-1607.

30. Matkovic V, Landoll JD, Badenhop-Stevens NE et al (2004) Nutrition influences skeletal development from childhood to adulthood: a study of hip, spine, and forearm in adolescent females. J Nutr 134:701S-705S.

31. Wiley AS (2005) Does milk make children grow? Relationships between milk consumption and height in NHANES 1999-2002. Am J Hum Biol 17:425-441.

32. Opotowsky AR, Bilezikian JP (2003) Racial differences in the effect of early milk consumption on peak and postmeno-pausal bone mineral density. J Bone Miner Res 18: 1978-1988.

33. Kalkwarf HJ, Khoury JC, Lanphear BP (2003) Milk intake during childhood and adolescence, adult bone density, and osteoporotic fractures in US women. Am J Clin Nutr 77: 257-265.

34. Leighton G, Clark ML. Milk consumption and the growth of school children. *BMJ*. 1929;1:23-25.

35. Budek AZ, Hoppe C, Michaelsen KF, Molgaard C (2007) High intake of milk, but not meat, decreases bone turnover in prepubertal boys after 7 days. Eur J Clin Nutr 61: 957-962.

36. Cadogan J, Eastell R, Jones N, Barker ME (1997) Milk intake and bone mineral acquisition in adolescent girls: ran-domised, controlled intervention trial. BMJ 315:1255-1260.

37. Cheng S, Lyytikainen A, Kroger H, et al. Effects of calcium, dairy product, and vitamin D supplementation on bone mass accrual and body composition in 10-12-y-old girls: a 2-y randomized trial. *Am J Clin Nutr*. 2005;82:1115-1126; quiz 1147-1148.

38. Du X, Zhu K, Trube A et al (2004) School-milk intervention trial enhances growth and bone mineral accretion in Chinese girls aged 10-12 years in Beijing. Br J Nutr 92:159-168.

39. Du X, Zhu K, Trube A et al (2005) Effects of school-milk intervention on growth and bone mineral accretion in Chinese girls aged 10-12 years: accounting for cluster randomisation. Br J Nutr 94:1038-1039.

40. Zhu K, Greenfield H, Du X, Zhang Q, Fraser DR. Effects of milk supplementation on cortical bone gain in Chinese girls aged 10-12 years. *Asia Pac J Clin Nutr.* 2003; 12(suppl):S47.

41. Zhu K, Du X, Cowell CT et al (2005) Effects of school milk intervention on cortical bone accretion and indicators relevant to bone metabolism in Chinese girls aged 10-12 y in Beijing. Am J Clin Nutr 81:1168-1175.

42. Zhu K, Greenfield H, Zhang Q et al (2004) Bone mineral accretion and growth in Chinese adolescent girls following the withdrawal of school milk intervention: preliminary results after two years. Asia Pac J Clin Nutr 13:S83.

43. Zhang Q, Ma GS, Greenfield H, Du XQ, Zhu K, Fraser DR. Effects of fortified milk consumption on regional bone mineral accrual in Chinese girls. *Asia Pac J Clin Nutr.* 2003; 12(suppl):S46.

44. Kristensen M, Jensen M, Kudsk J, Henriksen M, Molgaard C (2005) Short-term effects on bone turnover of replacing milk with cola beverages: a 10-day interventional study in young men. Osteoporos Int 16:1803-1808.

45. American Academy of Pediatrics Committee on School Health. Soft drinks in schools. *Pediatrics.* 2004;113:152-154.

46. Matkovic V, Kostial K, Simonovic I, Buzina R, Brodarec A, Nordin BE (1979) Bone status and fracture rates in two regions of Yugoslavia. Am J Clin Nutr 32:540-549.

47. Moore LL, Bradlee ML, Gao D, Singer MR (2008) Effects of average childhood dairy intake on adolescent bone health. J Pediatr 153:667-673.

48. Baker IA, Elwood PC, Hughes J, Jones M, Moore F, Sweetnam PM (1980) A randomised controlled trial of the effect of the provision of free school milk on the growth of children. J Epidemiol Community Health 34:31-34.

49. Lau EM, Lynn H, Chan YH, Lau W, Woo J (2004) Benefits of milk powder supplementation on bone accretion in Chinese children. Osteoporos Int 15:654-658.

50. Merrilees MJ, Smart EJ, Gilchrist NL et al (2000) Effects of dairy food supplements on bone mineral density in teenage girls. Eur J Nutr 39:256-262.

51. Orr JB. Influence of amount of milk consumption on the rate of growth of school children. *BMJ.* 1928;28:140-142.

52. Zhu K, Greenfield H, Zhang Q, et al (2008) Effects of two year's milk supplementation on site-corrected bone mineral density of Chinese girls. *Asia Pac J Clin Nutr* 17 suppl 1: 147–150

Protein Effects on Bone and Muscle in Elderly Women

R. L. Prince, X. Meng, A. Devine, D. A. Kerr, V. Solah, C. W. Binns, and K. Zhu

2.1 Introduction

Fractures continue to constitute a major public health problem of aging despite recent evidence that the age-specific rate may be falling.[1] The facts that before dying at a median age of approximately 83 years, 50% of women would have sustained a fracture with its consequent morbidity, and health care costs give some idea of the magnitude of the problem. As with other common health problems such as atherosclerotic cardiovascular disease, a combination of the whole of the population public health approach with pharmaceutical intervention for those at highest risk is recommended. In this regard, increased calcium supplementation to counteract reduced intestinal calcium absorption and increased renal excretion due to the loss of the effect of estrogen on these two mechanisms[2] is now widely accepted as is vitamin D supplementation due to a reduction in skin exposure to sunlight. Interestingly this latter factor, which in the absence of adequate sunlight can be replaced in the diet, has also been shown to play a significant role in falls prevention which together with osteoporosis constitute the pathological basis for fracture.

In recent years, there has been an increased interest in other nutrient deficiencies that may play a role in the increasing risk of fracture with age. In this regard, a research group, The Protein Intake Metabolic Outcome Study Collaborators, was formed in 2005. The basis of our interest was stimulated by early evidence that increased protein intake may be beneficial rather than being deleterious to the skeleton may be beneficial. In addition, there is

some evidence that muscle function may be enhanced by increased protein nutrition. It is possible that the magnitude of the effect could play a role in falls reduction and thereby reduce fracture risk. This chapter reviews recent ongoing work undertaken by our group in relation to the substantial work done by others in the area.

2.2 The Epidemiology of the Effects of Aging on Nutrition (Table 2.1)

There is a relative paucity of data on the effects of aging on nutrient intake. Indeed, it is not infrequent to consider that there is a greater problem from overnutrition than undernutrition, often based on studies of younger individuals. We have therefore recently reviewed data from a longitudinal study of 954 free-living elderly women aged 70–85 years at baseline who survived 7 years from a cohort of 1,500 elderly women recruited in 1998[3].

Compared to national data, this study population had a higher rate of overweight (44.2% vs. 35.6%), but a similar rate of obesity (21.9% vs. 22.9%).[4] This suggests that the increase in body size seen in Australia extends to older adulthood (>70 years), where the prevalence of chronic disease is already high and overweight and obesity remain as strong determinants of chronic disease.[5] The change in nutrient intake data is shown in Table 2.1. Over the 7 years, there was a reduction in energy intake and 68–76% of the population fell below the ideal Acceptable Macronutrient Distribution Range (AMDR) for energy intake[6] possibly related to declining appetite.[7] The reduction in energy intake extended to all three major classes of nutrients including protein, although protein intake was substantially above previously recommended levels.[8] In addition, it is clear that over the 7 years, there was a gradual

R.L. Prince (✉)
School of Medicine and Pharmacology, Sir Charles
Gairdner Hospital Unit, University of Western Australia,
Hospital Avenue, Nedlands WA 6009, Australia
e-mail: richard.prince@uwa.edu.au

P. Burckhardt et al. (eds.), *Nutritional Influences on Bone Health,*
DOI: 10.1007/978-1-84882-978-7_2, © Springer-Verlag London Limited 2010

Table 2.1 Anthropometric measurements of elderly women in the CAIFOS CARES cohort from baseline to 84 months

	Baseline ($n=949$)	60 months ($n=949$)	84 months ($n=949$)
Age (years)	74.9±2.6	79.9±2.6*	81.9±2.6*
Weight (kg)	68.7±11.9	67.9±12.0*	66.8±12.0*,**
Corrected tricep skinfold (cm)	0.86±0.26	0.85±0.25	0.70±0.26*,**
Corrected upper arm girth (cm)	1.03±0.12	1.02±0.13*	0.92±0.13*,**
Physical activity (kJ/day)[a]	498 (191, 866)	448 (122, 807)	382 (0, 782)*,***
Nutritional intake			
Energy (kJ/day)	7,206±2,134	6,866±2,307*	6,522±2,150*,**
All fats (g/day)	65±24	62±26*	62±24*
Protein (g/day)	81±27	78±31****	75±28*,***
Carbohydrates (g/day)	193±59	182±61*	176±59*,***

Results are mean±SD unless otherwise stated
*Significantly different from baseline ($p<0.001$)
**Significant differences between 60 and 84 months ($p<0.001$)
***Significant differences between 60 and 84 months ($p<0.05$)
****Significantly different from baseline ($p<0.05$)
[a]Median (interquartile range)

reduction in weight, fat mass as shown by triceps skin fold and muscle mass as shown by corrected upper arm girth. Thus it is possible that at least a proportion of the aging population may benefit from an increase in protein nutrition. This concept has been pursued in two further studies of the relation between protein nutrition and bone and muscle mass and function.

2.3 Epidemiology of the Effects of Protein Nutrition on Bone and Muscle Structure

The data on protein effects on bone and muscle have been published in two recent papers, both of which utilized data from the longitudinal study of aging in women which formed the basis for the report discussed above.

The subjects were recruited from the Western Australian general population of women over 70 years of age for a 10-year cohort study, where the first 5-year study was a prospective randomized controlled cohort trial of supplemental oral calcium to prevent osteoporotic fractures[3] and years 6–10 were a study of health outcomes with aging. Initially, a letter was sent to 24,800 individuals selected at random from the electoral roll,

which has the names and addresses of 98% of women of this age. Of the 4,312 women who responded to the letter, 34% joined the study. No subjects had any medical condition likely to influence the 5-year survival and subjects were not taking bone-related medication including calcium supplements, estrogen, bisphosphonates, and vitamin D at enrolment. Although women enrolled in this study were weighted in favor of those in higher socioeconomic categories, they did not differ from the whole population in health resource utilization.[9] During the intervention phase of the study (first 5 years), subjects were randomized to receive 1.2 g of calcium carbonate daily or matched placebo. At the commencement of the study, each subject completed a self-administered semiquantitative food frequency questionnaire developed by the Anti Cancer Council of Victoria (ACCV)[10–12,] from which the daily dietary intake of energy, carbohydrate, protein, fat, and calcium were derived. The dietary calcium was from food alone and did not include the amount from any supplement.

2.3.1 Study 1

The first report was of a cross-sectional study of protein intake effects on bone mass.[13] The demographics are shown in Table 2.2. Protein intake in Australian elderly women was found to be higher than previously recommended (0.94 g/kg). Furthermore, although there was a high correlation between protein intake and other nutrients, there was a low correlation with body weight emphasizing the fact that body composition is the result of past intake and not current nutrient intake.

Figures 2.1 and 2.2 show the relationship between protein intake in tertiles and bone structure at the heel site, measured by bone ultrasound attenuation (BUA) and hip areal BMD measured by DXA. After adjustment for age and BMI, individuals in the highest tertile of protein intake had the best bone structure at the heel and hip sites. Calcium intake was not significant in the model. A 50% increase in protein intake from the median 55 to 103 g was associated with a 2% increase

in bone structure. So, although the effect size was not large, nevertheless, it was possible to be demonstrate it in an epidemiological study.

2.3.2 Study 2

Next, we studied the protein intake effect on bone and muscle in a 5-year longitudinal design utilizing the data acquired as part of an RCT of calcium supplementation.[14] The study sample consisted of 862 community-dwelling women who had their nutritional intake assessed at baseline as indicated above and had a measurement of whole body DXA composition at 5 years. The baseline data is shown in Table 2.3. It is evident that individuals with a high protein intake were physically more active and had a higher calcium intake.

The relationship between baseline protein intake and bone mass at 5 years is shown in Fig. 2.3. It is clear that similar to the cross-sectional data, high protein intake was associated with high total body bone mass. There were insufficient individuals for heel ultrasound and hip DXA at 5 years to examine these endpoints. These data are consistent with some[13,15,16,] but not all[17] studies that have shown that a high protein intake is associated with reduced bone loss, and reduced risk of hip fracture.[18]

In addition to studying the effects of protein intake on bone mass, we were able to study the effects on muscle mass and fat mass. There was no relation between protein intake and fat mass. On the other hand, there was a substantial positive effect of baseline protein intake on muscle mass (Fig. 2.4). Thus subjects consuming 20% of kJ as protein as opposed to 17% of their kJ as protein had a 5.3% higher whole body lean mass, and 6.6% higher appendicular lean mass independent of age, body size, energy intake, and physical activity level.

These findings are consistent with the results of the Health ABC study in the US,[19] which showed that the community-dwelling older people in the highest quintile of protein intake lost 40% less lean mass and appendicular lean mass than did those in the lowest quintile of protein intake over a 3-year period, but are inconsistent with two cross-sectional studies.[20,21] Interestingly, the beneficial relationship between protein intake and whole body bone mass disappeared after adjustment for muscle mass effects. This raises the interesting possibility that the bone effect is dependent on the muscle effect.

Table 2.2 Baseline demographics of subjects in the study of protein consumption and lower limb bone mass

Variable	Value
Number	1,077
Age (years)	75±3
Weight (kg)	68.5±1.9
BMI (kg/m²)	27.1±4.5
Protein (g/day)	80.5±27.8
Protein (g/kg body weight/day)	1.19±0.44 (range 0.31–4.51)
Protein (% of energy)	19±2.9

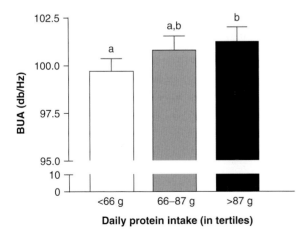

Fig. 2.1 Effects of differing habitual protein intake on heel ultrasound bone ultrasound attenuation (BUA). Results are mean±SE heel ultrasound BUA corrected for age and BMI. Bars with different letters differ at $p<0.05$ (reproduced from Devine et al[13])

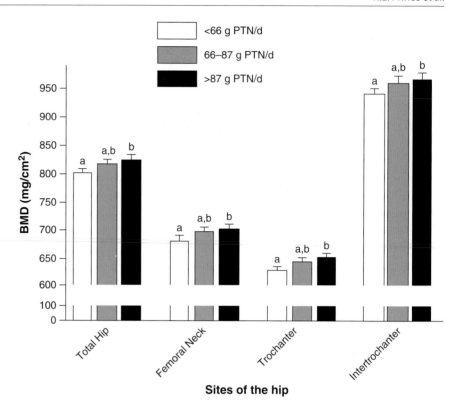

Fig. 2.2 Effects of differing habitual protein intake in DXA BMD. Results are mean ± SE hip DXA corrected for age and BMI. Bars with different letters differ at $p < 0.05$ (reproduced from Devine et al[13])

Table 2.3 Baseline demographics of a 5-year cohort study of the effects of high protein intake on lean mass and bone mineral content in elderly postmenopausal women

	First tertile protein <66 g/day ($n=287$)	Second tertile protein 66–87 g/day ($n=287$)	Third tertile Protein >87 g/day ($n=288$)
Age (year)	74.9 ± 2.5	75.0 ± 2.6	74.7 ± 2.7
BMI (kg/m²)	26.4 ± 4.2	26.7 ± 4.7	27.3 ± 4.3*
Physical activity (kJ/day)[a]	466 (0–808)	530 (207–897)*	614 (237–1,002)*
Protein (g/day)	54.4 ± 9.1	76.6 ± 6.2*	110.9 ± 23.4*,**
Protein (% of energy)	17.7 ± 2.7	19.0 ± 2.3*	20.4 ± 3.2*,**
Calcium (mg/day)	704 ± 202	973 ± 243*	1,220 ± 364*,**

Results are mean ± SD
*Significantly different from the first tertile, $p < 0.05$
**Significantly different from the second tertile, $p < 0.05$ (ANOVA with Tukey's test)
[a]Median and interquartile range

2.3.3 Conclusions

The nutritional epidemiology of body composition is a difficult area of study for a variety of reasons. First, there are substantial cocorrelations between nutrient intakes which make identification of a specific effect uncertain. Second, there are the problems of confounding of effects due to unrecognized baseline cocorrelates inherent in all epidemiological investigation. Third, there is the problem of the effects of nutrition on body size in cross-sectional

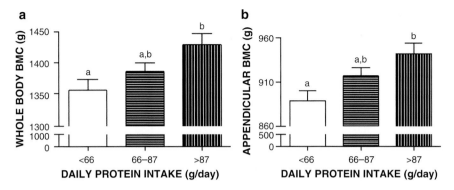

Fig. 2.3 Effects of baseline protein intake on DXA BMC of whole body and appendicular skeleton 5 years later. Results are mean±SE adjusted for baseline age, height, energy intake, physical activity, and calcium treatment. Groups with different lower case letters are significantly different, $p < 0.05$ (ANCOVA with Bonferroni test) (reproduced from Meng et al[14] with permission of the American Society for Bone and Mineral Research)

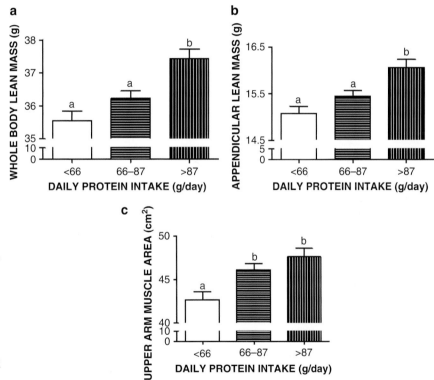

Fig. 2.4 Effect of baseline protein intake on DXA lean mass 5 years later. Results are mean±SE adjusted for baseline age, height, energy intake, and physical activity. Groups with different lower case letters are significantly different, $p < 0.05$ (ANCOVA with Bonferroni test) (reproduced from Meng et al[14] with permission of the American Society for Bone and Mineral Research)

studies. This is because body size is determined by many long-term factors including genetic effects in childhood and adolescence and nutritional intakes in the past. Given this complexity, it is surprising that the relationships outlined above are evident. Nevertheless, it is essential to subject observational studies of beneficial effects to controlled clinical trial interventions before cause and effect can be validly concluded. To this end, we have commenced a 2-year RCT of increased protein intake against identical placebo as outlined below.

2.4 A Population-Based, 2-Year Randomized, Double Blind and Placebo Controlled Trial of Protein Supplementation

In 2005, we commenced planning for an RCT of the effects of increased protein intake on body composition and metabolic outcomes, the PIMES (Protein Intake Metabolic Effect Study). Preliminary data on 1-year end points have been presented here.

The study design was to recruit community-dwelling ambulant women aged 70–80 years and offer them an intervention of a daily 250 mL drink. One contained a protein supplement group consisting of 30 g of whey protein isolate (Alacen 894, Fonterra NZ), 600 mg of calcium as calcium lactate, and 1,050 kJ of energy. The placebo contained 1.7 g protein, 600 mg of calcium as calcium lactate, and was isocaloric with the protein drink. Hundred women were recruited to the protein drink and 95 to the placebo drink. Body composition was measured at baseline and 1 year using whole body dual-energy X-ray absorptiometry and knee strength was assessed by isokinetic dynamometer.

The baseline demographics are shown in Table 2.4. There were no differences between the two groups for any of the factors assessed which were similar to the values obtained in the epidemiological studies. The effect of the intervention on lean mass, which is largely muscle mass in the appendicular regions including both arms and both legs and knee extensor and flexor strength is shown in Fig. 2.5. In essence, although there was an increase in lean mass and leg strength over 1 year there was no group difference.

2.5 Conclusions

The lack of a protein treatment effect must be regarded as preliminary as the study was designed to be a 2-year intervention, because the time course of a protein nutritional supplement was considered to be a long-term effect. Nevertheless, an alternate hypothesis that may be worth considering is that the increased calcium and caloric intake in both the groups may have induced a beneficial effect on muscle mass and function. Clearly, this concept suggests that nutritional intake in the ambulant elderly may not be optimal to maintain skeletal function.

Table 2.4 Baseline characteristics of the two test drink groups

	Protein group mean ± SD ($n = 100$)	Control group mean ± SD ($n = 95$)	p value
Age (year)	74 ± 3	74 ± 3	0.80
Height (m)	159.8 ± 6.3	159.8 ± 5.7	0.86
Weight (kg)	66.8 ± 11.1	69.6 ± 11.3	0.09
Dietary intakes assessed by 3-day food record			
Energy intake (kJ/day)	7,074 ± 1,595	7,307 ± 1,456	0.29
Protein intake (g/day)	76.6 ± 18.0	77.9 ± 21.6	0.65
Fat intake (g/day)	60.7 ± 19.6	64.0 ± 18.9	0.24
Carbohydrate intake (g/day)	188.6 ± 50.0	192.1 ± 44.0	0.61
Energy intake from protein (%)	19.0 ± 3.5	18.5 ± 3.4	0.28
Body composition			
Whole body lean mass (kg)	37.0 ± 4.7	37.7 ± 4.7	0.29
Appendicular lean mass (kg)	16.2 ± 2.4	16.6 ± 2.4	0.27
Total knee strength (kg)	25.2 ± 8.6	25.1 ± 8.7	0.93

Fig. 2.5 Change from baseline to 1 year for whole body and appendicular lean mass and total knee strength (knee extension strength and knee flexion strength). Results are the mean (SE). Paired sample t-test for within group change from baseline to 1 year

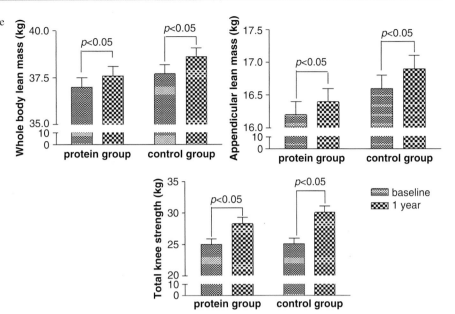

References

1. Leslie WD, O'Donnell S, Jean S, et al. Trends in hip fracture rates in Canada. *JAMA*. 2009;302:883-889.
2. Prince RL. Counterpoint: estrogen effects on calcitropic hormones and calcium homeostasis. *Endocr Rev*. 1994;15:301-309.
3. Prince RL, Devine A, Dhaliwal SS, Dick IM. Effects of calcium supplementation on clinical fracture and bone structure: results of a 5-year, double-blind, placebo-controlled trial in elderly women. *Arch Intern Med*. 2006;166:869-875.
4. Australian Bureau of Statistics & Commonwealth Department of Health and Aged Care. *National Nutrition Survey: Nutrient Intakes and Physical Measurements*. Canberra: Australian Bureau of Statistics catalogue no. 4805.0; 1998.
5. Australian Institute of Health and Welfare. *Australia's Health 2002*. Canberra: AIHW; 2002.
6. National Health and Medical Research Council (Australia), New Zealand. Ministry of Health, Australia. Department of Health and Ageing. *Nutrient Reference Values for Australia and New Zealand: Including Recommended Dietary Intakes*. Canberra, A.C.T.: National Health and Medical Research Council; 2006.
7. Omran ML, Morley JE. Assessment of protein energy malnutrition in older persons, part I: history, examination, body composition, and screening tools. *Nutrition*. 2000;16:50-63.
8. National Health and Medical Research Council. *Dietary Guidelines for Australians*. Canberra: Australian Government Publishing Service; 1991.
9. Bruce DG, Devine A, Prince RL. Recreational physical activity levels in healthy older women: the importance of fear of falling. *J Am Geriatr Soc*. 2002;50:84-89.
10. Ireland P, Jolley D, Giles G, et al. Development of the Melbourne FFQ: a food frequency questionnaire for use in an Australian prospective study involving an ethnically diverse cohort. *Asia Pac J Clin Nutr*. 1994;3:19-31.
11. Hodge A, Patterson AJ, Brown WJ, Ireland P, Giles G. The Anti Cancer Council of Victoria FFQ: relative validity of nutrient intakes compared with weighed food records in young to middle-aged women in a study of iron supplementation. *Aust N Z J Public Health*. 2000;24:576-583.
12. Hodge A, Patterson A, Brown W, Ireland P, Giles G. Erratum. *Aust N Z J Public Health*. 2003;27:468.
13. Devine A, Dick IM, Islam AF, Dhaliwal SS, Prince RL. Protein consumption is an important predictor of lower limb bone mass in elderly women. *Am J Clin Nutr*. 2005;81:1423-1428.
14. Meng X, Zhu K, Devine A, Kerr DA, Binns CW, Prince RL. A 5-year cohort study of the effects of high protein intake on lean mass and bone mineral content in elderly postmenopausal women. *J Bone Miner Res*. 2009;24(11): 1827-1834.
15. Hannan MT, Tucker KL, Dawson-Hughes B, Felson DT, Kiel DP. Effect of dietary protein on bone loss in elderly men and women: the Framingham Osteoporosis Study. *J Bone Miner Res*. 2000;15:2504-2512.
16. Promislow JHE, Goodman-Gruen D, Slymen DJ, Barrett-Connor E. Protein consumption and bone mineral density in the elderly: the Rancho Bernardo Study. *Am J Epidemiol*. 2002;155:636-644.
17. Rapuri PB, Gallagher JC, Haynatzka V. Protein intake: effects on bone mineral density and the rate of bone loss in elderly women. *Am J Clin Nutr*. 2003;77:1517-1525.
18. Wengreen HJ, Munger RG, Cutler DR, Corcoran CD, Zhang J, Sassano NE. Dietary protein intake and risk of osteoporotic hip fracture in elderly residents of Utah. *J Bone Miner Res*. 2004;19:537-545.
19. Houston DK, Nicklas BJ, Ding J, et al. Dietary protein intake is associated with lean mass change in older, community-dwelling adults: the Health, Aging, and Body Composition (Health ABC) Study. *Am J Clin Nutr*. 2008;87:150-155.
20. Starling RD, Ades PA, Poehlman ET. Physical activity, protein intake, and appendicular skeletal muscle mass in older men. *Am J Clin Nutr*. 1999;70:91-96.
21. Mitchell D, Haan MN, Steinberg FM, Visser M. Body composition in the elderly: the influence of nutritional factors and physical activity. *J Nutr Health Aging*. 2003;7: 130-139.

Dietary Protein and Bone Health: The Urgent Need for Large-Scale Supplementation Studies

3

Andrea L. Darling and Susan A. Lanham-New

Abbreviations

BMC	Bone mineral content
BMD	Bone mineral density
IGF-1	Insulin-like growth factor-1
IL-6	Interleukin-6
NRAE	Net renal acid excretion
PRAL	Potential renal acid load
RDA	Recommended daily allowance
TNF-α	Tumor necrosis factor-alpha

3.1 Introduction

There is a long-standing debate as to whether dietary protein is beneficial or detrimental to bone health. The proposed beneficial effects are due to the anabolic effects of protein on bone via hormones such as IGF-1 and possibly increased calcium absorption. This view is supported by epidemiological research showing benefits of increased protein intake on BMD and BMC within populations. However, high dietary protein intake has been shown to increase systemic acid load and thus could theoretically increase calciuria and bone resorption. Therefore, it has been suggested that dietary protein may be detrimental to bone health. Some cross-cultural studies support this hypothesis with increasing dietary protein intake being associated with increased fracture among populations. However, this is not supported by the majority of published epidemiological

studies within populations. Also, the hypothesis of a greater detriment caused by animal protein than vegetable protein is not likely to be valid as some vegetable proteins produce as high an acid load as animal proteins. The relationship between protein intake and bone health is indeed complex, with absolute intakes of protein and other aspects of the diet also modifying any effects seen, especially calcium and other acid-base relevant nutrients such as potassium and phosphate. A recent metaanalysis by our group assessed the effects of protein supplementation on BMD (presented at the ISNAO 2009 meeting and currently undergoing revisions for publication). This meta-analysis highlights the fact that more large-scale intervention studies are now urgently required to exactly assess the true influence of protein on bone health and are likely to be the only true way to resolve the protein debate.

3.2 Background

Bone is made, to a large extent, of protein and is continually being turned over. Not all protein can be reused by the body, so it requires a regular supply of new dietary protein for structure and maintenance.

Dietary protein has a variety of anabolic effects on bone. For example, it regulates the production of the growth factor IGF-1, which has a stimulatory effect on osteoblasts, promoting bone formation. Also, IGF-1 is important for the coupling of bone formation and resorption. Many research studies suggest that dietary protein also increases calcium absorption from the gut in humans[1] and rats.[2] Therefore, it may be important for the regulation of calcium balance. Therefore, the hypothesis has been put forward that a lack of dietary protein may be detrimental to bone.

A.L. Darling (✉)
Division of Nutritional Sciences, Faculty of Health
and Medical Sciences, University of Surrey, Stag Hill,
Guildford GU2 7XH, UK
e-mail: a.darling@surrey.ac.uk

P. Burckhardt et al. (eds.), *Nutritional Influences on Bone Health*,
DOI: 10.1007/978-1-84882-978-7_3, © Springer-Verlag London Limited 2010

The picture is, however, complicated by the long-term view that, theoretically, high protein intakes increase body acidity and thus may increase urinary calcium content which may detriment bone health. Different types of protein (animal, vegetable, soy) have slightly different sulfur amino acid contents. A hypothesis has been put forward that they may have different effects on bone, with claims that animal proteins have a higher sulfur amino acid content, and therefore, higher acidosis and higher calciuric effect than vegetable proteins. However, this hypothesis has been disputed by some authors as being flawed[3].

Elderly people in the western world and people of all ages in the developing world are at high risk of malnutrition due to poor dietary intakes of nutrients, including poor protein intake. Low protein intakes in older people have been linked to increased bone loss[4] and increased risk of fractures.[5] However, high intakes of dietary protein in adults and children in the western world mean that the potential impact of high protein intakes on bone has also become an issue of large importance. Thus, it is very important to examine the possible influence of high and low protein intakes on bone health.

The current debate over the impact of protein intakes on bone health will be discussed below, as well as how protein interacts with other dietary nutrients and also the evidence for and against any differential effects of different types of protein on bone.

3.3 The Potential Beneficial Effects of Protein on Bone

Dietary protein has been observed to be associated with increased production of the anabolic hormone, IGF-1,[6–8] and thus may influence bone health via the production and action of this hormone.

IGF-1 increases bone mass by increasing bone formation due to increased osteoblast activity. It also plays an essential role in the mineralization of bone matrix[9] and is involved in the control of phosphate metabolism.[10] Therefore, protein deficiency may decrease bone strength and alter bone microarchitecture.[3] It may also influence the release of cytokines (e.g., TNF-α, IL-6), which in some studies have been found to be detrimental to bone mass.[11]

Indeed, low protein diets have been shown to decrease the sensitivity of rat osteoblasts to IGF-1[12] and decrease intestinal calcium absorption,[1] which

therefore could lead to reduced bone density. Indeed, low protein diets have been linked to secondary hyperparathyroidism[13] and lower bone mass.[4]

The picture is further complicated by the fact that animal studies show that protein deficiency may affect some skeletal sites more than others. For example, Bourrin et al[12] found an influence of protein deficiency on cortical but not trabecular bone formation in rats. Therefore, protein influences may be site-specific.

3.3.1 Observational Studies Showing a Positive Association of Protein Intake and Bone Mineral Density

The effect of protein on bone health in pre and postmenopausal women has been widely studied in cross-sectional research. For example, Lacey et al[14] found a positive correlation between current protein intake and midradial BMC of Japanese pre and postmenopausal women. Also, in another study, protein intake had a significant positive impact on bone mass density.[15] A significant positive correlation between protein consumption and BMD of the distal radius and proximal femur was found in an observational study of pre and postmenopausal women by Cooper et al[16] Similarly, a study of the Framingham cohort found that low dietary protein was associated with increased femoral and spinal bone loss, with lowest intakes being most detrimental.[4] Also, Michaelsson et al[17] found a positive correlation between protein consumption and bone mass density of the femoral neck in Swedish pre and postmenopausal women. Last, Chiu et al[18] found a significant positive association between protein intake and lumbar spine BMD. However, in another study, no significant relationship was found between protein intakes and change in bone mass density in healthy postmenopausal New Zealand women over 2 years duration.[19]

Many positive associations between dietary protein intake and bone health have also been found in elderly populations. For example, a cross-sectional study in the USA of older postmenopausal women showed a positive relationship between protein intake and total body and hand BMD.[20] Beneficial effects of dietary protein were also found for BMD in an Australian study[21] and for BMC in a study of Seventh Day Adventists in the USA.[22] Last, Geinoz et al[23] found that elderly Swiss hospital patients consuming at least 1 g protein per kilogram ideal body weight had increased femoral neck bone mass density, with males also having higher lumbar spine bone mass density.

Protein may also have a synergistic role in respect to the beneficial effects of exercise on bone health. For example, Chevalley et al[24] found that higher dietary protein was correlated with a greater increase in BMC in pubertal boys undergoing exercise training than were lower dietary protein intakes. This would be as expected from physiology, as dietary protein is a substrate necessary for increased bone and muscle growth, so any changes in size stimulated by exercise are likely to manifest if adequate protein is present.

3.3.2 Supplementation Studies Showing a Benefit of Dietary Protein on Bone Mineral Density

Some supplementation studies have confirmed the results of the above cross-sectional and cohort studies. In a study by Dawson-Hughes et al[25], a high protein supplement was associated with increased IGF-1 and also lower urinary N-telopeptide.[25] Also, in hospitalized elderly patients, protein supplements (20 g/day) led to increased levels of IGF-1 and decreased bone loss of the proximal femur.[8] Tkatch et al[26] also found that a protein supplement of 20 g/day in elderly hospital patients led to a reduction in bone loss. These trials show the importance of adequate protein intake for bone health in hospitalized elderly populations, as well as reducing length of hospital stay and other morbidity.

3.3.3 Cohort Studies Showing Reduced Risk of Fracture with Increasing Dietary Protein Intakes

There have been few cohort studies examining the link between protein intake and fracture risk to draw firm conclusions, but there is some evidence that protein intake may be associated with decreased risk of fracture. For example, a prospective study of postmenopausal women aged 55–69 years old showed a negative association between protein intake and risk of hip fracture.[27] However, no link was found between self-reported current total protein intake and hip fractures in a study of the Nurses' health cohort.[28]

3.4 The Potential Detrimental Effects of Protein on Acid–Base Balance

Metabolic processes produce acid, (around 1 mEq/day) which must be excreted by the kidney to maintain a body pH of 7–35–7.45. Metabolic acid is produced from dietary sulfur, phosphorus, and chloride, while alkali is produced from sodium, calcium, potassium, and magnesium. Therefore, dietary composition may influence levels of systemic acidity.

Indeed, an imbalance of acid production over alkali increases net endogenous acid production (NEAP) and thus increases NRAE, the amount of acid excreted by the kidney. Such an imbalance between dietary induced acid and alkali may be harmful for bone. This is due to carbonate and citrate being released from bone to buffer the dietary induced acid load.[29] Calcium is released in this process and is then excreted in the urine. Acidosis also leads to decreased reabsorption of calcium in the kidney which worsens calciuria.

With age, the body becomes increasingly acidic due to decreased renal function.[30] There is thus concern in the literature that increasing dietary protein intake could cause more acid to be produced, which could compound the effect of increased acidity due to aging.

Much of the hypothesis of the potential detrimental effect of dietary protein-induced acid loads stems from research that shows increased cell-mediated bone resorption with increased acidity.[31] Conversely, there is also a stimulation of osteoblastic formation and reduction osteoclast activity with increasing alkalosis.[32]

Indeed, a large number of studies have found that high dietary protein consumers have increased calciuria than those consuming lower amounts of protein.[33–36] Indeed, it has been estimated that doubling protein intake increases calciuria by 50%.[29] However, as discussed by Bonjour[3] in his review of dietary protein and bone health, it is not necessarily the case that protein-induced acidosis would be detrimental to bone in vivo, due to the body's ability to use other mechanisms to buffer acidosis first.

Moreover, there has been much debate as to the source of the calciuria, in terms of whether it is due to increased intestinal calcium absorption[1] or has been lost from bone itself.[37] Indeed, Kerstetter et al[13] found that lower protein diets are associated with increased parathyroid hormone, which is contrary to what would be expected if protein increases bone resorption.

3.4.1 Observational Studies Showing a Negative Association Between Protein Intakes and Bone Mineral Density

Observational studies of populations consuming very high levels of protein have indicated that protein may lower BMC and BMD. For example, a cross-sectional survey of young American women found that high intakes of protein were associated with reduced radial bone density and BMC.[38] Also, a recent study in Croatian young men and women found a negative relationship between lumbar spine BMD and protein intake.[39] Last, an observational study by Mazess and Mather[40] of Alaskan Eskimos found that middle-aged adults had 10–15% less forearm BMC and earlier bone loss than Caucasians, presumably due to their high protein diets. However, dietary protein intake was not measured in this study, and it is clear that other factors such as other dietary, lifestyle, and genetic factors may also explain any associations between protein and bone health found.

However, some studies have found no adverse effect of high protein intakes. For example, an observational study of young Irish adults found no evidence of detrimental association between protein intake and BMD in men or women.[41] Last, a randomized control trial of high and low protein weight loss diets found no detrimental effect of a high protein diet on BMC after 6 months.[42]

3.4.2 Ecological and Cohort Studies Showing Increased Fracture Risk with Increasing Dietary Protein Intake

In terms of fracture risk, some cross-cultural studies of hip fracture incidence have found a relationship between increasing hip fracture and increasing protein intake. For example, Abelow et al[43] found an increased risk of hip fracture with increasing dietary animal protein intake. Also, Frassetto et al[44] found an increased risk of hip fracture with increasing total and animal protein, but not vegetable protein intake.

However, the results of cross-cultural comparisons have been criticized. For example, countries with high hip fracture rates have longer life expectancies and also vary in other dietary and lifestyle factors (e.g., exercise, calcium intake) that may affect bone health. Indeed, Meyer et al[45] found that high protein diets were only associated with increased fracture risk when calcium intake was low.

3.4.3 Intervention Studies Assessing the Effect of Protein Supplementation on Calcium Balance and Indices of Bone Health

Intervention studies have found conflicting results for the influence of protein on calciuria and bone markers. For example, Kerstetter et al[37] found that urinary N-telopeptide and calcium excretion were higher in young women consuming high protein diets, indicating a potential increase in bone resorption. Also, Ince et al[46] found that reducing dietary protein from unrestricted intakes to the USA RDA of 0.8 g/kg body weight per day reduced NRAE and calciuria in young, premenopausal women. However, an intervention study by Dawson-Hughes et al[25] randomized men and women over 50 years old to a high or low protein supplement. There was no difference in calciuria between the groups.[25] Kerstetter et al[47] compared the effect of high and low protein intakes on urinary calcium. It was found that the high protein diet was associated with a significant decrease in urinary calcium from bone.[47]

It must, however, be borne in mind that the studies by Ince et al[46] and Kerstetter et al[47] were of short duration and used few subjects, so the long-term effect of the interventions were not established. Indeed, some authors have discussed the possibility of adaption to long-term high protein intakes,[48] which could minimize calciuria in the long term.

Therefore, the relationship between protein intake and calciuria is not clear. Some researchers have discussed how some of these contradictory results for calcium balance may be explained by the fact that dietary protein increases calcium absorption, thus input of calcium, into the body, which could explain the increased calciuria.[3] Also, pure protein supplements may give different results from changes that would be seen in more realistic whole food diets.[29]

To summarize the debate so far, there does appear to be little observational evidence that increased protein intakes may be detrimental to bone health. The majority of observational evidence suggests a beneficial role of protein, however, it must be borne in mind that these studies are purely correlational. Indeed, other factors that are also associated with high protein diets may also be explanatory (e.g., consumption of other dietary nutrients such as sodium, calcium, phytate, and phosphorus, as well as social and lifestyle factors such as exercise levels and socioeconomic status). There have been no intervention studies of protein supplementation to the authors' knowledge that have shown a clear detriment to BMD or an increase in fracture risk.

An increase in fracture risk with increasing protein intake found in some cohort studies has been attributed to protein-induced calciuria. However, more intervention studies specifically examining protein and fracture are still required to confirm or refute this hypothesis. The issue is clearly complicated, especially when other aspects of the diet must also be considered, and also how the influence of protein may be dose-responsive.

It has been suggested that moderate protein intakes may be beneficial for bone health, whereby very high and very low intakes may be detrimental. For example, a study by Whiting et al[49] found that a moderate protein diet, adequate in calcium, phosphorus, and potassium, was associated with a beneficial effect on BMD. However, more research is required in this area; as to the author's knowledge, there are no supplementation trials looking at dosage of protein and effects on bone health.

3.5 Animal and Vegetable Protein: Effects on Bone

The proposed detrimental effect of protein intake on acid–base balance has led to much debate as to whether animal, vegetable, and soy proteins differ in their effects on bone. It has been suggested that some forms of vegetable protein may lead to a lesser degree of calcium excretion than animal protein, and thus less bone loss, due to the presence of less sulfur containing amino acids.

Some studies have supported this view. For example, Sellmeyer et al[50] found that a high animal-to-vegetable protein ratio in diets of elderly women was associated with increased bone loss at the femoral neck

and also increased risk of fracture. Also, Meyer et al[45] found that diets containing high amounts of nondairy meat protein were associated with increased fracture risk in Norwegian men and women when calcium intake was low. Feskanich et al[28] found an increase in forearm fracture risk with increasing animal protein intakes, but no relationship with vegetable protein. Last, Jenkins et al[51] found no negative impact of a high vegetable protein diet on calcium balance, despite increased calcium excretion, when calcium intake was high.

However, some studies have found no such detriment or even found a benefit of animal protein. For example, lower intakes of animal protein were associated with increased femoral and spine bone loss over 4 years.[4] Also, in a prospective study of older American women, animal protein was found to have a strong negative association with hip fracture.[27] A recent study by Ho-Pham et al[52] found that in Vietnamese Buddhist nuns, there was a positive relationship between the ratio of animal to vegetable protein in the diet and whole body BMD, but no significant relationship with lumbar spine or femoral neck BMD. Last, Dawson-Hughes and Harris[53] found no effect of the type of protein on the rate of bone loss in elderly women.

Indeed, some studies have found a detrimental effect of vegetable proteins. For example, a cross-sectional study of the elderly Rancho Bernardo cohort found a positive association between intake of animal protein and bone mass density in women, with a negative association of vegetable protein with bone mass density for both men and women.[54] Also, a cross-sectional study in elderly Chinese women found vegetarians had a lower bone mass density than omnivores, with energy, protein, and calcium intakes in the vegetarian group correlated with bone mass density.[55]

Thus, the evidence for differential effects of animal and vegetable protein is mixed, and many reasons for this have been proposed. It has been suggested that some vegetable proteins may produce an equal PRAL or even a higher PRAL than does animal protein,[56] and intakes of purified plant protein have also been found to increase calciuria.[29] Bonjour[3] discusses how consumption of vegetable proteins may not necessarily lead to reduced calciuria than animal protein consumption quoting a study by Massey and Kynast-Gales,[57] which showed no difference in calciuria when plant or beef proteins were consumed. Indeed, in calculations of PRAL by Remer and Manz,[58] cereal and rice products showed a higher PRAL than some meat products. This could partially explain the contradictory results in the literature.

The effect of animal and vegetable proteins on bone health may also be complex as they may affect the skeleton in different ways due to the other nutrients and constituents these proteins contain. For example, plant food often contains potassium, which decreases calciuria.[29] Also, dairy food (a form of animal protein) are not only high in not only protein, but also calcium, which as discussed previously may compensate for calcium losses.[53] Indeed, apart from hard cheese, dairy products have a low PRAL.[59] Moreover, as found in the study by Roughead et al,[48] when calcium intake is controlled for, the level of meat protein in diets is not found to influence calcium retention.

Overall, no consistency has been found in the studies of animal vs. plant protein,[29] and there is a lack of clear evidence that vegetable protein is healthier for bone than animal protein.[3] It may be the other constituents of animal and vegetable protein that cause any differences that have been found, not the protein itself.[29]

3.6 Soy Protein: Effects on Bone

It has been hypothesized that soy protein may have specific benefits for bone health. Some studies have found a beneficial effect of soy protein on bone. For example, Arjmandi, et al[60] found that supplementation for 1 year with 25 g soy protein reduced makers of bone resorption, but not lumbar and whole body bone loss.

However, a beneficial effect has not always been found. For example, the effect of substituting soy protein for meat protein on bone health in postmenopausal women was examined in a 7-week intervention study by Roughead et al[61] It was found that urinary calcium was not significantly lower on the soya diet, even though renal acid excretion was significantly lower, and there was no influence of protein type on markers of bone metabolism (e.g., N-telopeptide, hydroxyproline, osteocalcin).[61] Kreijkamp-Kaspers et al[62] and Potter et al[63] found no effect of soy on BMD. Dalais

et al[64] found no effect of soy on bone resorption markers. Last, a recent intervention study in older women by Kenny et al[65] found no difference in BMD between groups given soy protein vs. groups given a mixture of whey and egg protein. However, there was a significant negative association between bone turnover markers and total dietary protein intake.[65]

The relationship between soy protein and bone health is thus controversial and is complicated by the fact that soy protein based food contain other dietary components (e.g., isoflavones) that may affect bone. The recent research does suggest, however, that if any, effects of soy protein on bone health are minimal.

3.7 Other Dietary Constituents

3.7.1 Calcium Intakes

Much of the research has found that the influence of protein on calcium balance varies by dietary calcium intakes. Any benefit of calcium intake may be due to compensation for any protein-induced calcium loss[66] or due to its alkaline nature. Indeed, calcium salts include an anion that may act as a buffer to acidosis.[56]

In support of this view, a study by Vatanparast et al[67] found a beneficial effect of protein on bone mass in adolescents and young adult women when calcium was adequate, with less of a benefit when calcium was insufficient. A randomized control trial by Dawson-Hughes and Harris[53] found a beneficial effect of increased dietary protein on BMD in elderly individuals supplemented with vitamin D and calcium citrate malate. However, no effect was found of protein on bone in the placebo group,[53] indicating that calcium needed to be increased to show an effect of protein. In a recent study by Zhong et al[68] looking at the 1992–2002 NHANES data, it was found that when dietary protein was low at 46 g/day, high calcium intakes were actually associated with an increased risk of any fracture. Last, Rapuri et al[69] found that elderly women consuming the highest quartile of protein intake (over 72 g/day) had higher levels of bone mass density than those consuming less protein, but only when calcium intake was at least 408 mg/day. However, in the longitudinal aspect of this study there was no link between protein intake and loss of bone. The authors discuss whether this might have been due to the small sample size used, or due to the short duration of the study.[69]

However, not all studies have supported a protein-calcium link. In an intervention study of 35–65-year-old women, higher protein, energy, and calcium intakes were correlated with slower bone loss in the placebo group, with no differential effect found for the calcium supplemented group[70]. Also, Wang et al[71] found that the calcium-to-protein ratio of the diets of postmenopausal Mexican American women was not associated with bone mass density.

Overall, much research does support the theory that the link between protein and bone health may be mediated by calcium intake. Indeed, it has been proposed that protein and calcium may not affect bone optimally unless intakes of both are sufficient.[72] High calcium intakes may offset any detriment caused by high protein intakes, and low intakes may make protein-induced detriment worse.[73] Indeed, Heaney[74] suggests that the likely best ratio in the diet of calcium:protein for bone health is $\geq20{:}1$ (mg:g). Thus the low calcium:protein ratio due to high intakes of processed food and low dairy intake in the western world may be a significant problem for bone health.

3.7.2 Phosphorus, Sulfur, and Potassium

It must be borne in mind that high protein diets also contain high levels of phosphorus, which may exert positive or negative effects on bone.[75] They may also be lower in potassium, which may thus have a negative effect on bone. Indeed, high protein intakes may only be detrimental to bone if not enough potassium rich, alkaline food (e.g., fruit and vegetables) are consumed[59] and it may be that it is not protein that should be reduced, but fruit and vegetables that should be increased.[72]

Overall, protein, phosphorus, and calcium may have interactive effects on bone, making it difficult to separate out their individual effects. Protein and calcium, in particular, may act synergistically together to benefit bone health, but protein may be detrimental if calcium is insufficient.[76]

3.8 Methodology

It is important to note that there are some problems with study methodology and interpretation. For example, studies are usually short-term, which does not allow for adaption to high protein intakes[48]. Also, studies examining the effect of protein on urinary calcium excretion vary in terms of whether mixed composition diets are used, the levels of other nutrients also present, and whether protein intakes were in normal dietary ranges or not.[75] Indeed, many of the studies that show that protein increases calciuria used purified proteins in large quantities.[73]

As discussed above, much epidemiological research is based on cross-sectional surveys and cohort studies within populations. These studies can only give an indication of the association between protein intakes and bone indices. Some supplementation trials have been undertaken for BMD. However, more large-scale trials are now required to further assess if there is a causal effect of protein on bone indices, including BMD and fracture risk. Indeed, few, if any, studies have looked at differential effects of protein dosage. Most work on the separate effects of animal and vegetable proteins have looked at bone markers and calcium metabolism, not BMD and certainly not fracture risk. Indeed, a recent meta-analysis performed by the current authors (presented at the ISNAO 2009 meeting and currently undergoing revisions for publication) highlights the need for more homogeneous, large-scale supplementation studies to fully assess whether any association between dietary protein is in fact causal and if so, how this varies by dose and calcium intake. There is, in particular, an urgent need for supplementation studies that assess fracture risk as an outcome, this being the most important clinical end point.

3.9 Concluding Remarks

Overall, much evidence has been accumulated as to the effect of protein intakes on bone. Earlier experimental research showed that potentially high protein intakes may increase acidosis and thus calciuria, which could be detrimental to bone. It was also theorized that animal protein intakes could cause more acidosis than vegetable protein due to higher sulfur amino acid content and higher PRAL. However, this has been contended and more recent research has shown that this is not necessarily the case. It has been more recently emphasized that protein has important anabolic effects on bone, and there has been a recent trend in epidemiological studies toward showing a positive effect of protein on BMD, especially when calcium intakes are adequate. Apart from a few cross-cultural studies that show a positive association between protein intakes and hip fracture risk between countries, most epidemiological studies do not show an increased risk of fractures or low bone density with increased protein intakes. However, most research is still only observational and only assesses BMD, calcium metabolism, BMC, or bone markers. More research is needed into more important clinical outcomes such as fracture risk. Indeed, the influence of protein intake on the risk of fracture is unclear and more large-scale intervention studies are now needed into whether protein supplementation can increase bone mass and decrease fracture risk. There is still much debate as to the influence of the type of protein consumed on bone (e.g., animal, vegetable, soy) and how protein interacts with other dietary nutrients. There does not appear to be clear evidence that different types of protein have differential effects on bone health.

It is important that the link between protein intakes and bone health is clarified, to expand knowledge of the influence of macronutrients on bone health and how they interact with micronutrients. It would also inform the review of reference nutrient intakes and enable appropriate dietary advice to be given to the general population. The only valid way of finally establishing whether protein intake has a causal benefit or detriment for bone is via large scale, placebo controlled supplementation trials, looking at BMD and fracture risk, preferably with the establishment of potential differential effects of dosage, other dietary nutrients, and protein type.

References

1. Kerstetter JE, O'Brien KO, Insogna KL. Dietary protein affects intestinal calcium absorption. *Am J Clin Nutr.* 1998;68:859-865.
2. Gaffney-Stomberg E, Cucchi CE, Sun B, Simpson CA, Kerstetter JE, Insogna KL. A rodent model to evaluate the effect of dietary protein on intestinal calcium absorption. *Fed Am Soc Exp Biol.* 2009; 23:726.1.
3. Bonjour JP. Dietary protein: an essential nutrient for bone health. *J Am Coll Nutr.* 2005;24:526S-536S.
4. Hannan MT, Tucker KL, Dawson-Hughes B, Cupples LA, Felson DT, Kiel DP. Effect of dietary protein on bone loss in elderly men and women: the Framingham Osteoporosis Study. *J Bone Miner Res.* 2000;15:2504-2512.
5. WHO. Diet, nutrition and the prevention of chronic diseases. *World Health Organ Tech Rep Ser.* 2003;916:129-132.
6. Karl JP, Koenig C, Staab JS, et al. Dietary influences on free insulin-like growth factor-1. *J Am Diet Assoc.* 2007;107:A104.
7. Miura Y, Kato H, Noguchi T. Effect of dietary proteins on insulin-like growth factor-1 (IGF-1) messenger ribonucleic acid content in rat liver. *Br J Nutr.* 1992;67:257-2650.
8. Schurch MA, Rizzoli R, Slosman D, Vadas L, Vergnaud P, Bonjour JP. Protein supplements increase serum insulin-like growth factor-I levels and attenuate proximal femur bone loss in patients with recent hip fracture. A randomized, double-blind, placebo-controlled trial. *Ann Intern Med.* 1998; 128:801-809.
9. Zhang M, Xuan S, Bouxsein ML, et al. Osteoblast-specific knockout of the insulin-like growth factor (IGF) receptor gene reveals an essential role of IGF signaling in bone matrix mineralization. *J Biol Chem.* 2002;277:44005-44012.
10. Caverzasio J, Montessuit C, Bonjour JP. Stimulatory effect of insulin-like growth factor-1 on renal Pi transport and plasma 1, 25-dihydroxyvitamin D3. *Endocrinol.* 1990;127:453-459.
11. Ding C, Parameswaran V, Udayan R, Burgess J, Jones G. Circulating levels of inflammatory markers predict change in bone mineral density and resorption in older adults: a longitudinal study. *J Clin Endocrinol Metab.* 2008;93:1952-1958.
12. Bourrin S, Ammann P, Bonjour JP, Rizzoli R. Dietary protein restriction lowers plasma insulin-like growth factor I (IGF-I), impairs cortical bone formation, and induces osteoblastic resistance to IGF-I in adult female rats. *Endocrinology.* 2000;141:3149-3155.
13. Kerstetter JE, Caseria DD, Mitnick ME, et al. Increased circulating concentrations of parathyroid hormone in healthy, young women consuming a protein-restricted diet. *Am J Clin Nutr.* 1997;66:1188-1196.
14. Lacey JM, Anderson JJ, Fujita T, et al. Correlates of cortical bone mass among premenopausal and postmenopausal Japanese women. *J Bone Miner Res.* 1991;6:651-659.
15. Hirota T, Nara M, Ohguri M, Manago E, Hirota K. Effect of diet and lifestyle on bone mass in Asian young women. *Am J Clin Nutr.* 1992;55:1168-1173.
16. Cooper C, Atkinson EJ, Hensrud DD, et al. Dietary protein intake and bone mass in women. *Calcif Tissue Int.* 1996;58:320-325.
17. Michaelsson K, Holmberg L, Mallmin H, Wolk A, Bergstrom R, Ljunghall S. Diet, bone mass, and osteocalcin: a cross-sectional study. *Calcif Tissue Int.* 1995;57:86-93.
18. Chiu JF, Lan SJ, Yang CY, et al. Long-term vegetarian diet and bone mineral density in postmenopausal Taiwanese women. *Calcif Tissue Int.* 1997;60:245-249.
19. Reid IR, Ames RW, Evans MC, Sharpe SJ, Gamble GD. Determinants of the rate of bone loss in normal postmenopausal women. *J Clin Endocrinol Metab.* 1994;79:950-954.

20. Ilich JZ, Brownbill RA, Tamborini L. Bone and nutrition in elderly women: protein, energy, and calcium as main determinants of bone mineral density. *Eur J Clin Nutr.* 2003; 57:554-565.

21. Devine A, Dick IM, Islam AF, Dhaliwal SS, Prince RL. Protein consumption is an important predictor of lower limb bone mass in elderly women. *Am J Clin Nutr.* 2005;81:1423-1428.

22. Tylavsky FA, Anderson JJ. Dietary factors in bone health of elderly lactoovovegetarian and omnivorous women. *Am J Clin Nutr.* 1988;48:842-849.

23. Geinoz G, Rapin CH, Rizzoli R, et al. Relationship between bone mineral density and dietary intakes in the elderly. *Osteoporos Int.* 1993;3:242-248.

24. Chevalley T, Bonjour JP, Ferrari S, Rizzoli R. High-protein intake enhances the positive impact of physical activity on BMC in prepubertal boys. *J Bone Miner Res.* 2008;23:131-142.

25. Dawson-Hughes B, Harris SS, Rasmussen H, Song L, Dallal GE. Effect of dietary protein supplements on calcium excretion in healthy older men and women. *J Clin Endocrinol Metab.* 2004;89:1169-1173.

26. Tkatch L, Rapin CH, Rizzoli R, et al. Benefits of oral protein supplementation in elderly patients with fracture of the proximal femur. *J Am Coll Nutr.* 1992;11:519-525.

27. Munger RG, Cerhan JR, Chiu BC. Prospective study of dietary protein intake and risk of hip fracture in postmenopausal women. *Am J Clin Nutr.* 1999;69:147-152.

28. Feskanich D, Willett WC, Stampfer MJ, Colditz GA. Protein consumption and bone fractures in women. *Am J Epidemiol.* 1996;143:472-479.

29. Massey LK. Dietary animal and plant protein and human bone health: a whole foods approach. *J Nutr.* 2003;133: 862S-865S.

30. Frassetto L, Morris RC, Sellmeyer DE, Todd K, Sebastian A. Diet, evolution and aging–the pathophysiologic effects of the post-agricultural inversion of the potassium-to-sodium and base-to-chloride ratios in the human diet. *Eur J Nutr.* 2001;40:200-213.

31. Arnett TR, Dempster DW. Effect of pH on bone resorption by rat osteoclasts in vitro. *Endocrinol.* 1986;119:119-124.

32. Bushinsky DA. Metabolic alkalosis decreases bone calcium efflux by suppressing osteoclasts and stimulating osteoblasts. *Am J Physiol (Ren Fluid Electrol Physiol).* 1996;271: F216-F222.

33. Allen LH, Oddoye EA, Margen S. Protein-induced hypercalciuria: a longer term study. *Am J Clin Nutr.* 1979;32: 741-749.

34. Itoh R, Nishiyama N, Suyama Y. Dietary protein intake and urinary excretion of calcium:a cross-sectional study in a healthy Japanese population. *Am J Clin Nutr.* 1998;67:438-444.

35. Lutz J, Linkswiler HM. Calcium metabolism in postmenopausal and osteoporotic women consuming two levels of dietary protein. *Am J Clin Nutr.* 1981;34:2178-2186.

36. Margen S, Chu JY, Kaufmann A, Galloway DH. Studies in calcium metabolism. I. The calciuretic effect of dietary protein. *Am J Clin Nutr.* 1974;27:584-589.

37. Kerstetter JE, Mitnick ME, Gundberg MC, et al. Changes in bone turnover in young women consuming different levels of dietary protein. *J Clin Endocrinol Metab.* 1999;84: 1052-1055.

38. Metz JA, Anderson JJ, Gallagher PN Jr. Intakes of calcium, phosphorus, and protein, and physical-activity level are related to radial bone mass in young adult women. *Am J Clin Nutr.* 1993;58:537-542.

39. Avdagi SC, Bari IC, Keser I, et al. Differences in peak bone density between male and female students. *Arh Hig Rada Toksikol.* 2009;60:79-86.

40. Mazess RB, Mather W. Bone mineral content of North Alaskan Eskimos. *Am J Clin Nutr.* 1974;27:916-925.

41. Neville CE, Robson PJ, Murray LJ, et al. The effect of nutrient intake on bone mineral status in young adults: The Northern Ireland Young Hearts Project. *Calcif Tissue Int.* 2002;70:89-98.

42. Skov AR, Haulrik N, Toubro S, And MC, Astrup A. Effect of protein intake on bone mineralisation during weight loss: A 6 month trial. *Obes Res.* 2002;10:432-438.

43. Abelow BJ, Holford TR, Insogna KL. Cross-cultural association between dietary animal protein and hip fracture: a hypothesis. *Calcif Tissue Int.* 1992;50:14-18.

44. Frassetto LA, Todd KM, Morris RC Jr, Sebastian A. Worldwide incidence of hip fracture in elderly women: relation to consumption of animal and vegetable foods. *J Gerontol A Biol Sci Med Sci.* 2000;55:M585-M592.

45. Meyer HE, Pedersen JI, Loken EB, Tverdal A. Dietary factors and the incidence of hip fracture in middle-aged Norwegians. A prospective study. *Am J Epidemiol.* 1997;145:117-123.

46. Ince BA, Anderson EJ, Neer RM. Lowering dietary protein to U.S. Recommended dietary allowance levels reduces urinary calcium excretion and bone resorption in young women. *J Clin Endocrinol Metab.* 2004;89:3801-3807.

47. Kerstetter JE, O'Brien KO, Caseria DM, Wall DE, Insogna KL. The impact of dietary protein on calcium absorption and kinetic measures of bone turnover in women. *J Clin Endocrinol Metab.* 2005;90:26-31.

48. Roughead ZK, Johnson LK, Lykken GL, Hunt JR. Controlled high meat diets do not affect calcium retention or indices of bone status in healthy postmenopausal women. *J Nutr.* 2003;133:1020-1026.

49. Whiting SJ, Boyle JL, Thompson A, Mirwald RL, Faulkner RA. Dietary protein, phosphorus and potassium are beneficial to bone mineral density in adult men consuming adequate dietary calcium. *J Am Coll Nutr.* 2002;21:402-409.

50. Sellmeyer DE, Stone KL, Sebastian A, Cummings SR. A high ratio of dietary animal to vegetable protein increases the rate of bone loss and the risk of fracture in postmenopausal women. Study of Osteoporotic Fractures Research Group. *Am J Clin Nutr.* 2001;73:118-122.

51. Jenkins DJ, Kendall CW, Vidgen E, et al. Effect of high vegetable protein diets on urinary calcium loss in middle-aged men and women. *Eur J Clin Nutr.* 2003;57:376-382.

52. Ho-Pham LT, Nguyen PL, Le TT, et al. Veganism, bone mineral density, and body composition: a study in Buddhist nuns. *Osteoporos Int.* 2009;20:2087-2093.

53. Dawson-Hughes B, Harris SS. Calcium intake influences the association of protein intake with rates of bone loss in elderly men and women. *Am J Clin Nutr.* 2002;75:773-779.

54. Promislow JH, Goodman-Gruen D, Slymen DJ, Barrett-Connor E. Protein consumption and bone mineral density in the elderly: the Rancho Bernardo Study. *Am J Epidemiol.* 2002;155:636-644.

55. Lau EM, Kwok T, Woo J, Ho SC. Bone mineral density in Chinese elderly female vegetarians, vegans, lacto-vegetarians and omnivores. *Eur J Clin Nutr.* 1998;52:60-64.

56. Massey LK. Does excess dietary protein adversely affect bone? Symposium overview. *J Nutr.* 1998;128:1048-1105.

57. Massey LK, Kynast-Gales SA. Diets with either beef or plant proteins reduce risk of calcium oxalate precipitation in patients with a history of calcium kidney stones. *J Am Diet Assoc.* 2001;101:326-331.

58. Remer T, Manz F. Potential renal acid load of foods and its influence on urine pH. *J Am Diet Assoc.* 1995;95:791-797.

59. Barzel US, Massey LK. Excess dietary protein can adversely affect bone. *J Nutr.* 1998;128:1051-1053.

60. Arjmandi BH, Lucas EA, Khalil DA, et al. One year soy protein supplementation has positive effects on bone formation markers but not bone density in postmenopausal women. *Nutr J.* 2005;4:8.

61. Roughead ZK, Hunt JR, Johnson LK, Badger TM, Lykken GI. Controlled substitution of soy protein for meat protein: effects on calcium retention, bone and cardiovascular health indices in postmenopausal women. *J Clin Endocrinol Metab.* 2005;90(1):181-189.

62. Kreijkamp-Kaspers S, Kok L, Grobbee DE, et al. Effect of soy protein containing isoflavones on cognitive function, bone mineral density, and plasma lipids in postmenopausal women: a randomized controlled trial. *JAMA.* 2004;292:65-74.

63. Potter SM, Baum JA, Teng H, Stillman RJ, Shay NF, Erdman JW Jr. Soy protein and isoflavones: their effects on blood lipids and bone density in postmenopausal women. *Am J Clin Nutr.* 1998;68:1375S-1379S.

64. Dalais FS, Ebeling PR, Kotsopoulos D, McGrath BP, Teede HJ. The effects of soy protein containing isoflavones on lipids and indices of bone resorption in postmenopausal women. *Clin Endocrinol (Oxf).* 2003;58:704-709.

65. Kenny AM, Mangano KM, Abourizk RH, et al. Soy proteins and isoflavones affect bone mineral density in older women: a randomized controlled trial. *Am J Clin Nutr.* 2009;90:234-242.

66. Dawson-Hughes B. Interaction of dietary calcium and protein in bone health in humans. *J Nutr.* 2003;133:852S-854S.

67. Vatanparast H, Bailey DA, Baxter-Jones ADG, Whiting SJ. The effects of dietary protein on bone mineral mass in young adults may be modulated by adolescent calcium intake. *J Nutr.* 2007;137:2674-2679.

68. Zhong Y, Okoro C, Balluz L. Association of total calcium and dietary protein intakes with fracture risk in postmenopausal women: The 1999–2002 National Health and Nutrition Examination Survey (NHANES). *Nutrition.* 2008;25:647-654.

69. Rapuri PB, Gallagher JC, Haynatzka V. Protein intake: effects on bone mineral density and the rate of bone loss in elderly women. *Am J Clin Nutr.* 2003;77:1517-1525.

70. Freudenheim JL, Johnson NE, Smith EL. Relationships between usual nutrient intake and bone-mineral content of women 35-65 years of age: longitudinal and cross-sectional analysis. *Am J Clin Nutr.* 1986;44:863-876.

71. Wang MC, Luz Villa M, Marcus R, Kelsey JL. Associations of vitamin C, calcium and protein with bone mass in postmenopausal Mexican American women. *Osteoporos Int.* 1997;7:533-538.

72. Heaney RP, Layman DK. Amount and type of protein influences bone health. *Am J Clin Nutr.* 2008;87:1567S-1570S.

73. Ginty F. Dietary protein and bone health. *Proc Nutr Soc.* 2003;62:867-876.

74. Heaney RP. Excess dietary protein may not adversely affect bone. *J Nutr.* 1998;128(6):1054-1057.

75. Spencer H, Kramer L, Osis D, Norris C. Effect of phosphorus on the absorption of calcium and on the calcium balance in man. *J Nutr.* 1978;108:447-457.

76. Heaney RP. Protein and calcium: antagonists or synergists? *Am J Clin Nutr.* 2002;75:609-610.

4

Protein Intake During Weight Loss: Effects on Bone

Sue A. Shapses and Deeptha Sukumar

4.1 Introduction

Moderate weight loss will reduce the comorbidities associated with obesity. A 10% weight loss is also associated with loss of 1–2% of bone mass. Supplementation with specific nutrients, such as calcium,[1–3] may attenuate loss of bone mass during weight reduction. Recently, high-protein (HP) weight-loss diets have become more popular, and studies have shown that they are as effective as, or sometimes more effective than, standard high carbohydrate weight loss diets in reducing symptoms associated with metabolic syndrome.[4–6] The effect of higher protein diets on bone is important due to the greater acceptance among health care providers. Dietary protein has also been shown to have specific effects on the regulation of bone health.[7] Some large epidemiological studies have shown a beneficial impact of protein on bone health,[8–11] which is supported by intervention studies in patients with osteoporosis.[12,13] In contrast, others have suggested that a HP diet is associated with low bone mineral density (BMD) and greater fracture risk[14–16] and have attributed this to a greater acid load and increased urinary calcium excretion. Since lower calcium intake may mediate the negative effect of HP diets on bone,[17–20] controlled trials to study the effects of protein are important. During weight reduction, there is both a reduced calcium absorption and serum insulin-like growth factor-1 (IGF-1), which may contribute to bone loss, yet may be positively influenced by additional protein in the diet. The role of dietary protein during caloric restriction on bone health and potential mechanisms mediating these effects is reviewed.

4.2 Weight Loss and High-Protein Diets

Weight loss is often achieved by eliminating or reducing a specific food type or reducing intake of carbohydrate, protein, and fat. Diets that are high in protein and low in carbohydrate are popular and often result in greater short-term weight loss compared to high carbohydrate low fat (LF) diets. In addition, HP diets are associated with greater fat loss and preservation of lean mass that is supported by the evidence of a greater fat oxidation and higher protein balance.[5,21] The positive influence of dietary protein on weight loss may be mediated by its higher thermic effect and sleeping metabolic rate compared to carbohydrate and fat. These metabolic changes would be expected to increase total energy expenditure to ultimately promote a greater weight loss. In addition, higher protein (or dairy) diets also promote satiety, possibly mediated by higher postprandial cholecystokinin (CCK) levels, higher circulating concentrations of certain amino acids, or diet-induced thermogenesis.[22] Certain appetite regulatory hormones are also triggered by higher protein intake, including an increase in postprandial ghrelin, glucagon like peptide-1, and insulin secretion.[23] These mechanisms collectively may mediate the effect of higher protein intake on short-term weight loss and fat loss as compared to normal protein (NP) diets. The greater weight loss on a HP compared to a NP diet may contribute to the improved lipid profile, greater loss of fat, and improved insulin sensitivity.[24–26] Indeed, longer-term studies show that the greater weight loss on a higher protein diet is not

S.A. Shapses (✉)
96 Lipman Drive, New Brunswick, NJ 08901, USA
e-mail: shapses@aesop.rutgers.edu

P. Burckhardt et al. (eds.), *Nutritional Influences on Bone Health*,
DOI: 10.1007/978-1-84882-978-7_4, © Springer-Verlag London Limited 2010

sustained and is similar to that seen with a standard high carbohydrate diet after 1–2 years.[6]

Although HP diets have been shown to promote enhanced loss of body weight, some physiological concerns about the effect of such diets on different organs are still debated. For example, the long-term effect of HP weight loss diets may be detrimental to the kidneys. A 6-month weight-loss study showed greater glomerular filtration rate (GFR) and kidney volume on a HP (108 g/day) compared to NP diet (70 g/day).[27] However, the specific GFR, which is an expression of the filtration rate per unit kidney volume, and albumin levels were not altered by either treatment. The authors thus suggest that the changes in GFR were adaptations of the kidney to changes in protein load. In a large 11-year study examining 1,624 weight stable women with normal renal function, a HP intake of 93 g/day did not significantly alter GFR.[28] Most researchers agree that unlike renal patients, in healthy populations there is little evidence of adverse effects of HP diets on renal function.[27,28]

Overall, reports show that while HP diets do result in greater loss of body weight over a 6-month period, these diets do not result in any additional benefit to promote weight reduction or improve metabolic parameters compared to a high carbohydrate diet after 1–2 years. Since HP diets remain popular and prevalent among the diet choices, other outcome variables including bone should be addressed.

4.3 Weight Loss and Bone

A weight loss goal of ~10% is reasonable for most individuals and often has a positive effect on many of the comorbidities associated with obesity.[29] However, caloric restriction will increase bone mobilization and loss, showing about 1–2% at most sites, and this is largely observed in older women and men.[30] Caloric restriction may increase bone mobilization for a variety of reasons (Fig. 4.1), including a decrease in calcium intake and/or other nutrients,[1,2] a decrease in calcium absorption,[31] reduced weight bearing,[32,33] and/or hormonal changes.[30] For example, a reduction in adiposity has been shown to also reduce estrogen levels that may contribute to bone loss in postmenopausal women. In addition, caloric restriction is also associated with reduced serum IGF-1, which would negatively influence bone. Numerous adipocyte-derived hormones have been implicated in the regulation of bone during weight loss such as leptin, adiponectin, and resistin.[30,34] Gut peptides (i.e., ghrelin, incretins, CCK, peptide YY (PYY), and pancreatic polypeptide (PPY)) that regulate satiety are often altered in both obesity[35] and weight reduction.[36] Many of these hormones and peptides also regulate the osteoblast and/or osteoclast suggesting an interaction between the gut, brain, and bone. Other mechanisms such as reduced weight bearing due to a reduction in body weight may also play a role in mobilizing bone during caloric restriction. Exercise[32,33] and/or

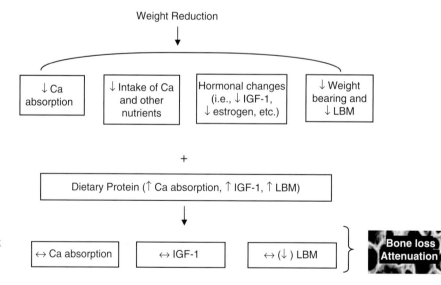

Fig. 4.1 Potential mechanisms regulating bone during caloric restriction with dietary protein

use of osteoporosis medications[37] have been shown to attenuate the bone loss associated with caloric restriction. In addition, we and others have shown that calcium supplementation will suppress bone turnover and loss during caloric restriction.[1-3] Whether or not other micro or macronutrients influence bone during caloric restriction remains unclear, yet some studies are currently underway.

4.4 High Protein Diets and Bone

Several observational and clinical studies have examined the influence of HP diets on bone. A higher protein intake (84–152 g/day) has been positively associated with change in femoral neck and spine BMD over a 4-year-period in the Framingham osteoporosis study.[9] Similarly, the NHANES III showed a positive association between femoral neck BMD and total protein intake (>75 g),[38] as did another study that found a decreased risk of hip fracture and wrist fracture[11] with higher protein intake. Intervention studies have shown that dietary protein supplementation in patients after hip fracture has a positive impact on serum levels of IGF-1, femur BMD, and a shorter hospital stay[12,13], although in one of these trials, the protein supplement group was also given more calcium and vitamin D.[13] On the other hand, a negative association of protein with BMD was found in a smaller study of young women.[16] In addition, in the Nurses Health Study, no association was observed between protein intake and the risk of hip fracture, yet the risk of forearm fractures was higher in women with a higher (>95 g) protein intake.[15] This is consistent with an epidemiological study showing that countries with higher protein intakes also have a greater fracture risk.[14] However, in all cross-sectional studies, protein intake was measured using self-assessed food frequency questionnaires and/or largely using diet recalls. It is important to note that no intervention studies to date have reported a negative influence of protein on bone, and there are potential mechanisms that would support either a positive or negative influence of protein on fracture risk.

Several mechanisms have been proposed by which a higher protein intake may improve bone mass including its positive effect on IGF-1 and calcium absorption. An increase in dietary protein intake has been shown to increase serum levels of IGF-1,[11,39] which promotes osteoblast proliferation and matrix formation[40] and may in turn increase bone mass and reduce fracture risk.[11,12] A higher protein intake (2.1 g/kg) has also been shown to increase intestinal calcium absorption that leads to a parallel increase in urinary calcium and decrease in bone turnover markers compared to a moderate intake (1.0 g/kg).[41] This 10-day study[41] and another 8-week isotopic tracer study examining protein intake[42] showed trends toward better calcium retention during HP intakes. It is interesting that one study found that with higher calcium intake, there was no protein-related increase in calcium absorption.[43] In addition, a higher protein intake is associated with an increase in muscle mass and promotes collagen synthesis, both of which may have a positive influence on acquisition of bone mass.[44]

In contrast, some epidemiological studies show that HP diets reduce bone mass, and this has been attributed to a higher acid load leading to a buffering response by the skeleton and greater urinary calcium excretion. It has been estimated that for every 1 g rise in dietary protein, approximately 1 mg calcium is lost in urine.[20] There has also been considerable debate on plant vs. animal protein sources, with some large epidemiological findings[14] attributing the negative effect on hip fracture to a higher content of sulfur containing amino acids in animal and some vegetable proteins. However, controlled intervention studies[42,43] have shown no adverse effects of animal protein on calcium retention. A metaanalysis[45] concluded that the calciuria associated with a higher net acid excretion from HP diets does not reflect a loss of whole body calcium. In addition, a normal to high calcium intake along with a HP diet will offset loss of urinary calcium, attenuate bone turnover,[18,20] and is associated with greater femoral neck and total body BMD, as measured in a 3-year study.[9] Consistent with this, a study[17] showed that HP diets (including meat) were associated with increased fracture risk only when the calcium intake was low (<400 mg/1,000 kcal).

Thus in light of the current available literature and in the absence of longer controlled intervention trials, most would agree that there is a beneficial effect of HP intake on bone in older individuals with a normal habitual low intake. In addition, a positive effect of dietary protein on bone is dependent on the presence of adequate calcium and vitamin D in the diet.

4.5 Weight Loss, Protein Intake, and Bone

4.5.1 Background and Previous Studies

HP weight-loss diets may preserve bone mass during caloric restriction by several mechanisms (Fig. 4.1). Caloric restriction leads to a decrease in IGF-1 levels and IGF-1/1GFBP-3 ratio,[46] whereas a HP intake raises these levels. Therefore, it is possible that a HP diet may attenuate the decrease in IGF-1 associated with caloric restriction. The rise in IGF-1 may also increase skeletal muscle mass and indirectly preserve bone mass.[12,44] In addition, a higher protein intake increases calcium absorption,[41] which may attenuate the decrease in absorption associated with caloric restriction.[31] Finally, due to reduced food intake during caloric restriction, protein intake may be compromised (<0.8 g/kg), and it is well established that low protein diets reduce IGF-1 production, which in turn has a negative effect on calcium and phosphate metabolism, and bone.[38,47]

Interestingly, several hormones that influence bone are also influenced by dietary protein intake. Following a HP meal, leptin sensitivity and levels are altered.[23] In addition, postprandial ghrelin secretion and incretins, specifically GLP-1 that eventually triggers insulin release, increase following a HP meal. Similarly, PYY concentrations also increase in response to a protein meal.[48] However, there is no evidence to show that such short-term influences of HP diets on these hormones will mediate its effects on bone.

Studies have examined the role of higher dietary protein on bone mass and turnover during caloric restriction (Table 4.1). In these studies[4,24–26,49–51] both a higher and NP diet produce similar weight loss except for one study,[47] showing greater weight loss in the HP compared to NP group. Some,[49,51] but not all,[4,24–26,50,51] of these studies demonstrate a positive impact of higher dietary protein on bone mass and turnover during caloric restriction, but none of these studies control for dietary calcium intake. The importance of dietary calcium on bone is well established,[52] as well as during weight loss.[1–3,50] Because studies that increase protein intake during dieting have accomplished this by increasing dairy intake, calcium levels are also higher in these diets. Hence, the HP diets (with adequate or high calcium) were compared to calcium insufficient (~600 mg/day) high carbohydrate diets.[49,51] Not surprisingly, high dairy and protein studies[49–51] have shown a positive impact of the diet on maintenance of bone mass during caloric restriction, similar to calcium supplementation studies without higher protein intake.[1–3] Thus the role of protein in the maintenance of bone mass during caloric restriction is unclear, and use of a high carbohydrate control group that is not deficient in calcium intake has not been previously examined.

4.5.2 Preliminary Findings

To understand whether dietary protein intake influences bone mass during caloric restriction while controlling for calcium intake and other nutrients, we examined overweight and obese postmenopausal women who were assigned to caloric restriction and 1.2 g Ca/day and a multivitamin supplementation with either a normal or higher protein intake and a LF intake for 1 year. Overweight and obese postmenopausal women were counseled weekly until 4 months, and then twice per month in a standard behavior-modification nutrition education weight loss program. In these preliminary findings, women who completed the protocol lost 6.6 ± 5.2% of their body weight after 1 year and did not differ significantly ($p < 0.001$) between groups. The average loss of fat mass was 4.3 ± 3.6 kg and of lean mass was 1.3 ± 1.1 kg, with no significant differences between groups. At baseline, there were no significant differences in nutrient intake between women assigned to HP or NP groups. During calorie-restricted diets, protein intake was higher at 85 ± 10 g protein/day (23% of calories, $n = 23$) in the HP group compared to 60 ± 11 g protein/day (18% of calories; $n = 20$) in the NP group ($p < 0.001$). There were no significant differences in calcium or vitamin D intake between the HP and NP groups, respectively. Results showed that the radius and lumbar spine (LS) BMD decreased in the NP as compared to the HP group. There were no significant differences between the groups at the femoral neck, total hip, or total body. In addition, there was a trend for a greater increase in serum IGF-1 levels in the HP compared to the NP group in a subset analyzed in this preliminary data.

Table 4.1 Studies examining higher protein intake during caloric restriction on bone mass and turnover

References	Population n, age, BMI	Groups (pro intake)	WL duration	Ca intake (mg/day)	Bone site and markers	Weight loss[a] (%)	Effect of HP diet
Skov et al[49]	n = 65 M & F 39 Years 30 kg/m^2	HP 102 g/day NP 71 g/day	6 Months	HP 936 NP 659	TB	8.1	Decreased loss of BMC
Farnsworth et al[24]	n = 57 M & F 50 Years 34 kg/m^2	HP (27%) NP (16%)	12 Weeks[b]	HP 1,600 NP 600	PYD, DPD	8.0	No effect
Bowen et al[50]	n = 50 M & F 50 Years 33 kg/m^2	2 HP groups Dairy (DP, 108 g/day) or mixed (MP 104 g/day)	12 Weeks[b]	DP 2,371 MP 509	Osteocalcin PYD, DPD	9.9	DP minimized bone turnover
Brinkworth et al[25]	n = 58 M & F 50.2 Years 34 kg/m^2	HP (30%) NP (15%)	12 Week[b]	NA	TB-BMC	8.9	No effect
Noakes et al[4]	n = 100 F 49 Years 32 kg/m^2	HP (31%) NP (18%)	12 Week[c]	HP 777 NP 594	Osteocalcin, PYD,DPD	8.4	No effect
Thorpe et al[51]	n = 130 M & F 46 Years 31 kg/m^2	HP 97 g/day NP 61 g/day	4 Months[d]	HP 1,120 NP 765	TB, LS, hip	8.2	Decreased loss of BMD at 12 months

PYD pyridinoline; *DPD* deoxypyridinoline; *BMD* bone mineral density; *BMC* bone mineral content; *HP* high protein; *NP* normal protein; *F* female; *M* males; *HF* high fat; *LF* low fat; *LS* lumbar spine; *TB* total body

[a]No difference in weight loss between HP and NP groups, except in Skovl et al.45 showing greater loss in HP (~10%) vs. NP (~6%) diet

[b]The weight loss was followed by a weight maintenance period of 4

[c]The weight loss was followed by a weight maintenance period of 1 year (this 1 year study showed no BMD difference between groups[26])

[d]The weight loss was followed by a weight maintenance period of 8 months

Confirmation of these preliminary findings has yet to be determined, but it is likely safe to conclude that a normal to higher intake of protein during dieting is not detrimental to bone and may be beneficial to avoid low protein intakes that might occur with low calorie diets.

4.6 Conclusion

Caloric restriction-mediated bone loss is an important health concern due to a high prevalence of dieting and a worldwide concern of osteoporosis. Although the benefits of calcium supplementation on bone have been studied in the dieting population, the effects of popular dietary macronutrient modifications, such as a higher protein on bone, require further study. Some weight reduction trials have addressed higher protein and dairy (or calcium) diets, and not surprisingly, found a positive effect on bone. Our preliminary data suggest that even without very high intakes of calcium and vitamin D, a HP diet is not detrimental to bone. It is possible that the mechanisms regulating bone with a higher protein intake include higher calcium absorption and serum IGF-1 or other hormones and a higher acid load, whereas their role when combined with caloric restriction is not known. Our understanding of the regulation of bone during weight loss has increased markedly over the past decade, and we are just beginning to understand how other nutrients, such as protein, may influence bone during caloric restriction.

Acknowledgments This work is supported by the NIH-NIA AG12161.

References

1. Jensen LB, Kollerup G, Quaade F, Sørensen OH. Bone minerals changes in obese women during a moderate weight loss with and without calcium supplementation. *J Bone Miner Res*. 2001;16(1):141-147.

2. Ricci TA, Chowdhury HA, Heymsfield SB, Stahl T, Pierson RN Jr, Shapses SA. Calcium supplementation suppresses bone turnover during weight reduction in postmenopausal women. *J Bone Miner Res*. 1998;13(6):1045-1050.

3. Riedt CS, Cifuentes M, Stahl T, Chowdhury HA, Schlussel Y, Shapses SA. Overweight postmenopausal women lose bone with moderate weight reduction and 1 g/day calcium intake. *J Bone Miner Res*. 2005;20(5):455-463.

4. Noakes M, Keogh JB, Foster PR, Clifton PM. Effect of an energy-restricted, high-protein, low-fat diet relative to a conventional high-carbohydrate, low-fat diet on weight loss, body composition, nutritional status, and markers of cardiovascular health in obese women. *Am J Clin Nutr*. 2005; 81(6):1298-1306.

5. Westerterp-Plantenga MS, Nieuwenhuizen A, Tome D, Soenen S, Westerterp KR. Dietary protein, weight loss, and weight maintenance. *Annu Rev Nutr*. 2009;29:21-41. doi: 10.1146/annurev-nutr-080508-141056.

6. Sacks FM, Bray GA, Carey VJ, et al. Comparison of weight-loss diets with different compositions of fat, protein, and carbohydrates. *N Engl J Med*. 2009;360(9):859-873.

7. Conigrave AD, Brown EM, Rizzoli R. Dietary protein and bone health: roles of amino acid-sensing receptors in the control of calcium metabolism and bone homeostasis. *Annu Rev Nutr*. 2008;28:131-155.

8. Thorpe DL, Knutsen SF, Beeson WL, Rajaram S, Fraser GE. Effects of meat consumption and vegetarian diet on risk of wrist fracture over 25 years in a cohort of peri- and postmenopausal women. *Public Health Nutr*. 2008;11(6):564-572.

9. Hannan MT, Tucker KL, Dawson-Hughes B, Cupples LA, Felson DT Kiel DP. Effect of dietary protein on bone loss in elderly men and women: the Framingham Osteoporosis Study. *J Bone Miner Res*. 2000;15(12):2504-2512.

10. Munger RG, Cerhan JR, Chiu BC. Prospective study of dietary protein intake and risk of hip fracture in postmenopausal women. *Am J Clin Nutr*. 1999;69(1):147-152.

11. Wengreen HJ, Munger RG, West NA, et al. Dietary protein intake and risk of osteoporotic hip fracture in elderly residents of Utah. *Bone Miner Res*. 2004;19(4):537-545.

12. Schürch MA, Rizzoli R, Slosman D, Vadas L, Vergnaud P, Bonjour JP. Protein supplements increase serum insulin-like growth factor-I levels and attenuate proximal femur bone loss in patients with recent hip fracture. A randomized, double-blind, placebo-controlled trial. *Ann Intern Med*. 1998;128(10): 801-809.

13. Delmi M, Rapin CH, Bengoa JM, Delmas PD, Vasey H, Bonjour JP. Dietary supplementation in elderly patients with fractured neck of the femur. *Lancet*. 1990;335(8696): 1013-1016.

14. Abelow BJ, Holford TR, Insogna KL. Cross-cultural association between dietary animal protein and hip fracture: a hypothesis. *Calcif Tissue Int*. 1992;50(1):14-18.

15. Feskanich D, Willett WC, Stampfer MJ, Colditz GA. Protein consumption and bone fractures in women. *Am J Epidemiol*. 1996;143:472-479.

16. Metz JA, Anderson JJ, Gallagher PN Jr. Intakes of calcium, phosphorus, and protein, and physical-activity level are related to radial bone mass in young adult women. *Am J Clin Nutr*. 1993;58(4):537-542.

17. Dargent-Molina P, Sabia S, Touvier M, et al. Proteins, dietary acid load, and calcium and risk of postmenopausal fractures in the E3N French women prospective study. *J Bone Miner Res*. 2008;23(12):1915-1922.

18. Dawson-Hughes B. Interaction of dietary calcium and protein in bone health in humans. *J Nutr*. 2003;133(3):852S-854S.

19. Dawson-Hughes B, Harris SS. Calcium intake influences the association of protein intake with rates of bone loss in elderly men and women. *Am J Clin Nutr*. 2002;75(4):773-779.

20. Heaney RP. Excess dietary protein may not adversely affect bone. *J Nutr*. 1998;128(6):1054-1057.

21. Krieger JW, Sitren HS, Daniels MJ, Langkamp-Henken B. Effects of variation in protein and carbohydrate intake on body mass and composition during energy restriction: a meta-regression. *Am J Clin Nutr*. 2006;83(2):260-274.

22. Westerterp-Plantenga MS, Rolland V, Wilson SA, Westerterp KR. Satiety related to 24 h diet-induced thermogenesis during high protein/carbohydrate vs high fat diets measured in a respiration chamber. *Eur J Clin Nutr*. 1999;53(6):495-502.

23. Weigle DS, Breen PA, Matthys CC, et al. A high-protein diet induces sustained reductions in appetite, ad libitum caloric intake, and body weight despite compensatory changes in diurnal plasma leptin and ghrelin concentrations. *Am J Clin Nutr*. 2005;82(1):41-48.

24. Farnsworth E, Luscombe ND, Noakes M, Wittert G, Argyiou E, Clifton PM. Effect of a high protein, energy restricted diet on body composition, glycemic control and lipid concentrations in overweight and obese hyperinsulinemic men and women. *Am J Clin Nutr*. 2003;78:31-39.

25. Brinkworth GD, Noakes M, Parker B, Foster P, Clifton PM. Long-term effects of advice to consume a high-protein, low-fat diet, rather than a conventional weight-loss diet, in obese adults with type 2 diabetes: one-year follow-up of a randomized trial. *Diabetologia*. 2004;47(10):1677-1686.

26. Clifton PM, Keogh JB, Noakes M. Long-term effects of a high-protein weight-loss diet. *Am J Clin Nutr*. 2008;87(1): 23-29.

27. Skov AR, Toubro S, Bülow J, Krabbe K, Parving HH, Astrup A. Changes in renal function during weight loss induced by high vs low-protein low-fat diets in overweight subjects. *Int J Obes Relat Metab Disord*. 1999;23(11):1170-1177.

28. Knight EL, Stampfer MJ, Hankinson SE, Spiegelman D, Curhan GC. The impact of protein intake on renal function decline in women with normal renal function or mild renal insufficiency. *Ann Intern Med*. 2003;138(6):460-467.

29. Wing RR, Phelan S. Long-term weight loss maintenance. *Am J Clin Nutr*. 2005;82(1 suppl):222S-225S.

30. Shapses SA, Riedt CS. Bone, body weight, and weight reduction: what are the concerns? *J Nutr*. 2006;136(6): 1453-1456.

31. Cifuentes M, Riedt CS, Brolin RE, Field MP, Sherrell RM, Shapses SA. Weight loss and calcium intake influence calcium absorption in overweight postmenopausal women. *Am J Clin Nutr*. 2004;80(1):123-130.

32. Villareal DT, Fontana L, Weiss EP, et al. Bone mineral density response to caloric restriction-induced weight loss or exercise-induced weight loss: a randomized controlled trial. *Arch Intern Med*. 2006;166(22):2502-2510.

33. Ryan AS, Nicklas BJ, Dennis KE. Aerobic exercise maintains regional bone mineral density during weight loss in postmenopausal women. *J Appl Physiol*. 1998;84:1305-1310.

34. Zhao LJ, Jiang H, Papasian CJ, et al. Correlation of obesity and osteoporosis: effect of fat mass on the determination of osteoporosis. *J Bone Miner Res*. 2008;23(1):17-29.

35. Crowell MD, Decker GA, Levy R, Jeffrey R, Talley NJ. Gut-brain neuropeptides in the regulation of ingestive behaviors and obesity. *Am J Gastroenterol*. 2006;101(12):2848-2856; quiz 2914.

36. Bueter M, le Roux CW. Sir David Cuthbertson Medal Lecture Bariatric surgery as a model to study appetite control. *Proc Nutr Soc*. 2009;29:1-7.

37. Gozansky WS, Van Pelt RE, Jankowski CM, Schwartz RS, Kohrt WM. Protection of bone mass by estrogens and raloxifene during exercise-induced weight Loss. *J Clin Endocrinol Metab*. 2005;90(1):52-59.

38. Kerstetter JE, Looker AC, Insogna KL. Low dietary protein and low bone density. *Calcif Tissue Int*. 2000;66(4):313.

39. Holmes MD, Pollak MN, Willett WC, Hankinson SE. Dietary correlates of plasma insulin-like growth factor I and insulin-like growth factor binding protein 3 concentrations. *Cancer Epidemiol Biomarkers Prev*. 2002;11(9):852-861.

40. Price JS, Oyajobi BO, Oreffo RO, Russell R. Cells cultured from the growing tip of red deer antler express alkaline phosphatase and proliferate in response to insulin-like growth factor-I. *J Endocrinol*. 1994;143(2):R9-R16.

41. Kerstetter JE, O'Brien KO, Caseria DM, Wall DE, Insogna KL. The impact of dietary protein on calcium absorption and kinetic measures of bone turnover in women. *J Clin Endocrinol Metab*. 2005;90(1):26-31.

42. Roughead ZK, Hunt JR, Johnson LK, Badger TM, Lykken GI. Controlled substitution of soy protein for meat protein: effects on calcium retention, bone, and cardiovascular health indices in postmenopausal women. *J Clin Endocrinol Metab*. 2005;90(1):181-189.

43. Hunt JR, Johnson LK, Fariba Roughead ZK. Dietary protein and calcium interact to influence calcium retention: a controlled feeding study. *Am J Clin Nutr*. 2009;89(5):1357-1365.

44. Ginty F. Dietary protein and bone health. *Proc Nutr Soc Nov*. 2003;62(4):867-876.

45. Fenton TR, Lyon AW, Eliasziw M, Tough SC, Hanley DA. Meta-analysis of the effect of the acid-ash hypothesis of osteoporosis on calcium balance. *J Bone Miner Res*. 2009;24: 1835-1840.doi:10.1359/JBMR.090515.

46. Oster MH, Fielder PJ, Levin N, Cronin M. Adaptation of the growth hormone and insulin-like growth factor-I axis to chronic and severe calorie or protein malnutrition. *J Clin Invest*. 1995;95(5):2258-2265.

47. Bourrin S, Ammann P, Bonjour JP, Rizzoli R. Dietary protein restriction lowers plasma insulin-like growth factor I (IGF-I), impairs cortical bone formation, and induces osteoblastic resistance to IGF-I in adult female rats. *Endocrinology*. 2000;141(9):3149-3155.

48. Batterham RL, Heffron H, Kapoor S, et al. Critical role for peptide YY in protein-mediated satiation and body-weight regulation. *Cell Metab*. 2006;4(3):223-233.

49. Skov AR, Haulrik N, Toubro S, Mølgaard C, Astrup A. Effect of protein intake on bone mineralization during weight loss: a 6-month trial. *Obes Res*. 2002;10(6):432-438.

50. Bowen J, Noakes M, Clifton P. High dairy-protein versus high mixed-protein energy restricted diets – the effect on bone turnover and calcium excretion in overweight adults. *Asia Pac J Clin Nutr*. 2003;12(suppl):S52.

51. Thorpe MP, Jacobson EH, Layman DK, He X, Kris-Etherton PM, Evans EM. A diet high in protein, dairy, and calcium attenuates bone loss over twelve months of weight loss and maintenance relative to a conventional high-carbohydrate diet in adults. *J Nutr*. 2008;138(6):1096-1100.

52. Dawson-Hughes B, Harris SS, Krall EA, Dallal GE. Effect of calcium and vitamin D supplementation on bone density in men and women 65 years of age or older. *N Engl J Med*. 1997;337(10):670-676.

A Comparison of Asian Asian and American Asian populations: Calcium and Bone Accretion During Formation of Peak Bone Mass

5

Warren T.K. Lee, Connie M. Weaver, and Lu Wu

5.1 Profiling Asian Asians vs. American Asians

Asian Asians. Osteoporosis has become one of the major public health problems in Asia attributed to the rise in aging populations. WHO has estimated that by the year 2050, 53 million people in Asia will reach the age of 65 years. It is projected that by this time, more than 50% of hip fractures will occur in Asia by 2050 – the incidence of fractures will be approximately 6.3 million per year of which 3.2 million per year will occur in Asia.[1] China has a vast population of 1.3 billion, and 7% (91 million) of the population have reached older than 65 years of age; with a growing life expectancy, osteoporosis is expected to become an epidemic in China.[1,2] It is estimated that almost 86 million people, i.e., 6.6% of the total population, are currently affected by the disease. The number is projected to increase to 232 million by the year 2050. Risk factors for osteoporotic fractures in China include population aging, low BMD, small body build, low calcium intake, physical inactivity and smoking.[3,4]

American Asians. The 2000 US Census Bureau indicates that Asians comprise 4.2% of the US population, but estimates that 10% of the US population will be of Asian descent by the year 2050.[5] Approximately one-fourth of these are Chinese which is the largest group of Asians living in the US.

Only 8% of the genetic variation separates the major races. It is not known which genetic markers distinguish among Asian populations. In a study of Americans,

genetic marker cluster analysis of 326 markers from the Family and Blood Pressure Program study showed that individuals were classified into four major racial groups that essentially completely matched their self classification of race completely.[6] Further subdivision of Asians by genetic marker cluster analysis was not possible.

American Asian children have lower aBMD and BMC than other racial groups.[7,8] Bone size accounted for most of these differences. In a six-state study of 326 white, 234 Hispanic, and 188 Asian sixth grade girls, the Asian girls had lower BMC of the total body, lumbar, spine, total hip, and radius than white and Hispanic girls. Race explained 10% of the variance in total body and total hip BMC. After adjusting for bone size, sexual maturity, calcium intake, and physical activity, racial differences disappeared. Dairy calcium explained 3.4% of total body BMC, and 0.07% of total hip BMC.[7]

5.2 Incidence of Osteoporosis

Asian Asians. When compared with Caucasian populations who have the highest rate of hip fracture, the hip fracture rate is intermediate in Asians and the lowest among the Black populations.[9] The Asian osteoporosis study is a multicountry survey conducted in 1997 to compare the age-adjusted incidence of hip fracture (per 100,000) in men and women respectively in four Asian countries, i.e., Hong Kong (180 and 459), Singapore (164 and 442), Malaysia (88 and 218) and Thailand (114 and 289). The Asian data were also compared to those of the US Caucasian counterparts (187 and 536) of 1989. Hip fracture rates were found to be higher among urbanized cities such as Hong Kong and Singapore, which were almost comparable to the rates in the US.[10] Latest

W.T.K. Lee (✉)
Division of Nutritional Sciences, Faculty of Health and Medical Sciences, University of Surrey, Guildford, Surrey GU2 7XH, UK
e-mail: w.t.lee@surrey.ac.uk

P. Burckhardt et al. (eds.), *Nutritional Influences on Bone Health*,
DOI: 10.1007/978-1-84882-978-7_5, © Springer-Verlag London Limited 2010

data from Beijing, China have shown that the age-adjusted incidence of hip fracture in Chinese women escalated from 87.4 to 243 per 100,000 from 1996 to 2006.[11] Such increases in hip fracture rate could be attributable to urbanization and affluent life-style changes in Asia.[10,12] However, the recent rate of hip fracture in Hong Kong has shown some signs of plateau as the rate ceased to increase between 2001 and 2006. The reasons for the secular decline in hip fracture incidence are unknown and might be related to the increase in body mass index and/or earlier diagnosis and treatment.[13]

American Asians. In the NORA study of 197,848 postmenopausal American women, Asians had an odds ratio (O.R) for osteoporosis (defined as Tscore < −2.5) of 0.55 (CI 0.48, 0.62) compared to the referent white population assigned an O.R. of 1.[14] In a 1-year follow-up of 82% of the women, the relative risk of fracture for Asian women was 0.52 (CI 0.38, 07.0) compared to 1.0 for white women.

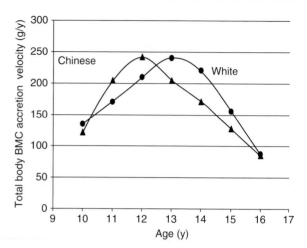

Fig. 5.1 Comparison of bone accretion between Chinese and white girls using the longitudinal data of Zhu et al[16] and Martin et al.[18] *Circles* represent white girls and *triangles* represent Chinese girls

5.3 BMC Accretion During Puberty

DXA is a highly accurate and precise technique to evaluate bone-mineral accrual and skeletal calcium-accretion longitudinally in children.[15,16] Bone-mineral content (BMC) increments throughout pubertal growth can be revealed by sequential total body bone scans. Skeletal calcium-retention rates can also be determined as the calcium fraction of BMC has been estimated to be 32.2%.[17] Few studies have measured bone accretion longitudinally throughout puberty. A classic study of annual DXA scans in Canadian white boys and girls throughout puberty allowed the investigators to plot total body BMC accretion velocity.[15,18] Recently, longitudinal total body BMC data in Chinese girls were reported.[16] Annual DXA scans were not taken, i.e., no DXA scans were taken during year 3 of the 5-year study, so the exact curve is less certain than that for the Canadian girls. Within this limitation, we plotted total body BMC accretion in the white Western girls and Asian Chinese girls (Fig. 5.1). This showed an earlier peak in bone accrual in the Chinese girls compared to white girls by more than 1 year. Peak velocity in BMC gains occurred approximately at the menarche for both cohorts. This is interesting since the age of menarche has been reported to be later in Asians compared to whites living in Hawaii.[19] Peak velocities

and similar total body BMC velocity at age 16 were similar in the two cohorts. Thus, despite average calcium intakes of about 444 mg/day in the Chinese girls compared to >1,000 mg/day in white Canadian girls, total bone-mineral accrual from age 10–15 years in the two cohorts was similar. This reflects a large difference in calcium retention efficiency (41% and 29.5%, respectively) for Chinese compared to white girls. It must be remembered that both environment (Western vs. Eastern) and race differed and there has been a decade time displacement between these studies which could influence the results.

5.4 Lifestyle Differences that Influence Bone

Asian Asians. Calcium intakes of Asian children and adolescents are relatively low in comparison to the Western counterparts[20–23] which could be *partly* attributable to the nonmilk based diets, inadequate knowledge and lower consumption of indigenous foods rich in bioavailable calcium, and/or poor dietary habits in some individuals.[24] In China, the adequate intakes (AIs) of calcium for children and adolescents are 800 mg/day for 4–10-year-old children and 1,000 mg/day for 11–17-year-old adolescents.[25] In the

Table 5.1 Average calcium intake (mg/day) in children and adolescents, China Nutrition and Health Survey (2002)[20]

	Age (years)			
	4–6	7–10	11–13	14–17
Calcium intake (mg/day) in boys	261	299	338	376
Calcium intake (mg/day) in girls	246	283	312	343

China Nutrition and Health Survey (2002), calcium intakes of children and adolescents in China were found to be low (Table 5.1), less than 2% children had their calcium intakes that reached the calcium AIs.[10] Although cow's milk is a good source of calcium, soy and soy products are traditional Chinese foods which also provide a good source of calcium. The national average consumption of cow's milk and soy and soy products was only 27 g/day (4% total calcium intake) and 11.8 g (13.9% total calcium intake) respectively.[20]

Children and adolescents in Asia are becoming physically less active than decades ago. In Malaysia, normal weight teenagers, both boys and girls, aged 13 spent on an average, 55 ± 4 min and 41 ± 2.8 min, respectively, on physical exercise and sports activities.[26] A recent China Health and Nutrition Survey conducted in 1997[27] showed that among 1,423 boys and 1,252 girls evaluated at 11.5 year, about 84% children actively commuted to school with an average of 100–150 min/week. Only 72% engaged in moderate to vigorous physical activities at school (90–110 min/week). Very few children (8%) participated in moderate to vigorous physical activities (90–110 min/week) outside schools. Less than 20% children actively participated in household chores. A cross-sectional study of 169 boys and 173 girls at aged 10–12-years in Hong Kong showed that body size and handgrip strength were significant determinants explaining the variation of BMC and BMD at the total hip, spine and whole body. However, physical activity and calcium intakes were also important predictors for BMC and BMD (Table 5.2).[28]

American Asians. American Asian children consume more calcium than those living in Asia, but intakes are much lower than that of white children. Using 24-h dietary recalls in 167 boys and girls aged 10–18 years across six states, median calcium intake was 868 mg/day for Asians, 896 mg/day for Hispanics, and 1,180 mg/day for whites.[29] In a sample of 748 sixth

grade girls across six states, Asian girls were 30.4% less active than white girls, but were similar to Hispanic girls (7). In this study, bone size explained most of the racial differences in BMC at the spine, total hip, and total body, but physical activity and dietary calcium were also significant predictors.

5.5 Calcium Metabolism

Asian Asians. We were the first to evaluate true fractional calcium absorption (TFCA) in Chinese children and adolescents. In an early study involving 7–8-years-old healthy Chinese children in Hong Kong and Southern China. TFCA was $54.8 \pm 7.3\%$ when consuming dietary calcium at 862 mg/day and with optimal plasma 25-OHD level (~33 ng/mL), whereas TFCA was higher ($63.1 \pm 10.7\%$) in those with an average calcium intake of 363 mg/day.[30] A further study in Beijing also revealed that TFCA of 12 adolescent girls aged 9–17-years was 57% with mean calcium intake of 600 mg/day and plasma 25-OHD level at 12.2 ± 3.9 ng/mL (Table 5.2). Mean 24-h urinary excretion of these girls was 80 mg/day.[31] The TFCA figures from our studies nearly doubled those of Caucasian children consuming a mean calcium intake of 925 mg/day (25–34%) using the same stable isotopic technique.[32] The findings of higher values of TFCA and lower urinary calcium excretion in Chinese children and adolescents suggested that calcium retention could be higher despite their lower habitual calcium intakes.

American Asians. We are the first to study calcium metabolism in Asian American children. Pubertal Chinese boys ($n = 16$) and girls ($n = 15$) aged 11–14 years were studied on controlled feeding studies run as a summer camp. Subject characteristics are given in Table 5.2. Each subject was studied on two calcium intakes for 3 weeks each separated by a washout period. Calcium intakes ranging from 600 to 1,800 mg/day were studied in order to determine the relationship between calcium intake and calcium absorption and calcium retention. Chinese adolescents, especially girls, were more efficient at utilizing calcium than previously studied white adolescents.[33–35] Black girls studied at one calcium intake[36] are also shown. The calcium load during the absorption test was one-third of the daily calcium intake. All races were studied under the same

Table 5.2 Comparison of regulators of calcium metabolism in Asian Asian and American Asian children/adolescents, X±SD

Location	Reference	Sex	Age (year)	Tanner score (mean or distribution)	Calcium intake (mg/day)	Serum 25(OH)D (ng/mL)	Serum PTH (pg/mL)	Total body BMC (g)	% Calcium absorption
Midwest USA		Boys	14.0±10.3	3.3±1.6	643±344	22.0±5.5	27.8±8.7	2,063±537	–
		Girls	13.3±1.26	3.3±1.4	628±317	19.9±6.6	41.1±18.7	1,897±332	–
Hong Kong and South China	19	Boys and girls (n=15)	7	T1: 100%	862±394	34.1±7.2	–	–	54.8±7.3
		Boys and girls (n=19)	7	T1: 100%	363±91	32.9±7.0	–	–	63.1±10.7
Beijing	20	Girls (n=12)	12.4±2.4	T1: 25%. T2–3: 58.3%	591±164	12.2±0.39		–	60.4±14.4
Hong Kong	18	Boys (n=169)	11.7±0.4	T1: 25.4%. T2–3: 74.6%	620±243	–	–	1,161±215	–
		Girls (n=172)	10.7±0.4	T1: 55%. T2–3: 43.6%	569±274	–	–	1,057±223	–

general protocol but at different times. The efficiency of calcium absorption is much higher for the Chinese girls at lower calcium intakes where habitual dietary intakes occur. The decreasing efficiency in fractional calcium absorption in Chinese girls, but not white girls, with greater calcium intakes suggests that skeletal calcium-accretion could be matched between the races at higher calcium intake. Indeed, Asians are getting taller, over time which has been attributed to improved nutrition.[37]

5.6 Summary

Asians have lower bone mass than other populations, and this is largely explained by smaller body and bone size. Despite the Asian's lower vitamin D status than whites, their calcium utilization rates are higher than that of many other races. Asian calcium-accretion rates are not lower throughout growth, and this suggest that low calcium intakes and smaller body and bone size may have strong roles in their observed reduced peak bone mass compared to other racial groups. As calcium content increases in the diets of Asians, their efficiency of calcium utilization will undoubtedly decrease, but nevertheless peak bone mass will increase. This will be important to reduce the risk of fracture in Asian populations around the world.

References

1. Cooper C, Campion G, Melton LJ III. Hip fractures in the elderly: a world wide projection. *Osteoporosis Int.* 1992;2:285-289.
2. WHO. The burden of musculoskeletal conditions at the start of the new millennium. *WHO Technical Report Series* 919; 2003, WHO, Geneva.
3. Lau EM, Woo J, Leung PC, Swaminthan R. Low bone mineral density, grip strength and skinfold thickness are important risk factors for hip fracture in Hong Kong Chinese. *Osteoporosis Int.* 1993;3:66-70.
4. Lau EM, Suriwongpaisal P, Lee JK, et al. Risk factors for hip fracture in Asian men and women: the Asian Osteoporosis Study. *J Bone Miner Res.* 2001;16:572-580.
5. Barnes J, Bennett CE. The Asian population: United States Census 2000 Brief. Available from http://www.census.gov/prod/2002pubs/C2kbr03-16.pdf; 2000.
6. Tang H, Quertermous J, Rodriguerez B, et al. Genetic structure, self-identified race/ethnicity and confounding in case-control association studies. *Am J Hum Genet.* 2005;76:268-275.
7. Weaver CM, McCabe LD, McCabe GP, et al. Bone mineral and predictors of bone mass in white, hispanic, and asian early pubertal girls. *Calcif Tissue Int.* 2007;81(5):352-363.
8. Bhudhikanok GS, Wang MC, Eckert K, et al. Differences in bone mineral in young Asian and Caucasian Americans may reflect differences in bone size. *J Bone Miner Res.* 2006;11:1545-1556.
9. Villa, ML, Nelson L. Race, ethnicity and osteoporosis. In: Marcus R, Fieldman D, Kelsey J, eds. *Osteoporosis.* San Diego, CA: Academic Press; 1996:435-447.
10. Lau EM, Lee JK, Suriwongpaisal P, et al. The incidence of hip fracture in four Asian countries: the Asian Osteoporosis Study (AOS). *Osteoporo Int.* 2001;12:239-243.
11. Xia W, He S, Liu A, Xu L. Epidemiology study of hip fracture in Beijing, China. *Bone.* 2008;43:S13.
12. Koh LK, Saw SM, Lee JJ, Leong KH, Lee J; National Working Committee on Osteoporosis. Hip fracture incidence rates in Singapore 1991-1998. *Osteoporos Int.* 2001;12(4):311-318.
13. Lau EM. The epidemiology of osteoporosis in Asia. *IBMS BoneKEy.* 2009;6:190-193.
14. Barrett-Connor E, Siris ES, Wehren LE, et al. Osteoporosis and fracture risk in women of different ethnic groups. *J Bone Miner Res.* 2005;20:185-194.
15. Bailey DA, Martin AD, McKay HA, Whiting S, Mirwald R. Calcium accretion in girls and boys during puberty: a longitudinal analysis. *J Bone Miner Res.* 2000;15:2245-2250.
16. Zhu K, Greenfield H, Zhang Q, et al. Growth and bone mineral accretion during puberty in Chinese girls: a five-year longitudinal study. *J Bone Miner Res.* 2008;23:167-172.
17. Ellis KJ, Shypailo RJ, Hergenroeder A, Perez M, Abrams S. Total body calcium and bone mineral content: comparison of dual-energy X-ray absorptiometry with neutron activation analysis. *J Bone Miner Res.* 1996;11:843-848.
18. Martin AD, Bailey DA, McKay HA, et al. Bone mineral and calcium accretion during puberty. *Am J Clin Nutr.* 1997;66:611-615.
19. Novotny R, Davis RPD, Wasnich RD. Adolescent milk consumption, menarche, birth weight, and ethnicity influence height of women in Hawaii. *J Am Diet Assoc.* 1996;96:802-804.
20. He Y, Zhai F, Wang Z, Hu Y, Yang X. Status of dietary calcium intake of Chinese residents. *J Hyg Res.* 2007;36:600-602.
21. Wu SJ, Pan WH, Yeh NH, Chang HY. Dietary nutrient intake and major food sources: the Nutrition and Health Survey of Taiwan Elementary School Children 2001-2002. *Asia Pac J Clin Nutr.* 2007;16(S2):518-533.
22. Ta TM, Nguyen KH, Kawakami M, Kawase M, Nguyen C. Micronutrient status of primary school girls in rural and urban areas of South Vietnam. *Asia Pac J Clin Nutr.* 2003;12:178-185.
23. Gibson RS, Manger MS, Krittaphol W, et al. Does zinc deficiency play a role in stunting among primary school children in NE Thailand? *Br J Nutr.* 2007;97:167-175.
24. Lee WTK, Jiang J. Calcium requirements for Asian children and adolescents. *Asia Pac J Clin Nutr.* 2008;17(S1):33-36.
25. Chinese Nutrition Society. Chinese dietary reference intakes, Beijing, China. Chinese Light Industry Press, 2000.

26. Zalilah MS, Khor GL, Mirnalini K, Norimah AK, Ang M. Dietary intake, physical activity and energy expenditure of Malaysian adolescents. *Singapore Med J*. 2006;47:491-498.

27. Tudor-Locke C, Ainsworth BE, Adair LS, Du S, Popkin BM. Physical activity and inactivity in Chinese school-aged youth: the China Health and Nutrition Survey. *Int J Obes Relat Metab Disord*. 2003;27:1093-1099.

28. Chan DCC, Lee WTK, Lo DHS, Leung JCS, Kwok AWL, Leung PC. Relationship between grip strength and bone mineral density in healthy Hong Kong adolescents. *Osteoporos Int*. 2008;19:1485-1495.

29. Novotny R, Boushey C, Bock MA, et al. Calcium intake of Asian, Hispanic, and white youth. *J Am Coll Nutr*. 2003;22: 64-70.

30. Lee WTK, Leung SSF, Fairweather-Tait SJ, et al. True fractional calcium absorption in Chinese children measured with stable isotopes (^{42}Ca and ^{44}Ca). *Br J Nutr*. 1994;72:883-897.

31. Lee WTK, Cheng JCY, Jiang J, Hu P, Hu X, Roberts DCK. Calcium absorption measured by stable calcium isotopes (^{42}Ca & ^{44}Ca) among Northern Chinese adolescents with low vitamin D status. *J Orthop Surg*. 2002;10:61-66.

32. Abrams SA, Stuff JE. Calcium metabolism in girls: current dietary intakes lead to low rates of calcium absorption and retention during puberty. *Am J Clin Nutr*. 1994;60: 739-743.

33. Jackman LA, Millane SS, Martin BR, et al. Calcium retention in relation to calcium intake and postmenarcheal age in adolescent females. *Am J Clin Nutr*. 1997;66:327-333.

34. Wastney ME, Martin BR, Peacock M, et al. Changes in calcium kinetics in adolescent girls induced by high calcium intake. *J Clin Endocrin Metab*. 2000;85:4470-4475.

35. Braun M, Palacios C, Wigertz K, et al. Racial differences in skeletal calcium retention in adolescent girls on a range of controlled calcium intakes. *Am J Clin Nutr*. 2007;85: 1657-1663.

36. Bryant RJ, Wastney ME, Martin BR, et al. Racial differences in bone turnover and calcium metabolism in adolescent females. *J Clin Endocrin Metab*. 2003;88(3):1043-1047.

37. Lau EMC. Osteoporosis in Asians-the role of calcium and other nutrition In: Heaney RP, Weaver CM, eds. *Nutritional Aspects of Osteoporosis '94. Challenges of Modern Medicine Ares Serono Symposia*; 1995;7:45-54.

Estimating Calcium Requirements

6

Connie M. Weaver and Kathleen M. Hill

6.1 Importance of Setting Appropriate Calcium Requirements

Nutrient requirements are used by many groups to determine food choices and meal plans for feeding people across the lifespan. They are used to evaluate sources of nutrients and for food labels to educate the consumer. Requirements also provide a guideline to determine whether supplements are needed. If calcium requirements are underestimated, inadequate intakes are more likely, which may compromise bone health and increase risk of chronic disease.

6.2 Approaches for Determining Calcium Requirements

The evidence supporting calcium requirements is stronger than for most other nutrients. Yet, we lack consensus on the appropriate approach for determining calcium requirements, the correct outcome measures, and the values for calcium requirements for population subgroups.[1] There are no status markers for calcium such as serum 25(OH)D for vitamin D or serum ferritin or transferrin for iron. Serum calcium is tightly regulated making serum calcium insensitive to calcium stores. Thus the indicator for calcium nutrition status

must be calcium intake, but assessing calcium intake in free living populations is fraught with error as is dietary assessment of other nutrients.[2]

A comparison of various approaches for determining calcium requirements will be reviewed. Calcium requirements have been determined largely based on calcium retention from short-term balance studies using well-controlled calcium intakes. In future, we may be able to assess calcium intakes sufficiently well to determine calcium intakes associated with optimal health or minimize disease risk for epidemiological approaches or trials using long-term outcome measures. Bone health is the primary consideration for adequate calcium nutrition because 99% of the body's calcium is in bone, which can be accessed for soft tissue needs when dietary calcium is inadequate. The few attempts to relate calcium intake to disease outcomes have not been very successful so far, possibly because of the difficulty in assessing calcium intakes, the wide fluctuations in calcium intakes from day to day within individuals, and the many additional factors which influence both calcium nutriture and any potential outcome measure. Even more problematic is the lack of good outcome measures for determining Upper Levels for calcium. Moreover, most studies do not use sufficiently high calcium intakes to evaluate potential consequences of calcium intake excess. It is revealing that all current calcium requirements for humans fall below animal chow levels for primates (150–300 mg Ca/100 kcal) and the intake of primitive humans (800–100 mg Ca/100 kcal) on an energy basis.[3] This gives some confidence that levels of calcium intake higher than current upper levels are safe, but gives less confidence that calcium requirements for contemporary man are optimal.

C.M. Weaver (✉)
Department of Foods and Nutrition, Purdue University,
700 West State Street, West Lafayette, IN 47907, USA
e-mail: weavercm@purdue.edu

P. Burckhardt et al. (eds.), *Nutritional Influences on Bone Health*,
DOI: 10.1007/978-1-84882-978-7_6, © Springer-Verlag London Limited 2010

6.3 Balance Studies for Estimating Calcium Requirements

Balance studies have been the most useful approach to setting calcium requirements because they offer a practical evaluation of the effect of a range of controlled calcium intakes on short-term outcome measures. Still, there have been several different applications of balance data for setting calcium requirements.

6.3.1 Factorial Method

The factorial method adds up losses of calcium from urine and skin with an estimate of growth during childhood and pregnancy or lactation and adjusts for absorption to determine required intake. Losses are usually determined as part of balance studies, but little attention has been given to the influence of calcium intake or calcium reserves of the subjects when estimating calcium requirements by this method. When the factorial method used values from feeding studies conducted on intakes near the requirement in adolescents, this approach gave values that were comparable to requirements based on the maximal calcium retention approach described below (Sect. 6.3.3).[4]

6.3.2 Neutral Balance Approach

The FAO/WHO report[5] plots calcium intake against net calcium absorption (intake minus fecal excretion) from 210 balance studies performed in 81 adults. The plot is a nonlinear relationship as shown in Fig. 6.1. Losses from urine and skin and increased excretion as a result of decreased absorption during menopause are added as lines of intersection, so that this approach is essentially a factorial method of accounting for calcium losses adjusted for absorption in order to determine calcium requirements. For adults, calcium requirement is assumed to occur where intake and output are equal. Nordin later acknowledged the need to adjust for decreasing calcium absorption efficiency with menopause.[6] Adjustments for various subgroups are shown in Fig. 6.2 with an estimate of a margin of safety of ±1 SD. The values for subgroups are not derived from balance studies performed using a range in calcium intakes to plot the relationship between calcium intake and net absorbed calcium as for nonpregnant adults. Rather, a single rate of skeletal calcium augmentation is assumed from skeletal calcium accretion with an allowance of 2 SD during pregnancy and puberty. A problem with using a calcium intake that equals excretion as an indicator of the requirement or as a starting point margin of safety is that it

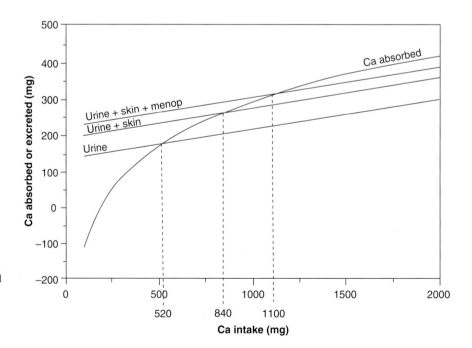

Fig. 6.1 Relationship between calcium absorption and calcium intake modified by calcium losses. The intercept suggests calcium requirement of postmenopausal women[5]

Fig. 6.2 Calcium intakes required to provide the absorbed calcium necessary to meet calcium requirements at different stages in the lifecycle used by the FAO/WHO.[5] The solid lines represent the mean and range of calcium absorption as a function of calcium intake derived from the regression depicted. The intercepted lines represented the estimated calcium require-ments for subpopulations

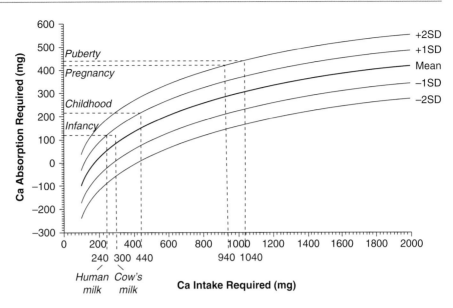

assumes bone calcium reserves are adequate. The inappropriateness of this approach has been argued by Heaney.[7,8] A steady-state positive balance more likely suggests that prior calcium intake has not maximized bone mass rather than that calcium intake is higher than the requirement.

6.3.3 Intakes for Maximal Retention

Calcium intake for maximal retention was the primary approach used to set calcium intakes for North America in 1997.[4] This is a modification of the FAO/WHO use of balance studies that overcame some of the limitations of that approach and made use of a wider data set. For each age group for which data were available, calcium intake was plotted against net calcium retention. Thus, each life stage was evaluated specifically, which allowed for adjustment for growth or bone involution. Basing cal-cium requirements on the intake for maximal retention is a better approach than the neutral balance approach because it makes no assumptions about the adequacy of the calcium reserves in the subjects. All adults should not necessarily be in neutral balance. This approach also inherently adjusts for changes in urinary calcium loss with increasing intake. The variation in calcium retention with calcium intake for each data set was given. In order to identify a specific value for the cal-cium intake for maximal calcium retention for each life

stage, the plot was converted to % maximal retention and the intake where the 95% confidence interval crossed 100% maximal retention was considered a good estimate of the lowest plausible value for the calcium requirement for maximizing bone mass. The two plots for adolescents are given in Fig. 6.3. Use of a plateau intake approach minimizes error associated with bal-ance studies because there is no need to know exact cal-cium retention. This is reassuring given the one-sided error associated with compliance of consumption and collection of excreta typically associated with balance studies and the tendency of the variance to increase at high calcium intake.[10] The approach presumed that cutaneous calcium losses were uniform across the range in calcium intakes in the absence of data on the effect of calcium intake on cutaneous calcium loss.

A limitation of all balance data sets used to set public health recommendations to date is the relative homoge-neity of the data. Almost all balance studies used to set calcium requirements have been determined on white subjects consuming Western diets. For several age groups, balance data were not collected on a significantly wide range of calcium intakes to determine a calcium intake plateau. Although others have pointed out the need to have considerable data points near the require-ments,[11] determining a plateau intake depends greatly on having sufficiently high intakes as well. These is still a deficiency of data at high calcium intakes in adult women. More recent data expanding our knowledge of subpopulation requirements are given below (Sect. 6.7).

Fig. 6.3 Calcium retention as a function of calcium intake (mean and 95% CI) expressed as retention in mg/day (**a**) or % maximal calcium retention (**b**). In (**a**), the shaded area is the 95% CI for mean maximal retention (taken from,[9] with permission from Springer)

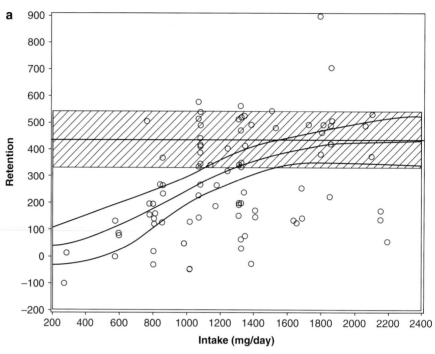

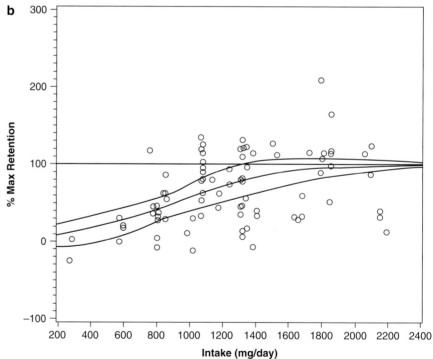

6.4 Challenges to Use of Balance Data

One of the concerns with balance data is that they may not reflect long-term skeletal calcium balance. This concern is due in part to the seeming continued adaptation to low calcium intakes over 21 months in male prisoners.[12] Also, the remodeling transient described by Heaney[7] that occurs in the first 6 months after shifting to a different calcium intake may prevent short-term studies from reflecting long-term effects on bone. In the short term, adaptation to controlled calcium intakes that are considerably different from habitual calcium intakes appears to take approximately 1 week. In children and young adults, calcium-to-PEG (a nonabsorbable fecal marker) ratios become constant after 6 days,[13] indicating steady state. In adults, ^{47}Ca retention stabilized after week 1–8 on both very high (2,000 mg/day) and very low (300 mg/day) calcium intakes, suggesting adaptation to new dietary calcium levels by week 2.[14]

To determine the ability of short-term balance studies to predict peak skeletal calcium accretion during puberty, we compared estimated calcium retention from our controlled metabolic balance studies in white girls aged 12–14 years[15] and white boys aged 13–15 year16 during their peak pubertal growth with skeletal calcium accretion calculated from longitudinal, annual DXA data in white Canadian boys and girls.[17] In girls, total body BMC accrual data[17] show a mean maximal calcium retention of 284 mg/day at a mean reported calcium intake of 1,113±378 mg/day. At the same calcium intake, the nonlinear regression model developed from our balance study data[15] predicts a mean maximal calcium retention of 238 mg/day. In boys, the reported calcium intake in the longitudinal DXA study of 1,140±392 mg/day coincidentally was the plateau intake we identified using our nonlinear regression model for determining the intake for maximal calcium retention.[16] Thus we could directly compare mean maximal calcium retention of the two approaches: 442 mg/day calculated by nonlinear regression model from balance study data compared to 359 mg/day from total body BMC accrual data from longitudinal study data which we reported previously.[18] The predicted yearly skeletal gain from the balance studies is 17.6% compared to the observed 14.3% gain in boys from the longitudinal study and 12.4% compared to the observed 14.8% in girls.[18] These comparisons suggest good ability of short-term balance studies to predict long-term skeletal calcium acquisition during growth.

Another concern with balance studies has been the ability to determine the appropriate plateau intake for maximal retention as the confidence interval depicted in Fig. 6.3b naturally reflects the size and heterogeneity of the studied cohort. A superficial look at Fig. 6.3a might suggest that increasing calcium intakes above 800 mg/day has questionable advantage. Taking advantage of our paired data on subjects studied on two calcium intakes in a cross-over design, we selected subjects who

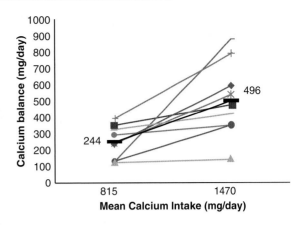

Fig. 6.4 Calcium retention in adolescent girls on paired low (~800 mg/day) and high (1,300 mg/day) calcium intakes. The mean is shown by the dark line

were studied on controlled calcium intakes of approximately 800 mg/day and close to the current calcium requirement for this age group (1,300 mg/day). Figure 6.4 shows calcium retention for ten adolescents. Calcium retention increased in all but one subject on the higher calcium intake and the relationship was highly significant. At a calcium retention of 496 mg/day on an intake of approximately 1,300 mg/day, annual skeletal gains in BMC would be a potential 25.8% compared to 12.6% with calcium retention of 243 mg/day on calcium intakes of approximately 800 mg/day. As an analogy, we present unpaired and paired data comparisons from 15 girls studied in our metabolic studies first during puberty at 12–14 years of age and a second time 3 years later in Fig. 6.5. By looking at the unpaired data, it is not especially convincing that all girls gain height, weight, lean body mass, or total body BMC after 13 or 14 years of age. It is very obvious that they do when paired data are inspected. Of note, even height has measurement error as one girl appears to shrink over the course of 3 years of puberty. The magnitude of growth during 3 years is similar to the impact of increasing calcium intake from 800 mg/day to ≥1,300 mg/day during puberty.

6.5 Controlled Trials

Randomized controlled trials (RCT) have long been considered the gold standard for testing drugs and other medical treatments. Use of evidence-based reviews that prioritize high quality RCTs is the current

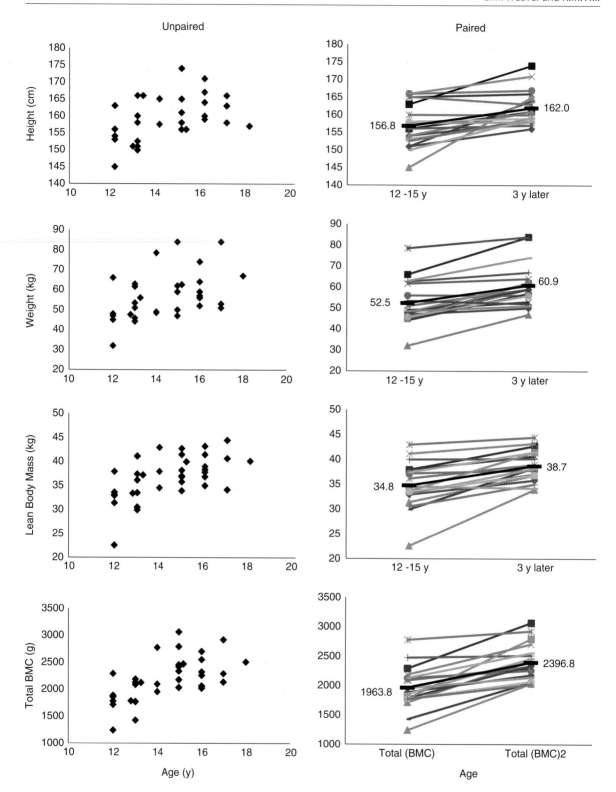

Fig. 6.5 Unpaired and paired data in pubertal girls restudied 3 years later. (**a**) height; (**b**) weight; (**c**) lean body mass; (**d**) total body BMC

favored strategy for setting public health policies.[19] RCTs do not require controlled feeding, so theoretically can be sufficiently long to determine changes in bone and risk of chronic disease. But setting calcium requirements using this approach is challenging. RCTs of calcium interventions through food or supplements can achieve higher calcium intakes to compare with calcium intakes of self-selected diets alone. But, the self-selected diet is likely to comprise at least a third of the total calcium intake of the calcium intervention group and all of the calcium intake of the placebo comparison group, giving considerable error to our ability to know actual calcium intakes of either group. Self-reported energy intakes compared to objective measures of energy needs using doubly labeled water or metabolizable energy balance using bomb calorimetry with balance studies show underreporting errors averaging $35 \pm 20\%$, and the error in underreporting increases as BMI increases.[20] Similarly, inaccurate self-reports of dietary intake lead to inaccurate assessments of individual nutrient intakes, like calcium.

Errors associated with compliance of the calcium intervention further compromise our ability to determine the relationship between calcium intake and any outcome measure. Additionally, RCTs typically compare only one level of supplemented calcium intake against a wide ranging, poorly defined comparison group. This does not allow for estimates of optimal calcium intake, which requires a range of calcium intakes. Outcome measures of disease end points are the preferred end points of RCTs. Use of disease end points for determining calcium requirements is less relevant because the calcium intakes relevant to prevent disease are likely in the years to decades preceding disease onset. Alternatively, measures of calcium absorption, calcium retention, and skeletal growth and maintenance are appropriate. Yet, few of these measures are available across a range of calcium intakes for most age groups from RCTs. The major argument against the RCT approach to defining the calcium intake requirement is that it is not feasible. RCTs must be large and carried out for ≥ 3 years to evaluate even a single calcium intake in a given segment of the population. It would take a prohibitively large number of trials to define effects of a series of different calcium intakes on change in BMC, BMD, fracture, or other indicators of chronic disease for each age, sex, and race group for whom it is needed. So, what may be the gold standard in drug and medical research may not be ideal for setting nutrient intake requirements.

6.6 Comparison of Controlled Feeding Studies and RCTs

Two examples will illustrate the comparison between information gained from controlled feeding studies and RCTs. In addition to having a known and stable intake of the nutrient of interest, controlled feeding studies eliminate many of the confounders in RCTs relating intake of a single nutrient to an outcome measure of interest, including other dietary variables, physical activity, season (vitamin D synthesis), etc. RCTs attempt to address confounders by assuming they are balanced across the treatment groups.

Our first example is of calcium intake and skeletal calcium excretion in pubertal girls. In 182 black and white adolescent girls from balance studies, we showed that calcium intake explained 12.3% of the variation in daily calcium retention, about the same as race which explained 13.7%.[21] This racial difference in net calcium retention during adolescence predicted the differences in femoral neck BMC and BMD observed in black and white adults in NHANES.[22,23] Yet, from epidemiological studies, racial effects appear much stronger than diet effects. Skeletal advantages in blacks compared to whites are frequently reported, whereas metaanalyses of RCTs of calcium supplementation show only modest benefits to bone.[19,24] One possibility is that race is more accurately assessed than diet and certainly does not fluctuate from day to day.

The second example is of calcium intake and bone health in adults. Controlled feeding studies and many smaller RCTs showed a benefit of increasing calcium intake above a g/day.[4] Yet, the large calcium and vitamin D trial in 36,282 postmenopausal women of the Women's Health Initiative showed no overall reduction in hip fracture.[25] Thus it could be concluded that calcium supplementation does not protect against hip fracture. However, a subanalysis suggested that subjects who were not already having calcium intakes near their requirement and were more compliant with the intervention benefited from calcium supplements with a significant reduction in hip fracture. As the placebo group's average intake was over 1,100 mg/day, a reasonable public health message would be that calcium supplementation is not to be recommended to protect against hip fracture when calcium intake is already adequate. In any nutrition intervention trial, the baseline nutritional status of the subjects should be taken into consideration; it may be that in many cases, the wrong people are studied in the first place – people who are already nutritionally adequate.

6.7 Further Refinements in Determining Calcium Requirements

Several important new data sets have become available since the last critical evaluations of calcium requirements have occurred. Calcium balance data are now available for young children.[26] Calcium balance data on a range of calcium intakes have been published on adolescent white boys[16] and African American girls.[21] In these studies, calcium intakes for achieving maximal calcium retention were not significantly different from white girls,[4,15] even though higher calcium retention was achieved on the same calcium intake for both black girls and white boys compared to white girls. A large new data set of balance studies in 155 white adults aged 20–75 year from the US Department of Agriculture Grand Forks Human Nutrition Research Center was reported.[27] Although there is adequate data around calcium intakes to achieve zero calcium balance, the range of calcium intakes was 415–1,740 mg/day, which apparently was inadequate to establish the plateau intake for either sex.

Early attempts to determine calcium requirements in Asians suggest that requirements may be lower than for other races, at least in females.[28,29] In girls, calcium absorption efficiency is much greater in Asians than Whites on lower calcium intakes.[28] In elderly Japanese men and women, calcium intakes to achieve zero calcium balance were estimated to be lower than those for Whites.[29] However, subjects were studied on only two calcium intakes so that the relationship between calcium intake and calcium retention is unknown if it is nonlinear as for White populations.

Several implications now suggest that calcium requirements may depend on size, including genetically programmed body size and excessive weight. The authors of the Japanese balance study described above[29] found that calcium requirements for men and women were similar if normalized on a per kg body weight basis at 18.1 mg/kg body weight. They also calculated that a 65 kg elderly white woman with a requirement of 1,200 mg Ca/day[4] would be similar on a weight-adjusted basis at 18.5 mg/kg body weight.

In growing girls, adult height seemed to influence calcium requirements. In a RCT of calcium supplementation from prepuberty to young adulthood with an estimated calcium intake difference at the end of 824 ± 351 mg/day for the placebo vs. $1,296 \pm 567$ mg/day for the intervention group,[30] girls destined to be taller at adulthood had higher proximal radius BMD than shorter girls of 18 years of age if they were in the intervention group, whereas shorter girls of 18 years of age in the placebo group appeared to catch up to the intervention group. Thus some girls needed more calcium than 800 mg/day on average and some did not. We recently reported that calcium retention increases with increasing BMI, especially at higher calcium intakes.[31]

6.8 Summary

Calcium requirements for North America and the FAO/WHO are based on short-term balance studies. Controlled feeding studies are efficacy studies which are best at showing the specific effect of calcium intake on an outcome variable related to health in a relatively short study period. And, because controlled feeding studies can be performed on a range of calcium intakes, plateau intakes can be determined. Comparison with longitudinal data shows that measures such as calcium retention and components of balance including calcium absorption and excretion can reflect long-term bone calcium accretion and retention. The advantage of using intakes to achieve maximal retention for setting calcium requirements is that no assumptions are made about adequacy of reserves in contrast to the approach of using intakes required to replace losses. Some additional balance study data sets are available in previously understudied populations for consideration by future committees.

The next revisions of calcium requirements for North America and Europe are considering evidence-based reviews of RCTs. RCTs of calcium supplementation and educational interventions are studying questions of effectiveness, rather than efficacy. Effectiveness research is valuable to assess how well various interventions work in translating the results of efficacy studies to the individual or community. But there are many obstacles to using effectiveness research to set calcium requirements such as fluctuating and unknown calcium intakes, other confounding factors, and the long latency between calcium intakes and disease outcomes. Also, RCTs are necessarily large and long for bone outcome measures, which limit their feasibility. Questions of effectiveness of interventions from RCTs may be more relevant to public health recommendations regarding calcium supplementation, rather than to determining calcium intake requirements. Determining calcium intake requirements is best done by efficacy studies including well-controlled feeding studies with a wide range of calcium intakes.

References

1. Atkinson SA, McCabe GP, Weaver CM, Abrams SA, O'Brien KO. Are current calcium recommendations for adolescents higher than needed to achieve optimal peak bone mass? The controversy. *J Nutr*. 2008;138:1182-1186.
2. Boushey CJ. Nutritional epidemiology: dietary assessment methods. In: Weaver CM, Heaney RP, eds. *Calcium in Human Health*. Totowa, NJ: Humana Press; 2006:39-63 [chapter 4].
3. Eaton B, Nelson DA. Calcium in evolutionary perspective. *Am J Clin Nutr*. 1991;S54:281S-287S.
4. Institute of Medicine, Standing Committee on the Scientific Evaluation of Dietary Reference Intakes, Food and Nutrition Board. *Dietary Reference Intakes for Calcium, Phosphorus, Magnesium, Vitamin D, and Fluoride*, Washington, DC: National Academy Press; 1997.
5. FAO/WHO Report of a Joint AAO/WHO Expert Consultation. Calcium. In: *Human Vitamin and Mineral Requirements*. Rome: FAO; 2002:151-179 [chapter 11].
6. Nordin BEC. Reflections on osteoporosis. In: Marcus R, Feldman D, Nelson DA, Rosen CJ, eds. *Osteoporosis*. 3rd ed. New York, NY: Elsevier; 2008:51-68 [chapter 4].
7. Heaney RP. The bone remodeling transient: interpreting interventions involving bone-related nutrients. *Nutr Rev*. 2001; 59:327-334.
8. Heaney RP. Mineral balance and mineral requirement. *Am J Clin Nutr*. 2008;87:1960-1962.
9. Weaver CM. Pre-puberty and adolescence. In: Weaver CM, Heaney RP, eds. *Calcium in Human Health*. Totowa, NJ: Humana Press; 2006:281-296 [chapter 17].
10. Weaver CM, McCabe GP, Peacock M. Calcium intake and age influence calcium retention in adolescents. In: Burkhardt P, Dawson-Hughes B, Heaney RP, eds. *Nutritional Aspects of Osteoporosis* (Proceedings of the Symposium on Nutritional Aspects of Osteoporosis 22-24 May, 1997, Lausanne Switzerland). New York, NY: Springer-Verlag; 1998:3-10.
11. Beaten GH. Statistical approaches to establishing mineral element recommendations. *J Nutr*. 1996;126:2320S-2328S.
12. Malm OJ. Calcium requirement and adaptation in adult men. *Scand J Clin Lab Invest*. 1958;10(suppl 36):1-280.
13. Weaver CM. Clinical approaches for studying calcium metabolism and its relationship to disease. In: Weaver CM, Heaney RP, eds. *Calcium in Human Health*. Totowa, NJ: Humana Press; 2006:65-81 [chapter 5].
14. Dawson-Hughes B, Harris S, Kramich C, Dallal G, Rasmussen HM. Calcium retention and hormone levels in black and white women on high- and low-calcium diets. *J Bone Miner Res*. 1993;8(7):779-787.
15. Jackman LA, Millane SS, Martin BR, et al. Calcium retention in relation to calcium intake and postmenarcheal age in adolescent females. *Am J Clin Nutr*. 1997;66:327-333.
16. Braun MM, Martin BR, Kern M, et al. Calcium retention in adolescent boys on a range of controlled calcium intakes. *Am J Clin Nutr*. 2006;84:414-418.
17. Bailey DA, Martin AD, McKay HA, Whiting S, Mirwald R. Calcium accretion in girls and body during puberty: a longitudinal analysis. *J Bone Miner Res*. 2000;15:2245-2250.
18. Hill K.M. Braun MM, Kern M, et al. Predictors of calcium retention in adolescent boys. *J Clin Endocrinol Metab*. 2008; 93(12):4743-4748.
19. The AHRQ Report. *Vitamin D and Calcium: A Systematic Review on Health Outcomes*. AARQ Publication No. OX-EOXX. Tufts. Boston, MA: Evidence-Based Practice Center; 2009.
20. Singh R, Martin BR, Hickey Y, et al. Comparison of self-reported energy intake and measured metabolizable energy intake with total energy expenditure in overweight teens. *Am J Clin Nutr*. 2009;89:1744-1750.
21. Braun M, Palacios C, Wigertz K, et al. Racial differences in skeletal calcium retention in adolescent girls on a range of controlled calcium intakes. *Am J Clin Nutr*. 2007;85:1657-1663.
22. Bryant RJ, Wastney ME, Martin BR, et al. Racial differences in bone turnover and calcium metabolism in adolescent females. *J Clin Endocrinol Metab*. 2003;88(3):1043-1047.
23. Looker AC, Wahner HW, Dunn WL, Calvo MS, et al. Updated data on proximal femur bone mineral levels of US adults. Osteoporos Int. 1998;8:468-489.
24. Winzenberg T, Shaw K, Fryer J, et al. Effects of calcium supplementation on bone density in healthy children: meta-analysis of randomised controlled trials. BMJ 2006;333: 775.
25. Jackson RD, LaCroix AZ, Gass M, Wallace RB, Robbins J, Lewis CE. Calcium plus vitamin D supplementation and the risk of fractures. *N Engl J Med*. 2006;354:669-683.
26. Lynch MF, Griffin IJ, Hawthorne KM, Chen Z, Hanzo M, Abrams SA. Calcium balance in 1-4-y-old children. *Am J Clin Nutr*. 2007;85:750-754.
27. Hunt CD, Johnson LK. Calcium requirements: new estimations for men and women by cross-sectional statistical analyses if calcium balance data from metabolic studies. *Am J Clin Nutr*. 2007;86:1054-1063.
28. Lee WT, Weaver CM, Wu L. *A comparison of Asian and American Asian Populations: Calcium and Bone Accretion During Formation of Peak Bone Mass* (This Book); 2010.
29. Uenishi K, Ishida H, Kamei A, et al. Calcium requirement estimated by balance study in elderly Japanese people. *Osteoporos Int*. 2001;12:858-863.
30. Matkovic V, Goel PK, Badenhop-Stevens NE, et al. Calcium supplementation and bone mineral density in females from childhood to young adulthood: a randomized controlled trial. *Am J Clin Nutr*. 2005;81:175-188.
31. Hill KM, Egan KA, Braun MK, et al. The relationship between calcium intake and calcium retention is dependent on BMI in adolescents bone, fat and brain. *J Bone Miner Res*. 2009;abstract M29.

Independent and Combined Effects of Exercise and Calcium on Bone Structural and Material Properties in Older Adults

7

Robin M. Daly and Sonja Kukuljan

7.1 Introduction

The ability of bone to resist fracture (or "whole bone strength") is dependent on the amount of bone (size and mass), its structure (spatial distribution – shape and microarchitecture) and the intrinsic properties of the materials that comprise the bone (porosity, matrix mineralization, collagen traits, microdamage).[1,2] With advancing age, bone strength decreases due to an imbalance in bone remodeling – the balance between the volume of bone resorbed and the volume formed in the basic multicellular unit is negative.[1,3] This leads to a reduction in BMD and cortical thickness, with accompanying increases in periosteal and endosteal areas. Thus, any factor that influences bone remodeling (disease, drugs, lifestyle) will impact upon whole bone strength.[1] Regular exercise and adequate nutrition, particularly calcium and vitamin D, are two widely recommended and prescribed lifestyle strategies that have been shown to independently have positive effects on bone in older adults. However, the mechanism by which exercise and calcium–vitamin D influence bone is different; exercise has a site-specific modifying effect, whereas nutrition has a permissive, generalized effect. Despite this, there are reports that the beneficial effects of exercise on bone may be dependent on adequate calcium (or nutrient) intake. In this chapter, we briefly review studies examining the independent and combined effects of calcium (or calcium and vitamin D) and exercise on bone strength and

its determinants in older adults. Specifically, we focus on studies which have used noninvasive 3D imaging techniques that can provide an assessment (or *estimate*) of bone material (e.g., apparent volumetric BMD or "tissue" density) and structural properties (e.g., total, cortical, and medullary area) that contribute to whole bone strength.

7.2 Effects of Calcium and/or Vitamin D on Bone Strength in Older Adults

Clinical trials in older women, and to a lesser extent, men have shown that calcium supplementation, with or without vitamin D, can reduce secondary hyperparathyroidism, slow down bone turnover, increase areal BMD (1–3%), or slow down bone loss.[4–9] The beneficial effects of supplementation on BMD result from a reduction in the bone remodeling space. That is, there is a decrease in the number of remodeling sites activated along the bone surface, which leads to a reduction in bone resorption. In addition, there is continued bone formation in the many resorption cavities formed during the remodeling cycle prior to the initiation of supplementation. The net effect is a gain in bone mass and continued mineralization (rapid primary and then slower secondary mineralization) of the newly formed and older bone.[10] Partial filling of the existing remodeling sites also reduces intracortical porosity and stress concentrations, which can further help restore (or improve) whole bone strength.[3] To date, however, there have been few long-term randomized controlled trials (RCTs) which have examined the effects of calcium and/or vitamin D supplementation on bone material and structural properties in older adults.

R.M. Daly (✉)
Department of Medicine (RMH/WH), Western Hospital, The University of Melbourne, Corner of Eleanor and Marion Street, Melbourne, VIC 3011, Australia
e-mail: rdaly@unimelb.edu.au

P. Burckhardt et al. (eds.), *Nutritional Influences on Bone Health*,
DOI: 10.1007/978-1-84882-978-7_7, © Springer-Verlag London Limited 2010

In a 4-year calcium or vitamin D supplementation RCT in adults aged over 60 years, Peacock et al[8] reported that calcium supplementation (750 mg/day) prevented bone loss at the hip and reduced medullary expansion at the midfemur, but had no effect on total femur width. However, these changes in bone structure were determined from radiographs, which cannot depict the true cross-sectional shape or geometry of bone. Preliminary data from the Women's Health Initiative (WHI), which assessed the effects of calcium (1,000 mg/day) and vitamin D (400 IU/day) on femoral bone strength (assessed by hip structure analysis (HSA)), revealed that supplementation improved femoral neck (FN) BMD, cortical thickness, and section modulus, but not neck diameter (which was reduced).[11] Several earlier studies have also reported that additional calcium can slow the age-related loss in cortical thickness in older adults.[12,13] In a more recent 2-year intervention in older men, Daly et al[4] reported that supplementation with calcium–vitamin D fortified milk (1,000 mg/day and 800 IU/day) maintained QCT-measured midfemur cortical area by slowing endocortical bone loss in men aged greater, but not less than, 62 years of age; there was no effect on bone size. Together, these findings indicate that calcium or calcium plus vitamin D supplementation may be effective for preserving cortical thickness by reducing endocortical bone loss.

Whether calcium and/or vitamin D can enhance the intrinsic material properties of bone, including the matrix mineralization and porosity, remains uncertain due, in part, to the lack of clinically available, noninvasive techniques to measure these properties. In the study by Daly et al[4] using QCT to assess midfemur cortical volumetric BMD (vBMD), which reflects both the degree of mineralization and the porosity of bone tissue, they found that calcium–vitamin D_3 supplementation significantly reduced the rate of bone loss in men aged over 62 years. Because QCT-derived cortical vBMD represents the "apparent" mineral density (e.g., including the pores) of cortical bone, it is not clear whether there was a reduction in intracortical porosity, increased bone mineralization, or a combination of these factors. However, the authors speculated that it was likely due to reduced cortical porosity since around 70% of the age-related decline in cortical vBMD is attributed to increased porosity. There is some evidence however, that calcium–vitamin D supplementation can improve bone mineralization. Transiliac bone biopsies taken before and after 2 years of raloxifene plus calcium–vitamin D_3 or calcium–vitamin D_3 supplemented placebo treatment showed a significant and similar 5–7% increase in the mean degree of mineralization of bone tissue in both the groups (assessed by quantitative microradiography).[14] Fratzl et al[15] also reported that individuals who had low matrix mineralization at baseline experienced greater increases following calcium–vitamin D supplementation. These findings highlight the importance of maintaining adequate calcium and vitamin D for proper bone mineralization. An increase in mineralization can improve the structural rigidity or stiffness of bone which may be advantageous for preventing fractures.

In summary, calcium and/or vitamin D supplementation has an acute antiresorptive effect on bone that acts systemically to downregulate bone remodeling to maintain BMD (or slow bone loss), preserve cortical thickness (by reducing endocortical resorption), and perhaps slow the increase in intracortical porosity and/or improve bone mineralization. There is no evidence that additional calcium–vitamin D supplementation can enhance periosteal apposition (bone size). However, the aforementioned skeletal benefits may be important for preserving the compressive strength of bone by maintaining a larger cross-sectional area on which axial loads can be distributed.[16] Whether these skeletal benefits translate directly into a significant reduction in fracture risk remains uncertain. However, the findings from a recent meta-analysis reported that supplementation with calcium or calcium and vitamin D was associated with a significant 12% risk reduction in fractures of all types.[17]

7.3 Effects of Exercise on Bone Strength in Older Adults

The majority of studies examining the effects of exercise on bone in older adults have measured changes in areal BMD by DXA. In general, the findings from RCTs ranging from 6 months to 3 years have shown that moderate to high-intensity exercise (including resistance training and/or weight-bearing exercise), results in site-specific gains in aBMD ranging from 1 to 3% in normally active older adults (for a recent review refer to Guadalupe-Grau et al[18]). However, since the introduction of peripheral QCT, there has been considerable interest in understanding whether exercise can enhance bone size, structure, and strength, as well as cortical and trabecular vBMD. Collectively, the findings from cross-sectional studies in older adults have generally shown that a higher level of physical activity (PA) (or athletic participation) is associated with greater cortical area (or thickness) and bone strength at loaded sites, largely due to an increase in bone size (periosteal apposition).[19–24] In contrast, these studies report either no effect of exercise on cortical or trabecular vBMD,[19,21] a small increase in trabecular vBMD[24] or a decrease in cortical vBMD at loaded sites in the active compared to inactive groups.[20] The decrease in cortical vBMD may be related to exercise-induced microdamage leading to targeted remodeling (increased intracortical porosity).[20] Nevertheless, the general consensus from these studies is that in older adults, the improvements in the mechanical competence of bone in response to exercise is related to bone structural adaptations and not to changes in vBMD. However, no definitive conclusions can be drawn from these studies because a causal relationship cannot be inferred from a cross-sectional design.

To date, there have been few long-term RCTs examining the effects of exercise training on bone geometry and strength in older adults, and nearly all trials have involved only women. In an early non-RCT using pQCT to assess bone geometric changes at the radius in response to a 6-month upper limb loading program in postmenopausal women, Adami et al[25] reported a significant training effect on cortical bone area (2.8%) and cortical BMC (3.2%), but a decrease in trabecular BMC (−3.4%). The authors speculated that increased loading resulted in reshaping of the bone cross-section (periosteal expansion) and a redistribution of bone mineral from the trabecular to the cortical component (e.g., corticalisation of the trabecular tissue). Similar findings were reported at the distal tibia in postmenopausal women who completed a 12-month exercise program involving 20 min of multidirectional jumping, 3 days per week.[26] In this study, exercise improved pQCT-derived estimated bone strength at the distal tibia by increasing the ratio of cortical to total area. There was no effect of exercise on total area, which suggests that exercise reduced endocortical bone loss. Contrary to these findings, other RCTs in older women conducted over 6–12 months have failed to observe any significant effect of resistance or impact training on pQCT-assessed bone structural properties at the tibia or radius,[27–29] but some beneficial effects on cortical vBMD at the

midshafts were observed.[29] A recent systematic review of pQCT studies examining the effects of exercise and PA of bone geometry in postmenopausal women concluded that exercise appears to have a modest, site-specific effect on bone mass and geometry at loaded sites, primarily affecting cortical rather than trabecular bone.[30] However, a limitation of this review is that it included cross-sectional and prospective studies and only a limited number of RCTs ($n = 4$).

In summary, we must await the outcome of further well-designed, long-term and adequately powered RCTs before any conclusion can be made about the effects of exercise on bone structural and material properties in older adults. However, we believe, based on the current data from the limited RCTs available, that training for up to 12 months results in modest gains in bone structure and strength. Any increase (or maintenance) in bone strength appears to be largely the result of an increase in tissue density and/or a reduction in endocortical bone loss, rather than an increase in bone size (periosteal apposition). However, to accurately determine whether exercise can enhance periosteal apposition during aging, further long-term (≥2 years) intervention trials are needed, because the changes which occur on the periosteal surface throughout adult life are reportedly very small (2–5 μm/year).[3]

7.4 Interaction Between Exercise, Calcium–Vitamin D Suplementation, and Bone Strength

There has been considerable interest in understanding whether combining exercise and calcium can produce additive or synergistic effects on bone. There is a sound physiological rationale for the existence of an interaction; exercise is needed to stimulate bone modeling and remodeling and calcium is an important substrate for bone mineralization.[31] In this section, we briefly review the evidence on whether the combination of exercise and calcium (or calcium–vitamin D supplementation) can enhance aBMD, bone structure, and strength in older adults. However, to fully appreciate the potential benefits of combining exercise and calcium (or optimal nutrition) on bone health, it is important to first understand interaction and the terms "additive" and "synergistic."

7.4.1 Understanding "Interaction": Additive or Synergistic?

The term interaction describes the combined effects of two or more variables as being *more* than the sum of their individual effects. That is, an "interaction" effect implies a result which is more than simply "additive"; it is multiplicative.[31] This is illustrated in Fig. 7.1, which provides a hypothetical example of both an "additive" and an "interactive" effect of exercise and calcium. In the left panel, the effects of both exercise and calcium supplementation on bone are shown to be additive, since exercise and calcium seem to work independently of each other. Here, FN BMC increases linearly with greater calcium supplementation *with* and *without* exercise; however, with exercise, the absolute increase is of a greater magnitude. That is, when exercise is included, its beneficial effect is *added* to that of calcium, but the difference between the groups remains the same at each level of calcium supplementation. In the case of an interaction (right panel), there is an exponential change in FN BMC when both exercise and calcium supplementation are present. Here, the osteogenic effect of exercise and calcium combined is greater than the sum of either factor alone because the effects are no longer parallel. Without exercise, the effect of increasing calcium on FN BMC is nil. Thus, in this example of "synergistic" interaction, exercise must be present in order for BMC to improve with calcium supplementation.

7.4.2 Effects of Exercise and Calcium–Vitamin D Supplementation on aBMD

Much of the interest in understanding whether there is an exercise-calcium interaction has stemmed from the findings of an early meta-analysis by Specker[32] involving 16 randomized and nonrandomized trials in peri- and postmenopausal women. The findings from this study showed that the beneficial effects of exercise on spine aBMD were apparent only at calcium intakes >1,000 mg/day; intakes below this level were insufficient to permit an osteogenic response. A subsequent meta-analysis involving six randomized and nonrandomized trials in postmenopausal women reported a significantly greater effect size of exercise on hip aBMD in women consuming more than, compared to less than, 1,000 mg/day of calcium.[33] These findings suggest that there may be a threshold of dietary calcium (~1,000 mg/day) necessary to attain the full osteogenic effects of exercise at loaded site.

In more recent years, there have been a number of large observational and prospective studies[21,22,34–36] and several RCTs[37,38] examining the effects of combined calcium and/or vitamin D supplementation with exercise on aBMD in older adults, with contrasting results. In a large population-based cross-sectional study of 1,497 Australian postmenopausal women, Devine et al[34] reported a significant synergistic interaction

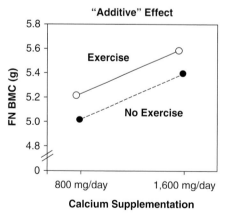
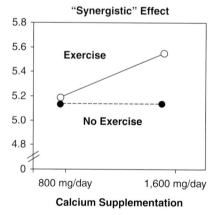
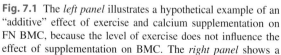

Fig. 7.1 The *left panel* illustrates a hypothetical example of an "additive" effect of exercise and calcium supplementation on FN BMC, because the level of exercise does not influence the effect of supplementation on BMC. The *right panel* shows a "synergistic" or "multiplicative" effect between exercise and calcium supplementation because BMC increases exponentially with exercise and calcium combined compared to calcium supplementation alone. Adapted from Specker and Vukovich[31]

between "high" PA levels (>169 kcal/day or around 4 h walking per week) and high calcium intakes (>792 mg/day) for FN aBMD (4.4%, $p < 0.05$). They also reported a trend for an interaction at the total hip, but this effect was additive and not synergistic. That is, high PA alone and high calcium alone were associated with increased total hip aBMD (+3.1% and +1.8% respectively, both $p < 0.05$), suggesting that calcium and exercise act independently. In a similar but smaller cross-sectional study of 422 women in three age categories (25–30, 40–45, and 60–65 years), divided into four groups by PA (high or low) and calcium intakes (>1,200 or <800 mg/day), Uusi-Rasi et al[22] reported that both high PA (defined as vigorous activity more than twice a week, at least 20 min/session causing enhanced breathing) and high calcium intakes were associated with improvements in a number of bone characteristics, but no interaction was detected for total body BMC, FN, and distal radius aBMD and selected dimensions and estimated strength variables (bone width, cortical thickness, section modulus). In a 10-year follow-up to this study involving 133 of the women in the 25–30 years age-group and 134 women in the 60–65 years age-group divided into four subgroups based on their concurrent levels of calcium and PA, no interactive effects were observed at any skeletal site; main effects of PA were reported for FN and trochanter BMC and strength estimates.[36]

In order to test the hypothesis that increased calcium can enhance bone's adaptive response to exercise, a 2×2 factorial design RCT with two factors is needed: (1) exercise (yes and no); and (2) calcium (yes and no). In one of the few published 2×2 trials, 41 sedentary and exercising women were recruited and randomly assigned to receive either a high-calcium milk drink (831 mg/day) or a low-calcium placebo drink (41 mg/day) for 12 months.[39] All participants were instructed to consume 800 mg/day of dietary calcium by consuming four daily serves of dairy foods. The exercising women were asked to participate in 4-weekly supervised walks (50 min sessions, wearing 3.1 kg weighted belts). For QCT-derived BMD at the lumbar spine and FN, main effects of exercise and high calcium were reported, but there was no exercise-by-calcium interaction. However, in this study, the small sample size most likely limited the ability to detect any interaction and exercise was not randomized. In one of only two RCTs in older adults specifically designed to test for an exercise-by-calcium interaction, Lau et al[38] randomized 50

postmenopausal Chinese women (age 62–92 years) with low baseline dietary calcium intakes (mean ~260 mg/day) into one of the following four groups: (1) load bearing exercise (bench stepping 4 times per week) plus a daily placebo tablet; (2) load bearing exercise plus calcium supplementation (800 mg/day); (3) calcium supplementation alone; and (4) placebo (no intervention). Despite the small sample size, a significant exercise-calcium interaction was detected for FN BMD after 10 months (+5.0%, $p < 0.05$) (Fig. 7 .2).[38] It is likely that the significant interaction observed in this study was related to the very low habitual calcium intakes of these women.

The only other factorial design RCT to address whether calcium (and vitamin D) can enhance the effects of exercise on bone was conducted in older Australian men. Kukuljan et al[37] reported that a 12-month high-intensity progressive resistance training and moderate impact weight-bearing exercise program performed 3 days per week combined with calcium–vitamin D_3 fortified milk (1,000 mg/day calcium and 800 IU/day vitamin D_3) did not lead to a synergistic response at the hip or spine in men ($n = 180$) aged 50–79 years. However, there was a main effect of exercise on FN aBMD (+1.8%, $p < 0.001$), but no effect of the fortified milk at any site. The lack of an interactive effect in this study was attributed to the relatively high baseline dietary calcium intakes (mean 1,002 mg/day) and serum 25-hydroxyvitamin D

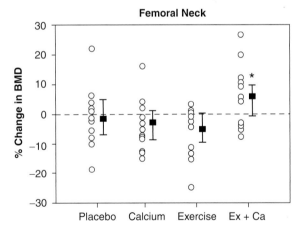

Fig. 7.2 Percentage changes in femoral neck BMD after 10 months for individual subjects (*open circles*) and the mean changes for the placebo ($n = 12$), calcium ($n = 12$), exercise ($n = 11$), and the exercise plus calcium ($n = 15$) groups (*square boxes* with 95% confidence intervals). The interaction between calcium supplements and exercise was significant (**p < 0.05*) (Adapted from Lau et al[38])

levels (mean 86 nmol/L) of the men. Therefore, based on the limited evidence from RCTs in older adults, it is likely that if an exercise-by-calcium interaction does exist, it may be limited to situations when a nutritional calcium insufficiency is corrected.

7.4.3 Effects of Exercise and Calcium–Vitamin D Supplementation on Bone Structure and Strength

Few studies have examined whether additional calcium can enhance the potential effects of exercise on bone structural properties in older adults. In a follow-up to their previous cross-sectional population-based study in Australian postmenopausal women, Nurzenski et al[35] reported no multiplicative effect between calcium and PA for HSA-derived bone geometry or strength estimates. There was however, an additive effect of the two factors. That is, women with combined high levels of PA (>65.5 kcal/day) and calcium (>1,039 mg/day) had greater bone cross-sectional area and section modulus than women with low PA and calcium. In a similar cross-sectional study in 218 pre- and 126 postmenopausal women using pQCT to assess bone geometry and vBMD at the radius and tibia, Uusi-Rasi et al[21] found that high PA (vigorous activity at least twice a week, ≥20 min per session) was associated with improvements in bone geometry and strength at the weight-bearing tibia, whereas high calcium (>1,200 mg/day) enhanced the mechanical competence of the nonweight-bearing radius; there was no physical activity–calcium interaction. Unfortunately, both these studies are limited by their cross-sectional design, but the findings indicate that calcium does not enhance the effects of exercise on geometric indices of bone strength in older adults. Preliminary data from the factorial design RCT in older men by Kukuljan et al[40] also indicates that combined calcium plus vitamin D_3 and exercise does not enhance bone structure, vBMD, or strength in older men. In this study of community dwelling men aged over 50 years, there was no exercise-by-calcium–vitamin D_3 interaction on DXA-derived FN HSA parameters or bone geometry, cortical or trabecular vBMD or strength estimates assessed by QCT at the midfemur, mid- or distal tibia, or lumbar spine. This was not unexpected since the men in this study had high habitual calcium intakes and sufficient circulating 25-hydroxyvitamin D levels.

Since calcium is a threshold nutrient, there is no reason to suggest that intakes exceeding the recommended requirements should enhance the structure or strength of bone in response to a given amount of loading. As previously indicated, a more likely explanation is that any potential skeletal adaptations to loading are likely to be compromised by inadequate intakes. In support of this notion, Lanyon et al[41] reported that calcium insufficiency attenuated the skeletal response to loading in the ulna of adult turkeys. Inman et al[42] also demonstrated that in the face of calcium deficiency, mechanical loading attenuated, but did not prevent, a decrease in bone strength (e.g., cross-sectional moment of inertia and bone stiffness) in mature female rats, compared with immobilized rats and ambulatory control rats.

7.4.4 Possible Interaction Mechanisms

If calcium does enhance the effect of exercise on bone in older adults, the mechanism to explain the interaction is not known. Studies in humans and animals have shown that exercise is associated with increased calcium absorption from the gut[43–45] which may help to meet any increased physiological requirement for calcium generated by increased exercise. However, this does not explain as to how additional calcium may enhance the effect of exercise on bone. There is some suggestion that calcium (nutrients) may modify the threshold of exercise needed to stimulate an osteogenic response.[46] This is consistent with Frost's observation that the "mechanostat" strain thresholds for bone formation or resorption may be moderated by nutritional parameters.[47] Despite initial reports that a calcium intake of around 1,000 mg/day may be needed for a positive skeletal response to exercise to occur,[32] further studies are still needed to determine and define if in fact a threshold exists. It is however unlikely that greater than adequate calcium intakes will enhance the adaptive responses to loading,[48] particularly, since calcium acts to downregulate bone remodeling and does not drive changes in bone geometry. As indicated by Frost, trying to significantly increase whole bone strength in healthy subjects by giving more calcium or vitamin D is like trying to make a car go faster by adding petrol to its tank.[49] It is more likely that if an interaction is detected, it is the result of additional calcium correcting a state of insufficiency, and thereby providing the necessary material (minerals) required to build a new bone.

7.5 Conclusion

In conclusion, the current evidence indicates that regular exercise (weight-bearing and/or resistance training) and adequate calcium (or calcium and vitamin D) are independently important for maintaining the mass, structure, and strength of bone in older adults. However, since bone is predominantly regulated by mechanical loading, exercise is a more important factor for optimizing whole bone strength. Nutritional factors, including calcium and vitamin D, have a permissive generalized effect on bone that act systemically to influence bone remodeling. There is no evidence that excess intakes will result in greater skeletal gains. In addition, in the absence of exercise, nutritional factors cannot adequately maintain bone mass, structure, or strength. Whether additional skeletal benefits from exercise can be achieved by increasing calcium (or nutrient) intakes remain uncertain, because there have been few well-designed 2×2 factorial design RCTs. From the limited data available, it would appear that additional calcium or calcium and vitamin D does not enhance the effects of exercise on bone structural or material properties in older adults with adequate calcium intakes or sufficient circulating vitamin D levels. However, there is some evidence that additional calcium can promote exercise-induced osteogenesis in older adults in a state of nutritional calcium insufficiency.[38] Furthermore, it has been suggested that there may be a threshold of calcium (around 1,000 mg/day) needed to optimize the skeletal response to loading,[32,33] but the evidence to support this threshold level is not strong. Further 2×2 factorial studies are needed to determine if indeed there is a threshold level of calcium necessary to maximize the mass, structure, and strength of bone. It is possible that in states of insufficiency, whole bone strength may not necessarily be compromised, if there is a change in bone structure (e.g., periosteal apposition) that increases bone strength without a corresponding net increase in bone mass. To address this question, future studies are needed that utilize state-of-the-art 3D bone imaging technology to increase our understanding of the structural basis by which exercise and nutrition influence whole bone strength.

References

1. Bouxsein ML. Determinants of skeletal fragility. *Best Pract Res Clin Rheumatol.* 2005;19:897-911.
2. Griffith JF, Genant HK. Bone mass and architecture determination: state of the art. *Best Pract Res Clin Endocrinol Metab.* 2008;22:737-764.
3. Seeman E, Delmas PD. Bone quality–the material and structural basis of bone strength and fragility. *N Engl J Med.* 2006;354:2250-2261.
4. Daly RM, Bass S, Nowson C. Long-term effects of calcium-vitamin-D3-fortified milk on bone geometry and strength in older men. *Bone.* 2006;39:946-953.
5. Daly RM, Brown M, Bass S, et al. Calcium and vitamin D3 fortified milk reduces bone loss at clinically relevant skeletal sites in older men: a 2-year randomised controlled trial. *J Bone Miner Res.* 2006;31:397-405.
6. Dawson Hughes B, Harris SS, Krall EA, et al. Effect of calcium and vitamin D supplementation on bone density in men and women 65 years of age or older. *N Eng J Med.* 1997;337:670-676.
7. Jackson RD, LaCroix AZ, Gass M, et al. Calcium plus vitamin D supplementation and the risk of fractures. *N Engl J Med.* 2006;354:669-683.
8. Peacock M, Liu GD, Carey M, et al. Effect of calcium or 25OH vitamin D-3 dietary supplementation on bone loss at the hip in men and women over the age of 60. *J Clin Endocrinol Metab.* 2000;85:3011-3019.
9. Zhu K, Devine A, Dick IM, et al. Effects of calcium and vitamin D supplementation on hip bone mineral density and calcium-related analytes in elderly ambulatory Australian women: a five-year randomized controlled trial. *J Clin Endocrinol Metab.* 2008;93:743-749.
10. Seeman E. To stop or not to stop, that is the question. *Osteoporos Int.* 2009;20:187-195.
11. Chen Z, Beck TJ, Wright NC, et al. The effect of calcium plus vitamin D supplement on hip geometric structures: results from the Women's Health Initiative CaD Trial. *J Bone Miner Res Suppl.* 2007;1:S59.
12. Elders PJ, Lips P, Netelenbos JC, et al. Long-term effect of calcium supplementation on bone loss in perimenopausal women. *J Bone Miner Res.* 1994;9:963-970.
13. Ettinger B, Genant HK, Cann CE. Postmenopausal bone loss is prevented by treatment with low-dosage estrogen with calcium. *Ann Intern Med.* 1987;106:40-45.
14. Boivin G, Lips P, Ott SM, et al. Contribution of raloxifene and calcium and vitamin D3 supplementation to the increase of the degree of mineralization of bone in postmenopausal women. *J Clin Endocrinol Metab.* 2003;88:4199-4205.
15. Fratzl P, Roschger P, Fratzl-Zelman N, et al. Evidence that treatment with risedronate in women with postmenopausal osteoporosis affects bone mineralization and bone volume. *Calcif Tissue Int.* 2007;81:73-80.

16. Seeman E. Reduced bone formation and increased bone resorption: rational targets for the treatment of osteoporosis. *Osteoporos Int.* 2003;14(suppl 3):S2-S8.

17. Tang BM, Eslick GD, Nowson C, et al. Use of calcium or calcium in combination with vitamin D supplementation to prevent fractures and bone loss in people aged 50 years and older: a meta-analysis. *Lancet.* 2007;370:657-666.

18. Guadalupe-Grau A, Fuentes T, Guerra B, et al. Exercise and bone mass in adults. *Sports Med.* 2009;39:439-468.

19. Daly RM, Bass SL. Lifetime sport and leisure activity participation is associated with greater bone size, quality and strength in older men. *Osteoporos Int.* 2006;17:1258-1267.

20. Wilks DC, Winwood K, Gilliver SF, et al. Bone mass and geometry of the tibia and the radius of master sprinters, middle and long distance runners, race-walkers and sedentary control participants: a pQCT study. *Bone.* 2009;45:91-97.

21. Uusi-Rasi K, Sievanen H, Pasanen M, et al. Associations of calcium intake and physical activity with bone density and size in premenopausal and postmenopausal women: a peripheral quantitative computed tomography study. *J Bone Miner Res.* 2002;17:544-552.

22. Uusi-Rasi K, Sievanen H, Vuori I, et al. Associations of physical activity and calcium intake with bone mass and size in healthy women at different ages. *J Bone Miner Res.* 1998;13:133-142.

23. Shedd KM, Hanson KB, Alekel DL, et al. Quantifying leisure physical activity and its relation to bone density and strength. *Med Sci Sports Exerc.* 2007;39:2189-2198.

24. Ma H, Leskinen T, Alen M, et al. Long-term leisure time physical activity and properties of bone: a Twin Study. *J Bone Miner Res.* 2009. doi:10.1359/JBMR.090309.

25. Adami S, Gatti D, Braga V, et al. Site-specific effects of strength training on bone structure and geometry of ultradistal radius in postmenopausal women. *J Bone Miner Res.* 1999;14:120-124.

26. Uusi-Rasi K, Kannus P, Cheng S, et al. Effect of alendronate and exercise on bone and physical performance of postmenopausal women: a randomized controlled trial. *Bone.* 2003;33:132-143.

27. Cheng S, Sipila S, Taaffe DR, et al. Change in bone mass distribution induced by hormone replacement therapy and high-impact physical exercise in post-menopausal women. *Bone.* 2002;31:126-135.

28. Karinkanta S, Heinonen A, Sievanen H, et al. A multi-component exercise regimen to prevent functional decline and bone fragility in home-dwelling elderly women: randomized, controlled trial. *Osteoporos Int.* 2007;18:453-462.

29. Liu-Ambrose TY, Khan KM, Eng JJ, et al. Both resistance and agility training reduce back pain and improve health-related quality of life in older women with low bone mass. *Osteoporos Int.* 2005;16:1321-1329.

30. Hamilton CJ, Swan VJ, Jamal SA. The effects of exercise and physical activity participation on bone mass and geometry in postmenopausal women: a systematic review of pQCT studies. *Osteoporos Int.* 2009. doi:10.1007/s00198-009-0967-1.

31. Specker B, Vukovich M. Evidence for an interaction between exercise and nutrition for improved bone health during growth. In: Daly RM, Petit MA, eds. *Optimizing bone mass and strength. The role of physical activity and nutrition during growth.* Basel: Karger; 2007.

32. Specker BL. Evidence for an interaction between calcium intake and physical activity on changes in bone mineral density. *J Bone Miner Res.* 1996;11:1539-1544.

33. Kelley GA. Aerobic exercise and bone density at the hip in postmenopausal women: a meta-analysis. *Prev Med.* 1998;27:798-807.

34. Devine A, Dhaliwal SS, Dick IM, et al. Physical activity and calcium consumption are important determinants of lower limb bone mass in older women. *J Bone Miner Res.* 2004;19:1634-1639.

35. Nurzenski MK, Briffa NK, Price RI, et al. Geometric indices of bone strength are associated with physical activity and dietary calcium intake in healthy older women. *J Bone Miner Res.* 2007;22:416-424.

36. Uusi-Rasi K, Sievanen H, Pasanen M, et al. Influence of calcium intake and physical activity on proximal femur bone mass and structure among pre- and postmenopausal women. A 10-year prospective study. *Calcif Tissue Int.* 2008;82:171-181.

37. Kukuljan S, Nowson CA, Bass SL, et al. Effects of a multicomponent exercise program and calcium-vitamin-D3-fortified milk on bone mineral density in older men: a randomised controlled trial. *Osteoporos Int.* 2009;20:1241-1251.

38. Lau EM, Woo J, Leung PC, et al. The effects of calcium supplementation and exercise on bone density in elderly Chinese women. *Osteoporos Int.* 1992;2:168-173.

39. Nelson ME, Fisher EC, Dilmanian FA, et al. A 1-y walking program and increased dietary calcium in postmenopausal women: effects on bone. *Am J Clin Nutr.* 1991;53:1304-1311.

40. Kukuljan S, Nowson CA, Bass S, et al. Effects of a targeted bone and muscle loading program on QCT bone geometry and strength, muscle size and function in older men: An 18 month RCT. *J Bone Miner Res.* 2008;23:S69.

41. Lanyon CE, Rubin CT, Baust G. Modulation of bone loss during calcium insufficiency by controlled dynamic loading. *Calcif Tissue Int.* 1986;38:209-216.

42. Inman CL, Warren GL, Hogan HA, et al. Mechanical loading attenuates bone loss due to immobilization and calcium deficiency. *J Appl Physiol.* 1999;87:189-195.

43. Yeh JK, Aloia JF. Effect of physical activity on calciotropic hormones and calcium balance in rats. *Am J Physiol.* 1990;258:E263-E268.

44. Zittermann A, Sabatschus O, Jantzen S, et al. Exercise-trained young men have higher calcium absorption rates and plasma calcitriol levels compared with age-matched sedentary controls. *Calcif Tissue Int.* 2000;67:215-219.

45. Zittermann A, Sabatschus O, Jantzen S, et al. Evidence for an acute rise of intestinal calcium absorption in response to aerobic exercise. *Eur J Nutr.* 2002;41:189-196.

46. Iwamoto J, Takeda T, Ichimura S. Effect of exercise training and detraining on bone mineral density in postmenopausal women with osteoporosis. *J Orthop Sci.* 2001;6:128-132.

47. Frost HM. Bone's mechanostat: a 2003 update. *Anat Rec.* 2003;275A:1081-1101.

48. Heaney RP. The importance of calcium intake for lifelong skeletal health. *Calcif Tissue Int.* 2002;70:70-73.

49. Frost HM, Schonau E. The "muscle-bone unit" in children and adolescents: a 2000 overview. *J Pediatr Endocrinol Metab.* 2000;13:571-590.

The Bone Benefits of Calcium and Exercise in Children

8

Joan M. Lappe

8.1 Introduction

During growth, bone strength, defined as the ability to resist fracture, develops through the adaptation of skeletal mass and geometry in response to mechanical loads. Bones have a tremendous potential to respond to mechanical loading by changing shape, and this adaptive ability is much greater during growth than after growth ceases. Throughout childhood and adolescence, the skeleton is adapting to changes in mechanical loads to become strong enough to support body weight and current physical activity. Furthermore, at the completion of growth, the bones must be of sufficient strength to meet the lifetime load-bearing demands of adulthood. Bone mass, size, and strength are regulated by daily mechanical loads, but the relative response to loads is dependent upon other factors: genetics, lifestyle choices, and health, hormonal and nutritional status. This chapter focuses on the role of mechanical loading (physical activity) and calcium nutrition in childhood skeletal development.

8.2 Bone Physiology During Growth

Data from a cohort of Canadian children followed since 1991 have contributed greatly to our understanding of bone development during childhood and adolescence. Those data indicate that peak height velocity (PHV) in girls occurs at a mean age of 11.9 ± 0.89 years at a maturation point equivalent to 92% of adult height.[1] Peak bone area (BA) velocity is seen at a mean age of 12.19 ± 0.89 years, while peak bone mineral content (BMC) velocity occurs at a mean age of 12.67 ± 0.99 years, coincident with menarche.[1] In boys, PHV occurs at 13.57 ± 0.92 years while peak BA is seen at 13.69 ± 0.96 years. Peak BMC velocity occurs at 14.14 ± 1.05 years.

Appendicular growth is more rapid than axial growth before puberty, while axial growth predominates during early puberty.[2] Growth of both the regions decelerates in late puberty. Size-corrected bone mineral density (BMD) increases significantly until about 4 years after PHV.[1]

Parfitt et al[3] described structural and cellular changes during bone growth based on iliac crest bone biopsies from 58 healthy white subjects aged 1.5–23 years. Between 2 and 20 years, in the ilium, as noted in iliac crest biopsies, the bone enlarges by periosteal apposition and endocortical resorption on the outer cortex, and net periosteal resorption and net endocortical formation on the medial cortex. The researchers estimated that endocortical apposition continues until the age of 30 years. In girls, a considerable degree of increase in cortical width in the metacarpal occurs in early puberty due to the production of estrogen, but after menarche, this stabilizes. Endocortical apposition at the metacarpal is not seen in boys.[2,4] Also during growth, lateral modeling drift of the inner cortex results in a larger marrow cavity, and the new trabeculae in this space arise from the cancelization of unresorbed cortical bone.[3] Based on the biopsy analyses, Parfitt et al concluded that iliac bone growth (core width) is completed by late adolescence, but the cortical thickness further increases during the period of consolidation, up until the age of peak bone mass.[3]

J.M. Lappe
Departments of Nursing and Medicine, Creighton University,
601 North 30th Street, Omaha, NE 68131, USA
e-mail: jmlappe@creighton.edu

P. Burckhardt et al. (eds.), *Nutritional Influences on Bone Health*,
DOI: 10.1007/978-1-84882-978-7_8, © Springer-Verlag London Limited 2010

Modeling, persistence of bone formation or resorption at one location, is the primary mode of bone turnover in the prepubertal skeleton. However, remodeling, the cyclical replacement of bone by resorption and formation, becomes the dominant mode of turnover after longitudinal growth ceases.[4] The outcome producing ideal bone structure in the ilium is both macrostructural (large outer dimension of the ilium and increased cortical thickness), and microstructural (trabeculae that are adequate in numbers, thickness, and connectivity). In the case of tubular bone such as the tibia, the macrostructural and microstructural modeling changes are similar to that of the ilium. Mechanical loading is the key element for the development of maximal bone strength.

8.3 Mechanical Loading and Bone Responses

Mechanical loads create bone bending or strain. They work at the cellular level to alter bone metabolism and thereby adapt bone size, shape, and strength to reduce strains and to prevent fracture. The magnitude of the bone stimulus is dependent upon strain magnitude, strain rate, number of cycles, and frequency.[5] When activity and bone strains are in the normally adapted range, cellular activity is in a steady state and bone mass maintained. However, when strains increase to create a mild overload, then local osteoblast formation is stimulated and local bone resorption decreased for a net gain in bone mass. Loading also increases periosteal circumference and cortical thickness which results in increased strength.[6]

In animal studies, bone formation response to loading is activated immediately with biochemical and mRNA changes detected within minutes and hours of loading.[7] The modeling response is independent of prior osteoclast activation and results in net bone formation. Osteoblasts appear on the surface within 48 h of loading and bone formation rate is accelerated by day five.[8] If loads are maintained, then maximal bone formation rates are achieved within 3 weeks and may be complete within 12–18 weeks.[9] Generally, the response is relative to strain (deformation) magnitude and localized to surfaces with the greatest strain. The net effect of this modeling response is to increase bone size and mass quickly to reduce strain. In studies using the ulna loading model, Robling et al[10] showed that a small percent increase in BMC significantly increased bone strength. For each 1% increase in BMC in the loaded ulna, ultimate strength increased by 11.5%.

Animal studies have also shown that the frequency of mechanical stimulus is critical to the degree of adaptation, i.e., more frequent loading results in greater bone formation.[10] Rest periods, but not longer duration of the loading stimulus, result in greater bone accrual. Also, larger initial loading stimuli produce greater gains in bone strength, and after a few weeks of loading, the bone stops responding so that the amount of adaptation is proportional to the initial peak magnitude of load.[11]

Warden et al found that exercising in growing rodents resulted in improved bone structure that remained after detraining and into senescence.[12] Exercise, using the forearm axial compression loading model, increased both bone quantity and structure. However, after 2 years, when the animals were elderly, the bone structure changes persisted, but the bone quantity changes did not. In the aged animals, the exercised ulnas had greater ultimate force, i.e., greater fracture resistance. If we could directly apply this in vivo work to humans, we could conclude that exercise during growth reduces the incidence of fractures in old age.

8.4 Human Exercise Studies

Although no exercise studies have prospectively followed humans from childhood into old age, numerous studies support the positive effect of weight-bearing physical activity, i.e., mechanical loading during childhood and adolescence on the development of a stronger skeleton.

The majority of studies of exercise in children have assessed bone effects with DXA, which measures areal density. Although DXA provides valuable information about bone responses to exercise, it is important to note that DXA has limitations when used in children. Furthermore, as DXA software has improved for measurement in children, comparison of older studies with more recent ones is difficult. For example, early software had limited ability to detect bone edges in children because of their incompletely mineralized bone, while newer software is much better at edge detection. Because of the ability of the newer software to improve the detection of low-density bone, there is greater increase in identified BA than in BMC. Thus, the BMD values obtained with the newer software are systematically lower than those obtained with the older versions.[13]

DXA values are more difficult to interpret in children than in adults because children are changing in body size and composition, skeletal maturation, and pubertal stage. For example, areal BMD underestimates volumetric BMD in children who are short for their age.[14] Also DXA is unable to distinguish between cortical and trabecular bone or to differentiate between changes in bone dimensions and bone density. Increases in areal BMD may actually indicate increases in the size of the bone rather than in the bone density. Lastly, studies of DXA in children are challenging to compare because variable hardware and software were used, and a variety of outcomes were reported – BMD, BMC, and both BMD and BMC adjusted for age, tanner stage, height, weight, etc.

Despite the challenges of assessing bone changes, the positive effect of exercise on the skeletons of children and adolescents has strong support in the literature. Cross-sectional studies have shown that bone mass is higher in active compared to sedentary children[15,16] and in athletes than in nonathletes[17,18] For example, Kannus et al assessed the effect of training with side-to-side comparison in sports with unilateral loading.[18] Female tennis and squash players had significantly higher BMC at every measured site in the arm compared to controls. BMC at the upper arm was 23.5% higher than in the controls for those who started sport participation greater than 5 years before menarche. The benefit of playing was 2 times greater if started before menarche. Retrospective studies have shown that retired dancers and long-term athletes have greater bone mass than controls,[19] while prospective studies show greater increases in bone mass in active children than in those who are less active.[20]

A recent review of controlled trials concluded that weight-bearing physical activity enhances bone mineral accrual in children.[21] The evidence from the trials suggests that early puberty may be the stage of maturity at which exercise has the maximum benefit; however, there are not enough data to make a definite conclusion. In one of the largest randomized trials, which included approximately 400 boys and girls, Canadian researchers conducted a 10–12-min moderate impact circuit training program 3 times per week in an elementary school setting.[22] After 20 months, both boys and girls had a nearly 5% greater increase in bone accrual than controls ($p < 0.05$). To put this gain into perspective, it has been estimated that increasing the bone mass of the elderly population by five percent would decrease hip fracture incidence by 50%.[23]

In the above-mentioned review, the trial by Fuchs et al[24] was rated as one of the strongest trials with a low risk of bias. In that study, boys and girls between 5.9 and 9.8 years were randomly assigned to a 7-month jumping intervention or control group. The jumping group performed 100, two-footed jumps from a 61-cm box 3 times per week in a supervised school setting. The control group performed stretching exercises. At the end of the study, the jumping group had 4.5% and 3.1% greater increase in BMC at the femoral neck ($p < 0.001$) and the lumbar spine, respectively, than the controls ($p < 0.05$). Thus, short bouts of moderate activity in prepubertal children can result in a considerable benefit to bone.

Gunter et al later combined data from the Fuchs study with data from an identical study and followed the children for 8 years.[25] In the combined analysis, BMC of the total hip increased in jumpers over controls by 3.6% ($p < 0.05$) by the end of the intervention. After follow-up with 47% of the original sample for 8 years after the end of the intervention, the jumping group had a 1.4% greater hip BMC than controls. These findings demonstrate that bone quantity gains due to a simple jumping intervention during childhood are sustained, albeit decreased, for quite a while after exercise stops. Based on the animal studies of Warden et al[12] mentioned earlier, these children may have had even greater advantages in bone structure that weren't measurable by DXA.

Because of the limitations of DXA, research efforts have increased to assess bone size and structure during growth and in response to physical activity using magnetic resonance imaging (MRI) and peripheral quantitative computed tomography (pQCT). Studies of racket sport players have shown that bending strength is increased by the apposition of relatively small amounts of bone at specific loaded sites on the periosteal surface rather than by increased bone mass over the entire skeleton.[26,27] For example, Bass et al[28] studied the effect of mechanical loading on the size and shape of bone in competitive female tennis players aged 8–17 years using MRI combined with DXA. The loaded arms demonstrated 11–14% greater BMC and moment of inertia ($p < 0.01$) compared to the nonloaded arms. The higher BMC reflected a 7–11% greater cortical area due to greater periosteal expansion. Nikander et al [26] recently reported a study of 113 female Finnish national athletes (mean age 20.9 years) using peripheral pQCT. They were volleyball players, hurdlers, swimmers, racket players, soccer players, and a volunteer control group. The weight-bearing lower extremities of the athletes (except swimmers) were characterized by larger diaphyses, thicker cortices, and denser cortical bone compared to controls. Specifically, at the distal tibia, the athletes had significantly higher trabecular BMC and polar moment of inertia and thicker cortical walls than controls. These structural advantages contribute to increased bone strength. Further evidence that physical activity during growth increases bone strength includes studies showing that military recruits are less likely to have stress fractures during basic training if they have a history of being physically active.[29,30]

Thus, strong evidence supports the notion that short-term exercise programs during childhood and early adolescence provide long-term benefits to skeletal health.

8.5 Importance of Adequate Calcium Nutrition for Bone Development

Calcium is essential for bone mineralization, and a positive calcium balance is necessary for maximal bone adaptation to mechanical loading. In their chapter of this book, Daly and Kukujan describe this as a "synergistic" interaction between calcium and exercise (see Chap. 7 for definitions of the terms "interaction," "additive," and "synergistic" in relation to the effects of calcium and exercise). Growing children and adolescents are depositing large amounts of calcium in their skeletons, and their calcium requirements are substantially higher than those of young adults (calcium requirements during growth are discussed in Chap. 6). Both for younger children and those going through puberty, supplemental calcium can have significant positive effects on skeletal mineral content. Evidence suggests that calcium intake may positively affect peak bone mass by as much as 5–10%,[31] an amount equal to about 0.5–1.0 standard deviations in peak skeletal mass. Although peak mass is not achieved

until about age 30, at least 90% of the adult mass is accrued by the age of 19 or 20.[31] Thus, adequate calcium intake during childhood and adolescence is critical.

Calcium is a critical nutrient for metabolic functioning as well as for bone health. Ionized calcium plays a vital role in mediating numerous cellular processes. The skeleton serves as a reservoir of calcium to maintain plasma calcium ion (Ca++) levels. When dietary sources of calcium are not adequate to maintain essential Ca++ levels, bone is resorbed to provide the needed extracellular calcium. Thus, the strength of the skeleton may be sacrificed to maintain plasma Ca++ homeostasis. During puberty, there is an increased bone turnover to meet the high demand for calcium associated with growth. When calcium intake is suboptimal, calcium is taken from the cortical bone resulting in cortical porosity and greater risk of appendicular fractures.[4]

Interestingly, a recent report indicates that forearm fracture rates in children have increased considerably over the past three decades.[32] Age-adjusted fracture rates increased by 32% in males and 56% in females. This may be due, in part, to decreased consumption of milk, which is a major source of dietary calcium. Milk consumption by children has decreased in the recent past,[33] and low milk intake in children has been associated with a greater number of fractures.[34]

8.6 Studies of Calcium and Skeletal Development

One of the first studies to demonstrate the importance of dietary calcium for the promotion of bone health was a classic cross-sectional study in which bone density and fracture rates were evaluated in two Croatian populations, one of which had twice the intake of dietary calcium of the other (940 ± 27 mg/day vs. 445 ± 30 mg/day).[35] There was a significantly higher fracture rate in the low than the high calcium district. Young adults in the district with higher calcium intake also had significantly higher bone mass than young adults in the district with low calcium intake. Since the greater bone mass in the high calcium district was evident in all age groups, the authors concluded that the greater bone mass achieved in childhood was maintained throughout life.

Strong evidence exists for the effect of calcium supplementation on increase in bone mass at different stages of maturation. Generally, studies report a positive short-term effect of increased calcium intake, whether from supplements, fortified foods, or dairy products, on various bone measures. Calcium supplementation produces the greatest increase in bone mass in children with the lowest habitual dietary calcium intake.[36] The stage of development at which calcium supplementation may have the greatest effect on bone health is not clear. One review concluded that the effect is greater in prepubertal children,[37] while another review concluded that the effects were the greatest during puberty.[38] Findings from follow-up studies to determine the long-term effect of calcium supplementation are also not consistent. Some have found no long-term effect,[39–41] while others have shown that the positive effect on bone is detectable for as long as 7.5 years after the end of supplementation.[42–44]

Welch et al studied the effects of a moderately low vs. adequate dietary calcium intake along with impact exercise on bone development in a highly controlled study of growing rodents[45] (see Fig. 8.1). They found that both impact exercise and dietary calcium increased the density and structure of cortical and trabecular bone; however, impact loading resulted in greater effects than calcium. A recent review of human studies also concluded that the effects of exercise on bone are greater than the effects of calcium.[46] In the growing

rodent study, impact exercise and dietary calcium had additive effects for cortical BA in the proximal ulna and for trabecular volumetric BMD, total BA, and periosteal circumference in the distal tibia. Mechanical testing showed that the animals subjected to impact loading had greater mechanical strength, indicated by force to breaking, regardless of diet. However, it is important to note that the higher calcium group was given adequate calcium, but not high doses of supplementation.

Although no randomized human trials have reported the effect of calcium supplementation on fracture incidence in growing children, cross-sectional data show that children who avoid drinking milk have a higher incidence of fracture.[34] Also, one trial has shown that calcium supplementation during periods of intense physical activity, at the end of adolescence and longitudinal growth, can dramatically reduce the incidence of stress fracture.[47] In this study, 5,201 female military basic trainees were randomly assigned to supplementation with calcium and vitamin D3 or identical placebo during the 8 weeks of US Navy basic training. During basic training, recruits participate in rigorous activities including running, jumping, and walking long distances. For many of the recruits (mean age 20 years), basic training involves physical activity levels that are much higher than those to which they are accustomed. Thus, calcium intake is essential not only for supporting adaptation to exercise but also for the repair of microdamage. In this study, supplementation with calcium 2,000 mg/day and vitamin D3 800 IU/day decreased the incidence of stress fracture by 20%. This study shows that calcium intake is important for maintaining bone strength in young persons, who on an average have reached about 95% of their peak bone mass.

8.7 Combined Effects of Calcium and Exercise

Although there are only a few randomized trials of the effect of exercise and calcium combined on bone accrual in children, there is evidence that the effect of exercise is enhanced in the presence of adequate calcium intake. For example, in a study of prepubertal and pubertal girls, participants were assigned to one of the four groups: moderate impact exercise with or

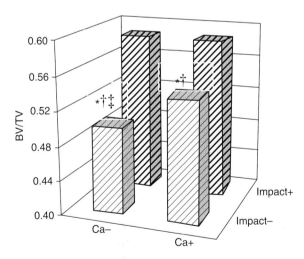

Fig. 8.1 The effects of calcium and freefall impact on bone volume/tissue volume in the trabecular fraction of the proximal ulna. Different from Impact⁺, Ca⁺ : *$p<0.05$. Different from Impact⁺, Ca⁻: $p<0.05$. Used with permission

without calcium supplementation or low-impact exercise with or without calcium. Those assigned to moderate impact exercise and calcium supplementation experienced a greater increase in BMC of the femur, a loaded site, than the other three groups.[48] In a randomized study of calcium supplementation and physical activity in children aged 3–5 years,[49] there was a significant interaction between physical activity and calcium supplementation. Positive effects on changes in leg bone mass occurred only in children consuming high calcium intakes (≥1,100 mg/day). However, there were increases in periosteal and endosteal tibial circumferences in the physical activity group independent of calcium intake.

Another study evaluated gain in BMC in prepubertal girls after a 1-year rope jumping intervention in which three groups were compared: exercise, exercise plus intake of at least 1,500 mg of calcium from foods/day, and a control group who continued with their usual activity and dietary intake.[50] The group that exercised and had a high calcium intake had a 27% gain in femoral neck BMC ($p<0.05$), while in the control group it increased by 20% (NS), and in the group that exercised, but did not increase their calcium, by 19% (NS). Iuliano-Burns used a similar design and found a significant calcium/exercise interaction in femur BMC accrual[48] (see Fig. 8.2). The main effect of exercise was at the tibia/fibula, where BMC increased by 3% more in

the exercise than the nonexercise group ($p<0.05$). In the forearm, a nonloaded site, there was no exercise effect, but there was the main effect of calcium supplementation. The BMC of the radius/ulna increased by 4% more in the supplemented girls than in the control group ($p<0.01$). The authors concluded that exercise confers region-specific effects while dietary calcium confers generalized effects to the skeleton. Thus, evidence suggests that greater gains in bone mass at loaded skeletal sites are achieved when exercise is combined with increased calcium intake.

8.8 Bone Development and Fractures in Adulthood

It is well established that peak bone mass is an important predictor of osteoporotic fracture. However, no prospective studies have followed individuals from childhood into old age to determine the importance of bone development for the prevention of fractures in the elderly. It has been shown that higher bone density is associated with fewer fractures in young adult women, who should have attained about 95% of their peak bone mass. In this study,[51] bone density was determined in a large cohort of female US Army recruits at the start of military basic training. The recruits were

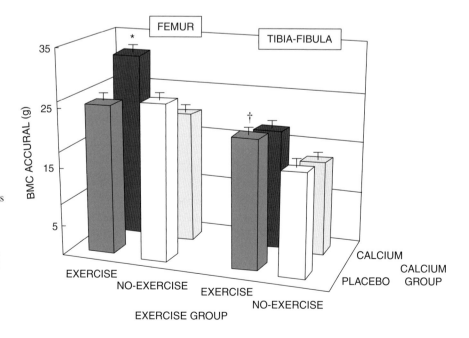

Fig. 8.2 Changes in humerus and radius-ulna BMC after 8.5 months in the Ex+Ca ($n=16$), Ex+placebo ($n=18$), No-Ex+Ca ($n=14$), and No-Ex+placebo ($n=18$) groups. The main effect was detected at the humerus and radius-ulna: $p<0.1$; $p<0.01$ calcium vs. placebo groups

followed for the ascertainment of stress fractures. The relative risk of stress fracture for those in the lowest quintile of bone density was 6.7. In recruits without a history of regular exercise, those in the lowest quintile of bone density had nearly a 10-times greater risk of fracture than those in the highest quintile. This provides evidence that bone development during childhood is important for the prevention of fractures in at least the early years of adulthood.

8.9 Summary

Strong evidence supports the importance of adequate calcium and physical activity for building strong bones during childhood and adolescence. Evidence suggests that exercise has greater effect than calcium and that the combination of calcium and exercise has a synergistic effect, particularly at loaded skeletal sites. Higher bone density is associated with fewer fractures at the end of adolescence. Also, those who exercise during childhood and adolescence have a lower risk of fractures at the end of adolescence. Cross-sectional data show that children who drink milk have a lower incidence of fractures. Calcium and vitamin D supplementation dramatically decreases fractures in highly active females at the end of adolescence.

It is likely that adequate dietary calcium intake is necessary for full adaptation to mechanical loading in growing children. The optimal amount of exercise has not been delineated, but the level is greater than that currently obtained by most children. Now, the emphasis should be on finding ways to assure that children ingest recommended levels of calcium and participate in regular weight-bearing physical activity.

References

1. Faulkner R, Davison K, Bailey D, Mirwald R, Baxter-Jones A. Size-corrected BMD decreases during peak linear growth: implications for fracture incidence during adolescence. *J Bone Miner Res.* 2006;21:1864-1870.
2. Bass S, Delmas P, Pearce G, Hendrich E, Tabensky A, Seeman E. The differing tempo of growth in bone size, mass, and density in girls is region-specific. *J Clin Invest.* 1999; 104:795-804.
3. Parfitt A, Travers R, Rauch F, Glorieux F. Structural and cellular changes during bone growth in healthy children. *Bone.* 2000;27:487-494.
4. Parfitt A. The two faces of growth: benefits and risks to bone integrity. *Osteoporosis Int.* 1994;4:382-398.
5. Rubin C, Lanyon L. Regulation of bone mass by mechanical strain magnitude. *Calcif Tissue Int.* 1985;37:411-417.
6. Kirmani S, Christen D, van Lenthe GH, et al. Bone structure at the distal radius during adolescent growth. *J Bone Miner Res.* 2009;24:1033-1042.
7. Raab-Cullen D. In-vivo bone cell histology and biochemical responses to mechanical loading. In: Maughan R, ed. *Biochemistry of Exercise.* Champaign IL: Human Kinetics; 1996:543-554.
8. Boppart M, Kimmel D, Yee J, Cullen D. Time course of osteoblast appearance after in-vivo mechanical loading. *Bone.* 1998;23:409-415.
9. Raab-Cullen D, Akhter M, Kimmel D, Recker R. Bone response to alternate-day mechanical loading of the rat tibia. *J Bone Miner Res.* 1994;9:203-211.
10. Robling A, Hinant F, Burr D, Turner C. Shorter, more frequent mechanical loading sessions enhance bone mass. *Med Sci Sports Exerc.* 2001;34:196-202.
11. Schriefer JL, Warden SJ, Saxon LK, Robling AG, Turner CH. Cellular accommodation and the response of bone to mechanical loading. *J Biomech.* 2005;38:1838-1845.
12. Warden S, Fuchs R, Castillo AB, Nelson IR, Turner CH. Exercise when young provides lifelong benefits to bone structure and strength. *J Bone Miner Res.* 2007;22: 251-259.
13. Leonard M, Feldman H, Zemel B, Berlin J, Barden E, Stallings V. Evalaution of low density spine software for the assessment of bone mineral density in children. *J Bone Miner Res.* 1998;13:1687-1690.
14. Prentice A, Parsons TJ, Cole TJ. Uncritical use one bone mineral density in absorptiometry may lead to size-related artifacts in the identification of bone mineral determinants. *Am J Clin Nutr.* 1994;60:837-842.
15. Daly RM, Rich PA, Klein R. Influence of high impact loading on ultrasound bone measurements in children: a cross-sectional report. *Calcif Tissue Int.* 1997;60:401-404.
16. Haapasalo H, Kannus P, Sievanen H, et al. Effect of long-term unilateral activity on bone mineral density of female junior tennis players. *J Bone Miner Res.* 1998;13:310-319.
17. Nevill AM, Holder RL, Stewart AD. Modeling elite male athletes' peripheral bone mass, assessed using regional dual x-ray absorptiometry. *Bone.* 2003;32:62-68.
18. Kannus P, Haapasalo H, Sankelo M, et al. Effect of starting age of physical activity on bone mass in the dominant arm of tennis and squash players. *Ann Intern Med.* 1995;123: 27-31.
19. Khan KM, Bennell KL, Hopper JL, et al. Self-reported ballet classes undertaken at age 10-12 years and hip bone mineral density in later life. *Osteoporosis Int.* 1998;8:165-173.
20. Gunnes M, Lehmann EH. Physical activity and dietary constituents as predictors of forearm cortical and trabecular bone gain in healthy children and adolescents: a prospective study. *Acta Paediatrica.* 1996;85:19-25.
21. Hind K, Burrows M. Weight-bearing exercise and bone mineral accrual in children and adolescents: a review of controlled trials. *Bone.* 2007;40:14-27.
22. MacKelvie K, McKay H, Khan K, Crocker PRE. A school-based exercise intervention augments bone mineral accrual in early pubertal girls. *J Pediatr.* 2001;139:501-508.

23. Melton J. Osteoporosis: a worldwide problem. In: *The Proceedings of the Third International Symposium: Osteoporosis–Research Advances and Clinical Applications*; 1994:23.

24. Fuchs R, Bauer JJ, Snow CM. Jumping improves hip and lumbar spine bone mass in prepubescent children: a randomized controlled trial. *Bone Miner Res*. 2001;16:148-156.

25. Gunter K, Baxter-Jones A, Mirwald R, et al. Impact exercise increases BMC during growth: an 8-year longitudinal study. *J Bone Miner Res*. 2007;23:986-993.

26. Nikander R, Sievanen H, Uusi-rasi K, Heinonen A, Kannus P. Loading modalities and bone structures at non-weight-bearing upper extremity and weight-bearing lower extremity: a pQCT study of adult female athletes. *Bone*. 2006;39:886-894.

27. Liu L, Maruno R, Mashimo T. Effects of physical training on cortical bone at midtibia assessed by peripheral QCT. *J Appl Physiol*. 2003;95:219-224.

28. Bass S, Saxon L, Daly R, et al. The effect of mechanical loading on the size and shape of bone in pre-, peri-, and postpubertal girls: a study in tennis players. *J Bone Miner Res*. 2002;17:2274-2280.

29. Rauh M, Macera C, Trone D, Shaffer R, Brodine S. Epidemiology of stress fracture and lower-extremity overuse injury in female recruits. *Med Sci Sports Exerc*. 2006;38: 1571-1577.

30. Lappe J, Stegman M, Recker R. The impact of lifestyle factors on stress fractures in female army recruits. *Osteoporos Int*. 2001;12:35-42.

31. Matkovic V, Ilich J, Skugor M. Calcium intake and skeletal formation. In: Burchhardt P, Heaney R, eds. *Nutritional Aspects of Osteoporosis '94*. Rome, Italy: Ares-Serono Symposia Pub; 1995:129-145.

32. Khosla S, Melton III L, Dekutoski M, Achenback S, Oberg A, Riggs B. Incidence of childhood distal forearm fractures over 30 years. *JAMA*. 2003;1479-1485.

33. Borrud L, Wilkinson Enns C, Mickle S. What we eat: USDA surveys food consumption changes. *Community Nutr Inst Newslett*. 1997;1997:4-5.

34. Goulding A, Rockwell J, Black R, Grant A, Jones I, Williams S. Children who avoid drinking cow's milk are at increased risk for prepubertal bone fractures. *J Am Diet Assoc*. 2004;104: 250-253.

35. Matkovic V, Kostial K, Simonovic I, Buzina R, Nordin B. Bone status and fracture rates in two regions of Yugoslavia. *Am J Clin Nutr*. 1979;32:540-549.

36. Dibba B, Prentice A, Ceesay M, Stirling D, Cole T, Poskitt E. Effect of calcium supplementation on bone mineral accretion in Gambian children accustomed to a low-calcium diet. *Am J Clin Nutr*. 2000;71:544-549.

37. Vatanparast H, Whiting SJ. Calcium supplementation trials and bone mass development in children, adolescents, and young adults. *Nutr Rev*. 2006;64:204-209.

38. Wosje K, Specker B. Role of calcium in bone health during childhood. *Nutr Rev*. 2000;58:253-268.

39. Lee W, Leung S, Leung D, Cheng J. A follow-up study on the effect of calcium-supplement withdrawal and puberty on bone acquisition in children. *Am J Clin Nutr*. 1996; 64:71-77.

40. Lee WT, Leung SS, Leung DM, et al. Bone mineral acquisition in low calcium intake children following the withdrawal of calcium supplement. *Acta Paediatrica*. 1997;86: 570-576.

41. Slemenda CW, Peacock M, Hui S, Zhou L, Johnston CC. Reduced rates of skeletal remodeling are associated with increased bone mineral density during the development of peak skeletal mass. *J Bone Miner Res*.1997;12:676-682.

42. Bonjour J, Chevalley T, Ammann P, Slosman D, Rizzoli R. Gain in bone mineral mass in prepubertal girls 3-5 years after discontinuation of calcium supplementation: a follow up study. *Lancet*. 2001;358:1208-1212.

43. Chevalley T, Rizzoli R, Hans D, Ferrari S, Bonjour J. Interaction between calcium intake and menarcheal age on bone mass gain: an eight-year follow-up study from prepuberty to postmenarche. *J Clin Endocrinol Metab*. 2005;90:44-51.

44. Dodiuk-Gad R, Rozen G, Rennert G, Ish-Shalom S. Sustained effect of short-term calcium supplementation on bone mass in adolescent girls with low calcium intake. *Am J Clin Nutr*. 2005;81:168-174.

45. Welch JM, Turner CH, Devareddy L, Arjmandi BH, Weaver CM. High impact exercise is more beneficial than dietary calcium for building bone strength in the growing rat skeleton. *Bone*. 2008;42:660-668.

46. Specker B, Vukovich M. Evidence for an interaction between exercise and nutrition for improved bone health during growth. *Med Sport Sci*. 2007;51:50-63.

47. Lappe J, Cullen D, Haynatzki G, Recker R, Ahlf R, Thompson K. Calcium and vitamin D supplementation decreases incidence of stress fractures in female Navy recruits. *J Bone Miner Res*. 2008;23:741-749.

48. Iuliano-Burns S, Saxon L, Naughton G, Gibbons K, Bass S. Regional specificity of exercise and calcium during skeletal growth in girls: a randomized controlled trial. *J Bone Miner Res*. 2003;18:156-162.

49. Specker B, Binkley T. Randomized trial of physical activity and calcium supplementation on bone mineral content in 3- to 5-year-old children. *J Bone Miner Res*. 2003;18:885-892.

50. Lappe J, Stubby J, Davies K, Recker R. Exercise without sufficient calcium does not increase rate of bone mass accrual in pubertal females. *J Bone Miner Res*. 2001; 16:138.

51. Lappe J, Davies K, Recker R, Heaney R. Quantitative ultrasound: use in screening for susceptibility to stress fractures in female army recruits. *J Bone Miner Res*. 2005;20: 571-578.

Calcium Supplementation Plays a Positive Role in Bone and Body Composition in Chinese Adolescents

9

Guansheng Ma, Qian Zhang, Jing Yin, Ailing Liu, Weijing Du, Xiaoyan Wang, and Xiaoqi Hu

Abbreviations

CNNHS   China National Nutrition and Health Survey
RCT   Randomized controlled trial
BMC   Bone mineral content
BMD   Bone mineral density
CV   Coefficient of variation
BMI   Body mass index

9.1 Introduction

Adolescence is a period of rapid skeletal growth and nearly half of the adult skeletal mass is accrued during this period. Impaired achievement of bone mass in puberty is an important risk factor for the development of osteoporosis in later life.[1] Adolescence is therefore a window of opportunity for improving peak bone mass and reducing the risk of osteoporosis later in life.[2] Calcium intake may be an important modifiable factor influencing the attainment of peak bone mass within the genetic potential in an individual.[3] Skeletal development may be at risk if calcium intake falls short of the required levels.[4,5]

It is now well accepted that bone mineral mass is largely controlled by familial and genetic factors. However, environmental factors, such as diet and lifestyle, are also important contributors to the population variance in bone mineral mass.[6–8] Some studies indicated that differences in calcium intakes, dietary pattern, calcium absorption and retention, physique and bone physiological structure, and the incidence rate of bone fracture might exist under different genetic and environmental backgrounds.[9–12] Most of these studies were carried out in western countries. Till now, some studies of calcium supplements have been carried out in Chinese adolescents,[13–16] but they only compared the effects of calcium intakes at two levels, or effects within a short period which could not compare the long-term effect of calcium supplementation.

The 2002 China National Nutrition and Health Survey (CNNHS) found that the daily calcium intakes was 376 mg for boys aged 14–17 of years, and 343 mg for their female counterparts,[17] which was only about 30% of the current recommendation on adequate calcium intakes (1,000 mg/day). The aim of this study was to evaluate the effects of calcium supplementation at different levels on bone mineral accretion and body composition in Chinese adolescents with low habitual calcium intakes.

9.2 Materials and Methods

9.2.1 Supplementation

We performed a double-blind randomized controlled trial (RCT) of four doses of calcium supplementation

G. Ma (✉)
National Institute for Nutrition and Food
Safety, Chinese Center for Disease Control and Prevention,
7 Pan Jia Yuan Nan Li, Beijing 100021, China
e-mail: mags@chinacdc.net.cn

Conflict of Interest and Funding Disclosure

The authors declare that they have no conflict of interest or disclosures.
This research was supported by China National Natural Science Foundation (Project No. 30471453).

given for 24 months to 257 (135 boys and 122 girls) healthy adolescents aged 12–15 years. We recruited adolescents from two junior middle schools in Beijing. They were randomly assigned to one of the four doses stratified by sex; the doses of calcium carbonate per day provided elemental calcium of 63, 354, 660, or 966 mg/day. The calcium carbonates were given as three chewable tablets and were distributed by the teacher of each class every week in each term. To cover weekends and holidays, calcium carbonate tablets were given to participants beforehand by teachers. Trained investigators monitored compliance by calling participants and asking them to record the amounts they took in diary. Compliance, defined as the number of tablets consumed relative to the number allocated, was monitored with the diary and by counting the tablets remaining at the end of intervention. We also asked the participants to recall the actual intake of tablets in an interview at the end of intervention. Actual calcium intake from supplements was calculated based on these records. Subjects with adequate data were reclassified into three groups based on actual total calcium intakes, including those from diet and calcium tablets supplied in this study; cut-off points were 500 mg/day and 800 mg/day. The average calcium intakes were 386, 629, and 984 mg/day in three groups, respectively, and the dose of calcium supplements were 85, 230, and 500 mg/day.

Subjects were excluded if they had a family history of bone disease or arthropathy, taking medicines that could affect bone, cartilage or calcium metabolism, or if they refused to have their blood taken. The study was approved by the Ethical Committee of the National Institute for Nutrition and Food Safety, Chinese Center for Disease Control and Prevention. A written consent form was obtained from each participant and his/her parents or guardian. Data collection was conducted at baseline and after 24 months of supplementation.

9.2.2 Bone Mineral and Body Composition Measurement

A Norland XR-36 (DXA) scanner (Norland, Fort Atkinson, WI) was used both at baseline and 24 months to measure the BMC and BMD of the total body and lumbar spine and total body composition. Quality

control was performed every day during the study period according to the manufacturer's instructions. The coefficient of variation (CV) value for repeated measurements was 0.56–0.65%.

9.2.3 Assessment on Physical Activity Level and Dietary Intake

Information on physical activity for the previous 1 year was collected by validated questionnaire[18] by trained interviewers. Energy expenditure and duration of physical activity were calculated. Dietary intake was assessed with a consecutive 3-D food recall questionnaire (including 2 weekdays and 1 weekend). The Chinese Food Composition Tables were used to calculate nutrient intakes.[19]

9.2.4 Anthropometric Measurements and Pubertal Stage

Height and weight were measured in standing position while wearing light clothing and no shoes. Participants were weighed to the nearest 0.1 kg with an electronic digital scale (Thinner, Fairfield, WI). Height was measured by the same observer (QZ). The subjects were measured in bare feet to the nearest 0.1 cm by stadiometer (TG-III Type, No. 6; Machinery Plant, Beijing, China). Body mass index (BMI) was calculated (kg/m^2). Female breast or male genitalia development, pubic hair development was ascertained according to Tanner's definitions of five stages of puberty[20] during an interview.

9.2.5 Statistical Analysis

Descriptive statistics are reported as means±SDs unless otherwise indicated. ANOVA, Kruskal–Wallis test, and Chi square analysis were used to compare differences in baseline characteristics between supplemented groups. Intervention effects on differences indicators between the three groups were investigated by multiple linear regression or ANCOVA models after adjustment for baseline values and for potential confounders. All statistical analysis was done with SAS (SAS 8.2e for Windows, SAS Institute, Inc.).

9.3 Results

A total of 197 subjects completed 2 years of supplementation (101 boys, 96 girls), and the response rate was 77%. There were no significant differences between subjects who completed 2 years of supplements and those were lost to follow-up except in dietary calcium intake, included participants were higher than excluded.

Males in Group 3 had higher dietary intakes of energy (2,211 kcal/day) and calcium (532 mg/day) and performed less physical activity (6.5 h/w) compared with other groups ($p < 0.05$). Females in Group 2 and Group 3 had higher dietary intakes of energy and calcium compared with group 1. A higher percentage of females in group 3 had a tanner stage $\geq$IV. There were no other significant differences between the three groups (Table 9.1).

At baseline, there were no significant differences among the three groups on BMC and BMD of total body and lumbar spine. After 2 years of calcium supplements, total body BMC in males in Group 2 (2,464 g)

and Group 3 (2,437 g) were significantly higher than that in Group 1 (2,321 g), adjusted for baseline value ($p < 0.05$) (Table 9.2). This persisted after additional adjustment for age, pubertal development, BMI, physical activity, and energy intake. Also in males, increases in total body BMC after 2 years were higher in Group 2 and Group 3 than Group 1 ($p < 0.05$). There were no statistically significant differences in the BMD of total body or lumbar spine between the groups after 2 years. There were no significant effect differences among groups in case of females.

At baseline, total body composition was not different in 3 groups. After 2 years, in males, lean body mass and body weight were significantly higher in Group 2 (49.1 and 62.3 kg, respectively) and Group 3 (48.8 and 61.7 kg) than in Group 1 (46.7 and 58.9 kg), adjusted for baseline value ($p < 0.05$) (Table 9.2), and this difference persisted after additional adjustment for age, pubertal development, BMI, physical activity, and energy intake ($p < 0.05$). In males, changes in lean body mass was significantly higher in Group 2 and Group 3 than in Group 1($p < 0.05$), but there were no significant differences between groups in the changes of body fat and body fat percentage. In females, there were no significant differences in the changes of body composition among groups over 2 years.

Table 9.1 Comparison of characteristics among three groups

	Male			p	Female			p
	Group 1	Group 2	Group 3		Group 1	Group 2	Group 3	
n	38	40	23		35	39	22	
Age (years)	13.5±0.5	13.6±0.5	13.5±0.5	0.801	13.4±0.6	13.2±0.5	13.3±0.5	0.525
Height (cm)	156.9±9.3	158.0±8.1	161.6±9.8	0.133	155.5±8.7	155.7±6.2	156.7±5.0	0.800
Weight (kg)	48.5±14.9	48.7±11.1	48.2±10.7	0.988	46.8±9.9	48.5±10.7	49.9±12.3	0.565
Energy intake (kcal/day)	1,790±370	1,818±428	2,212±640	0.002*	1,369±292	1,541±350	1,639±354	0.009*
Calcium intakes from food (mg/day)	311±67	397±127	532±250	0.000*	290±84	401±131	430±159	0.000*
Calcium intakes from tablets (mg/day)	76±60	232±130	496±298	0.000*	95±74	229±119	508±231	0.000*
Total Calcium intakes (mg/day)	387±17	629±16	1,028±22	0.000*	385±18	630±17	938±22	0.000*
Time of physical activity (h/w)[a]	10.8(13.3)	12.4(11.5)	6.7(5.9)	0.008*	9.5(9.2)	10.2(7.2)	9.8(9.7)	0.935
Tanner stage ≥IV (%)[b]	50	63	61	0.499	49	51	82	0.029*

[a]Med (Q3-Q1), Kruskal–Wallis Test
[b]Chisq test

Table 9.2 Effect of calcium intervention on bone measures and body composition

		Male			Female		
		Group 1	Group 2	Group 3	Group 1	Group 2	Group 3
Total body BMC (g)	Baseline	1,821±436	1,872±357	1,893±374	1,864±348	1,902±292	1,885±265
	2 Years later	2,321±460	2,464±365*,**,***	2,437±442*,**,***	2,172±325	2,216±249	2,208±308
Total body BMD (g/cm²)	Baseline	0.75±0.10	0.76±0.09	0.75±0.09	0.78±0.09	0.80±0.08	0.79±0.08
	2 Years later	0.86±0.12	0.90±0.10	0.88±0.10	0.85±0.08	0.88±0.07	0.87±0.08
Lumbar spine BMC (g)	Baseline	28.97±8.74	29.43±6.74	30.79±7.81	32.57±8.93	32.79±6.57	32.07±6.38
	2 Years later	40.97±9.33	41.93±6.44	43.03±9.05	39.14±6.98	39.65±5.69	37.88±6.53
Lumbar spine BMD (g/cm²)	Baseline	0.73±0.13	0.74±0.12	0.718±0.11	0.84±0.16	0.84±0.13	0.81±0.13
	2 Years later	0.93±0.16	0.94±0.12	0.91±0.13	0.97±0.12	0.98±0.11	0.93±0.12
Lean body mass (kg)	Baseline	38.3±10.1	38.5±7	38.7±8.1	32.9±5.7	32.8±4.8	33.8±5.3
	2 Years later	46.7±8.6	49.1±5.8*,**,***	48.8±8*,**,***	35.1±5.8	35.1±5.4	35.9±6.9
Body fat (kg)	Baseline	9.9±6.3	9.9±5.8	9.4±4.5	13.6±4.9	15.3±6.8	15.8±7.5
	2 Years later	11.2±7.5	11.7±6.4	11.7±7.2	17.9±6.1	18.7±6.3	20±7.3

Comparison at baseline $p > 0.05$
Comparison 2 years later:
*Adjusted for the baseline value, $p < 0.05$
**Additional adjustment for age, pubertal development, and bmi, $p < 0.05$
***Additional adjustment for physical activity and energy intake, $p < 0.05$

Table 9.3 Multivariable stepwise regression on influencing factors of bone mineral accretion of the total body

Variables	β	p	R^2	R_c^2
Gender (females>males)	−0.607	0	0.389	0.429
Tanner stage (IV+V)>(I–III)	−0.181	0.001	0.026	
Time of physical activity	0.136	0.013	0.013	
Groups of calcium supplementation	0.115	0.036	0.012	

Independent variables were sex, groups of calcium supplementation, energy intakes, time of physical activity; dependent variable was change of total body BMC
Standard of enter model was 0.10, remove model was 0.15

After supplementation, body weight of Group 2 (62.3 kg) and Group 3 (61.7 kg) in males was significantly higher than Group 1 (58.9 kg) after adjustment ($p < 0.05$). There were no significant differences among groups in height before and after intervention.

Factors associated with the changes in total body BMC were sex, pubertal stage, physical activity, and calcium intakes in adolescents ($R_c^2 = 0.429$) (Table 9.3). Sex explained about 39% of variation in bone mineral accretion with males having greater increases than females. Pubertal stage was negatively associated, while physical activity and calcium intakes were positively associated with total body BMC change.

9.4 Discussion

A recent meta-analysis of RCTs of calcium supplementation found that there was a small effect of calcium supplementation in the upper limb,[7] but raised doubts as to whether calcium supplementation in children benefits BMD. However, in our study, total body BMC in male adolescents with low habitual calcium intakes benefited from calcium supplementation of 230 and 500 mg/day lasting for 2 years. Our study may have demonstrated an effect, because male subjects in this study were at the peak stage of bone mineral accretion since BMC velocity peak is at 13.3 years for boys.[21] In addition, at baseline, dietary calcium intake of our sample was very low at 382 mg/day and supplementation may have had an effect because of this. Our results also show that tanner stage was one of the most important potential factors affecting bone mass gain. During puberty, bone turnover is increased and sex steroids, the GH-IGF-I axis and $1,25(OH)_2D$ play major roles in bone mass change.[22] Dietary calcium intake in midpuberty was strongly associated with young adult bone mass.[23] Similar significant results were found in white adolescents at the age of 16–18 years who supplemented 600 mg calcium per day lasting for 13 months.[24]

Sex was another important determinant of bone mineral accretion and no significant effects of supplementation were found in females in this study. The BMC velocity peak in girls is at 11.4 years, earlier than in boys. Within 3 years, on either side of BMC velocity peak, boys had consistently higher BMC velocity compared with girls and the discrepancy increased steadily through puberty.[21] Subjects in this study were 13–15 years old during the supplementation of 2 years, which might explain as to why males benefited from calcium supplementation and females did not.

Dietary calcium intake is a potential factor influencing weight gain and may reduce body weight,[25] but the evidence for this in children is conflicting. A meta-analysis was performed recently in children; no statistically significant effects of calcium supplementation were found on weight or body fat.[6] However, most studies on the effects of calcium or milk supplementation on body composition have been in girls.[26–28] Our finding that calcium supplementation had no effect on body composition in female is consistent with this, but our data also suggest that male adolescents may have benefits in terms of lean body mass and body weight from calcium supplementation. Similar significant results on lean body mass were found in white adolescents at the age of 16–18 years.[24] A plausible mechanism for the effect of calcium supplements on increase in male's lean mass might be through increases in mechanical loading and muscle forces.[29]

In conclusion, calcium supplementation of more than 230 mg/day for 2 years can enhance total body bone mineral accretion and increase lean body mass in Chinese male adolescents with low habitual calcium intakes, but not in females. Sex, tanner stage, physical activity, and calcium intakes are important determinants of bone mineral accretion.

Acknowledgments   The authors wish to thank all subjects for their participation in this study. A special thanks to Dr Tania Winzenberg for assistance on English reviewing.

References

1. Suuriniemi M, Mahonen A, Kovanen V, et al. Association between exercise and pubertal BMD is modulated by estrogen receptor alpha genotype. *J Bone Miner Res.* 2004;19: 1758-1765.
2. Weaver CM. The growing years and prevention of osteoporosis in later life. *Proc Nutr Soc.* 2000;59:303-306.
3. Matkovic V. Diet, genetics and peak bone mass of adolescent girls. *Nutr Today.* 1991;26:21-24.
4. Report of a joint FAO/WHO expert consultation. *Human Vitamin and Mineral Requirements*;2002:59-93.
5. Prentice A, Bates CJ. An appraisal of the adequacy of dietary mineral intakes in developing countries for bone growth and development in children. *Nutr Res Rev.* 1993;6:51-69.
6. Winzenberg T, Shaw K, Fryer J, et al. Calcium supplements in healthy children do not affect weight gain, height, or body composition. *Obesity.* 2007;15:1789-1798.
7. Winzenberg TM, Shaw K, Fryer J, et al. Calcium supplementation for improving bone mineral density in children. *Cochrane Database Syst Rev.* 2006;19:CD005119.
8. Prentice A. The relative contribution of diet and genotype to bone development. *Proc Nutr Soc.* 2001;60:45-52.
9. Anderson JB. The important role of physical activity in skeletal development:how exercise may counter low calcium intake. *Am J Clin Nutr.* 2000;71:1384-1385.
10. Bryant RJ, Wastney ME, Martin BR, et al. Racial differences in bone turnover and calcium metabolism in adolescent females. *J Clin Endocrinol Metab.* 2003;88:1043-1047.
11. Horlick M, Thornton J, Wang J, et al. Bone mineral in prepubertal children:gender and ethnicity. *J Bone Miner Res.* 2000;15:1393-1397.
12. Wu L, Martin B, Braun M, et al. Calcium retention as a function of calcium intake in Asian adolescents. *J Faseb.* 2007;21:548.
13. Cheng J, Leung S, Lee W. Determinants of axial and peripheral bone mass in Chinese adolescents. *Arch Dis Child.* 1998;78:524-530.
14. Du X, Zhu K, Trube A, et al. School-milk intervention trial enhances growth and bone mineral accretion in Chinese girls aged 10-12 years in Beijing. *Br J Nutr.* 2004;92:159-168.
15. Ho SC, Guldan GS, Woo J, et al. A prospective study of the effects of 1-year calcium-fortified soy milk supplementation on dietary calcium intake and bone health in Chinese adolescent girls aged 14 to 16. *Osteoporos Int.* 2005;16:1907-1916.
16. Li J, Li H, Wang S. Effects of calcium supplementation on bone mineral accretion in adolescents. *Wei Sheng Yan Jiu.* 2002;31:363-366.
17. Zhai FY, Yang XG, Ge KY. *Report of Chinese National Survey of Nutrition and Health in 2002, Dietary Intake.* Beijing: People's health Press; 2006.

18. Liu AL, Ma GS, Zhang Q, et al. Reliability and validity of a 72day physical activity questionnaire for elementary students. *Chin J Epidemiol*. 2003;24:901-904.

19. Yang Y, Wang G, Pan X. *Chinese Food Composition Table*. Bejing: Medical Press of Beijing University; 2002.

20. Tanner JM (1962) *Growth at Adolescence*. 2nd ed. London: Oxford, Blackwell.

21. Martin AD, Bailey DA, McKay HA, et al. Bone mineral and calcium accretion during puberty. *Am J Clin Nutr*. 1997;66: 611-615.

22. Saggese G, Baroncelli GI, Bertelloni S. Puberty and bone development. *Best Pract Res Clin Endocrinol Metab*. 2002; 16:53-64.

23. Wang MC, Crawford PB, Hudes M, et al. Diet in midpuberty and sedentary activity in prepuberty predict peak bone mass. *Am J Clin Nutr*. 2003;77:495-503.

24. Prentice A, Ginty F, Stear SJ, et al. Calcium supplementation increases stature and bone mineral mass of 16- to 18-year-old boys. *J Clin Endocrinol Metab*. 2005;90: 3153-3161.

25. Zemel MB. Role of calcium and dairy products in energy partitioning and weight management. *Am J Clin Nutr*. 2004; 79:907S-912S.

26. Cheng S, Lyytikäinen A, Kröger H, et al. Effects of calcium, dairy product, and vitamin D supplementation on bone mass accrual and body composition in 10-12-y-old girls:a 2-y randomized trial. *Am J Clin Nutr*. 2005;82:1115-1126.

27. Lorenzen JK, Mølgaard C, Michaelsen KF, et al. Calcium supplementation for 1 y does not reduce body weight or fat mass in young girls. *Am J Clin Nutr*. 2006;83:18-23.

28. Merrilees MJ, Smart EJ, Gilchrist NL, et al. Effects of diary food supplements on bone mineral density in teenage girls. *Eur J Nutr*. 2000;39:256-262.

29. Ruff C. Growth in bone strength, body size, and muscle size in a juvenile longitudinal sample. *Bone*. 2003;33: 317-332.

Effects of High Calcium and Vitamin D Diets on Changes in Body Fat, Lean Mass, and Bone Mineral Density by Self-Controlled Dieting for 4 Months in Young Asian Women

10

Takako Hirota, Izumi Kawasaki, and Kenji Hirota

10.1 Introduction

An inadequate calcium intake among Japanese youth has been commonly observed and it has been associated with lower bone mineral density (BMD).[1,2] Moreover, the increasing prevalence of unhealthy dieting practices is seen among young women in most industrialized countries. In fact, more frequent dieting has been associated with lower BMD in Japanese young women.[1] The increasing prevalence of unhealthful dieting practices may also adversely affect dairy food consumption.

Research indicates that young women may reduce dairy food consumption due to fears about weight gain and erroneous beliefs that milk and other dairy foods are fattening.[3] However, recent research suggests an inverse relation of dairy food and calcium consumption with weight or fatness. This new evidence and review of studies conducted in Caucasians and African–Americans support the view that calcium plays a role in adipocyte lipid kinetics and in moderating fatness.[4–7] Longitudinal analyses in adults have shown that increased levels of calcium or dairy foods are negatively associated with changes in body weight.[4–7] More recently, no relation was observed between the intake of calcium or dairy products and the accumulation of BMI by several intervention studies.[8,9] Both the mechanism and magnitude of the calcium-body weight effect remain uncertain as well. Other components in dairy products may also play a role in body weight regulation. Most studies that report longitudinal change in body composition measures are limited to Caucasians and Africans, but not Asians, whose body weight and fat mass are smaller, and whose habitual calcium and dairy intakes are much lower than those reported for Caucasians and Africans in the United States and Europe.[5–7] Also, few data about lean mass change were available in relation to such weight loss. Therefore, further study in Asian subjects on dieting may provide a new viewpoint and evidence of calcium function for the regulation of not only body fat but also lean mass.

Unnecessary dieting appears to be increasing in popularity among young women in many industrialized countries, and weight loss may be accompanied by loss of bone and lean mass.[1,10]

In this study, we examined the relation of increased intake of milk to lean body mass, fat mass, and BMD during a 4-month, moderate, self-controlled dieting regimen in Asian young women of normal weight. In addition, the effect of vitamin D on changes in fat and muscle mass was investigated. We tried to find the healthiest and most comfortable dieting method that would decrease body fat and increase lean mass without decreasing BMD.

10.2 Materials and Methods

10.2.1 Subjects

One hundred and forty-eight new college students had voluntarily attended this program. Two students who were obese (BMI > 30) and two students who were very short (body height < −2 SD) were excluded from

T. Hirota (✉)
Department of Health and Nutrition, Kyoto Koka Women's University, 38 Kadono-cyo, Nishikyougoku, Kyoto, Japan
e-mail: tsujiken@tec-tsuji.com

P. Burckhardt et al. (eds.), *Nutritional Influences on Bone Health*,
DOI: 10.1007/978-1-84882-978-7_10, © Springer-Verlag London Limited 2010

this study. The students were randomly assigned to drink a glass of milk (≥200 mL) daily ($n=77$; milk group) or drink freely (whatever they wanted, $n=71$; control group). Of the 77 subjects in the milk group, 18 students preferred to switch to the control group due to their distaste for milk. Of the 71 subjects in the control group, 11 students preferred to switch to the milk group. Thirty seven subjects (12 in milk and 25 in control) could not keep a diary of body weight, diet, and physical activity which was essential for this program. Eleven subjects (6 in milk and 5 in control) could not get blood test at the end of this program. Finally 100 subjects (52 in milk and 48 in control) could complete this dieting program of 4-months (Table 10.1).

10.2.2 Study Design

Subjects were instructed either to drink more than 200 mL milk before dinner (milk group) or to drink freely with no obligations (control). Subjects were advised by a registered dietician on ways to decrease energy intake and increase physical activities in order to lose body fat. All the subjects were asked to keep a diary of daily body weight, dairy intake, physical activity, and any other changes related to body weight thought to be important for successful dieting program.

10.2.3 Bone Density and Body Composition Measurement

Body fat, lean mass, bone mineral content (BMC), and bone mineral density (BMD at the lumbar spine (L2–L4), femoral neck, Ward's triangle, trochanter) were measured by DXA (DPX; GE Lunar, Madison, Wisconsin, USA) at baseline and after 4-months of dieting. Measurements were completed between 1 and 3 weeks after conclusion of dieting.

10.2.4 Assessment of Dietary Intake and Other Lifestyle Factors

Three-day dietary records at the start and the end of the study for all subjects were reviewed and analyzed by a trained dietitian using software (DELTIS; Olympus

Table 10.1 Baseline characteristics of the subjects who completed the study[a]

	($n=100$)
Age (year)	23±5 (18–37)[b]
Height (cm)	159±6 (148–174)
Body weight (by scale) (kg)	54.1±6.4(38.4–75.3)
BMI (kg/m²)	21.5±2.3(16.0–28.6)
Circumference (cm)	
Waist	67.1±5.3 (56.5–86.0)
Hip	93.6±5.1 (80.4–108.5)
DXA measure	
Body weight (kg)	54.20±6.39 (37.63–76.04)
Body fat mass (kg)	17.46±5.22 (4.25–34.56)
Lean mass (kg)	34.34±3.16 (27.10–41.24)
BMC (kg)	2.39±0.26 (1.81–3.22)
BMD (g/cm²)	
Lumber spine (L$_2$–L$_4$)	1.189±0.121 (0.903–1.443)
Femoral	
Neck	0.961±0.116 (0.677–1.273)
Ward's triangle	0.942±0.144 (0.585–1.311)
Trochanter	0.830±0.119 (0.548–1.158)
Intake of	
Energy (kJ/day)	7,755±1,679 (3,660–12,132)
Carbohydrate (g/day)	238.0±51.6 (59.5–426.5)
Protein (g/day)	65.2±16.8 (26.8–113.2)
Fat (g/day)	67.9±21.1 (24.7–128.0)
Cholesterol (mg/day)	376±146 (95–884)
Calcium (mg/day)	474±196 (101–968)
Vitamin D (µg/day)	5.8±4.3 (0.4–21.7)
Milk (mL/day)	116±115 (0–600)
Duration of	
Sunbathing (min/day)	42±24 (0–120)
Walking (min/day)	40±22 (0–90)
Physical activity (min/month)	155±345 (0–1920)

BMI body mass index; *DXA* dual-energy X-ray absorptiometry; *BMC* bone mineral content; *BMD* bone mineral densities
[a]x±SD (all such values)
[b]Numbers in parentheses represented range (all such values)

Optical Co. Ltd., Tokyo). Fourteen subjects (8 in control and 6 in milk group) did not report the records at 4-months. Lifestyle questionnaires assessed previous and current sports activities and medical history at baseline and 4-months for all subjects.

10.2.5 Statistical Analyses

Descriptive and univariate statistics were assessed for all variables. All statistical analyses were carried out using the Statistical Package for Social Sciences (SPSS 12.0, SPSS, Chicago, IL, USA). Student's t-test was used to identify significant differences between milk and control groups at baseline and at 4-months. The statistical significance of the differences among multiple groups was studied with analysis of variance (ANOVA). If the ANOVA was significant, we performed the Tukey test for comparisons within all groups. Equality of two correlation coefficients was evaluated by Excel. p values of <0.05 were considered statistically significant.

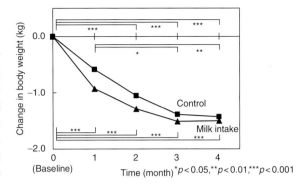

Fig. 10.1 Mean ($\pm$SD) change in body weight by assignment to control and milk groups through 4 months. Time course changes are presented as body weight loss measured by electronic scale. There were significant differences in the mean changes of body weight at 1 month ($p<0.01$) and 2 months ($p<0.05$, Student's t-test) between control and milk groups. Significantly different decreases in body weight from baseline were observed at 3 and 4 months in control and 1, 2, 3, and 4 months in the milk group ($p<0.05$, one-way ANOVA and Tukey's test)

10.3 Results

10.3.1 Baseline Characteristics of the Subjects Between Control and Milk Groups

There were no significant differences in baseline characteristics of anthropometric measurements, physical activities, and duration of sunbathing between the control and the milk groups. Baseline intake of milk (59 ± 75 and 169 ± 120 mL/day, respectively), protein, and calcium and BMD of the lumbar spine and femur were significantly lower in the control group. It is because some subjects in each group, after being randomly assigned, who disliked (in milk group) or liked milk (in control group) transferred from one to another as described in material and methods.

10.3.2 Nutritional Intake, Physical Activity, and Body Weight During Dieting

Daily intakes of milk and calcium were significantly greater in milk (198 ± 85 mL/day) than control group (71 ± 70 mL/day) throughout the intervention. Actual mean intake of milk in the milk group was not more than 200 mL/day. Only 22 subjects drank more milk

than 200 mL/day in the milk group. Total calcium intakes during dieting were significantly different between the groups (557 ± 248 mg/day vs. 382 ± 143 mg/day). The mean intake of energy, carbohydrate, and fat were significantly decreased in the both control and milk groups; however, intakes of vitamin D and duration of physical activities and sunbathing were not significantly different from baseline in both the groups.

The curves of monthly changes in body weights measured by scale were similar in both the control and milk groups (Fig. 10.1).

10.3.3 Changes in Body Fat Mass, Lean Mass, and BMD After 4 Months of Dieting

Mean body weight, waist and hip circumferences, and lumbar spine BMD after 4-months of dieting were significantly decreased from baseline in both milk and control groups.

Body fat mass was significantly decreased only in the milk group (-1.2 ± 2.6 kg) but not in the control group (-0.4 ± 3.0 kg), and change in body lean mass was $+0.3\pm2.0$ kg in milk group and -0.5 ± 2.6 kg in the control group (Fig. 10.2).

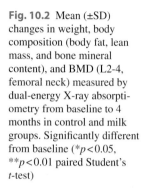

Fig. 10.2 Mean (±SD) changes in weight, body composition (body fat, lean mass, and bone mineral content), and BMD (L2-4, femoral neck) measured by dual-energy X-ray absorptiometry from baseline to 4 months in control and milk groups. Significantly different from baseline (*$p<0.05$, **$p<0.01$ paired Student's t-test)

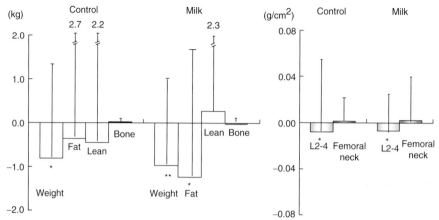

**$p < 0.001$, *$p < 0.01$ (Student t-test); Significantly different from baseline

The changes in lean mass in the milk group were correlated with changes in L2-L4 BMD ($p=0.05$), and the subjects in the highest quartile of lean mass gain did not indicate any decrease in L2-L4 BMD.

10.3.4 Effect of the Amount of Milk Intake on Body Fat Loss and Lean Mass Gain

Significantly higher body fat loss (-2.0 ± 2.8 kg) and higher lean mass gain (0.8 ± 2.0 kg) were observed only in those who drank more milk than 200 mL/day ($n=22$) than the control group.

10.3.5 Effect of Vitamin D Intake on the Changes in Body Fat and Lean Mass

When the subjects were subgrouped by the median intake (4.7 µg/day) of vitamin D, a significantly larger decrease in body fat (-1.7 ± 2.8 kg) and larger increase in lean mass (0.58 ± 2.2kg) were observed in milk subjects with higher vitamin D intake than the controls (Fig. 10.3). However, changes in body composition were not associated with the levels of vitamin D in the control group (Fig. 10.3).

10.3.6 Effect of Higher Intake of Milk and Vitamin D

When the subjects were subgrouped by the median (4.7 µg/day) intake of vitamin D along with milk (200 mL/day), the highest decrease in body fat (-2.5 ± 3.0 kg) and the highest increase in lean mass ($+0.9\pm2.2$ kg) were observed in the subjects with higher intake of milk (>200 mL/day) along with higher vitamin D intake (≥4.7 µg/day).

10.3.7 Association Between Lean Body Mass Gain and Fat Loss

The changes in lean body mass gain were strongly associated with changes in body fat loss in both milk ($r=-0.79$) and control ($r=-0.76$) groups, while such association was significantly stronger in the subjects who had higher intake of vitamin D (≥4.7 µg/day; $y=-0.726\times-0.628, r=-0.85$) than in those with a lower intake (<4.7 µg/day; $y=-0.520\times-0.555, r=-0.68$).

10.4 Discussion

Our study had two major findings. First, daily milk intake did not increase body fat mass, but decreased body fat and increased lean mass during moderate

Fig. 10.3 Mean (±SD) changes in weight and body composition (body fat and lean mass) measured by dual-energy X-ray absorptiometry from baseline to 4 months in control and milk subjects subgrouped by the median intake (4.7 µg/day) of vitamin D. Significantly different from baseline (**$p<0.05$, ***$p<0.01$; paired Student's t-test). Significantly different between groups (*$p<0.05$; Student's t-test)

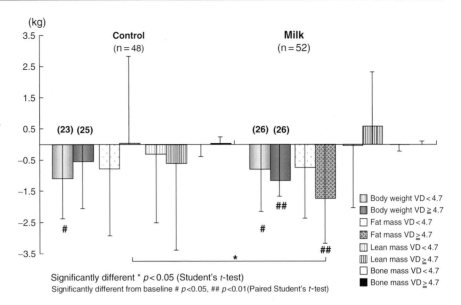

Significantly different * $p<0.05$ (Student's t-test)
Significantly different from baseline # $p<0.05$, ## $p<0.01$ (Paired Student's t-test)

weight loss (Fig. 10.2). Second, higher intake of vitamin D could enhance such milk effects on fat loss and lean mass gain (Fig. 10.3). The higher vitamin D intake likely helps to effect a change from fat to lean mass. Another finding was that the significant milk effects on body fat loss and lean gain were found in the subjects who ingested more than 200 mL of milk daily.

Although much of the clinical data supports a negative relation between calcium or dairy intake and body weight or fat mass,[4-7] some researchers have found little evidence for an effect of dairy or calcium supplementation in reducing body weight or fat mass.[8,9] Most of these data did not demonstrate the change in lean body mass with calcium intake during weight reduction. Our study succeeded in demonstrating for the first time that a daily intake of a glass of milk (>200 mL) along with a higher intake of vitamin D was associated with, not only a decrease in body fat mass, but also an increase in lean mass during dieting. The stronger associations between lean mass gain and fat mass loss in the subjects with higher intake of vitamin D were clearly found in our study.

The baseline calcium intake in our subjects was quite low, 474 ± 196 mg/day including calcium from milk (about 116 mL/day) (Table 10.1), which are quite similar to the mean value of Japanese women in the national nutrition survey,[11] while the reported basal calcium intake in the US populations was as much as 700–1,000 mg/day.[5,6] What's more, dairy foods, whose

absorption rate of calcium is presumably the highest among foods, provided only 24% of total calcium intake in the diets of Japanese. Sixty-three percent of calcium intake was from vegetables,[11] the calcium absorption rate of which is quite low. Thus increased intake of just a glass of milk (>200 mL), a highly bioavailable calcium source, resulted in about 47% increase in calcium intake in young Asian subjects in this study, which might lead to significant changes of body composition. Therefore, a similar amount of milk may not necessarily have a similar effect in Western subjects.

We also found that higher intake of vitamin D along with higher milk intake was associated with a greater decrease in body fat mass and increase in lean mass during weight reduction (Fig. 10.3). This finding may prove the additive effects of vitamin D to calcium on the body fat mass and lean mass. As we have indicated that the association between body lean mass gain and fat mass loss was stronger in the subjects with higher intake of vitamin D, Vitamin D may play important roles in muscle metabolism in addition to calcium absorption.

Zemel et al previously proposed that consumption of dairy products had greater effect on fat loss than calcium supplements, owing to other nutrients in milk, such as branched chain amino acids.[6] These researchers did not discuss the effect of natural vitamin D or dairy fortified vitamin D, but did suggest a calcium effect on lipolysis operating through serum 1,25-dihydroxy vitamin D [1,25(OH)$_2$D] in adipocytes.[12] Similarly, most investigators did not demonstrate an effect of native vitamin D intake on body fat reduction or lean mass gain followed by dairy or calcium intake.[4-9] It is noteworthy that dairy products are not fortified with vitamin D in our country in contrast to usual vitamin D fortification in the United States. This lack of vitamin D fortification in milk in this study offers some clarification of the independent effect of vitamin D intake from dairy products on body composition. Interestingly, obese adults have been found to have low serum 25-hydroxy vitamin D [25(OH)D], a reflection of endogenous vitamin D nutrition, and a negative correlation of serum 25(OH)D with body fat mass.[13,14]

In addition to the optimal intake of vitamin D for maximal calcium absorption, recent data have shown that higher intake of vitamin D is associated with increased muscle strength, potentially leading to reduced falls and decreased incidence of bone fracture.[15,16] These data related to poor nutrition among the elderly agree with our data on gain of lean mass among our milk subjects who have a higher intake of vitamin D during dieting.

We believe that this is the first longitudinal study that helps clarify the relation of the intake of calcium and vitamin D on gain of lean body mass and fat loss. A limitation of our study is that we did not measure serum 25(OH)D levels, which would have provided an accurate indication of vitamin D levels. Another limitation of our study is that basal calcium intakes between the control and milk groups were significantly different owing to the eight subjects who finally completed in each group but switched from one group to another in order to obtain informed consent. Still, all of the milk subjects did not drink milk above 200 mL/day. It shows that unfortunately, dairy food is not so popular among young Asian females.

Anthropometric measurements and bone mineral densities are lower and mean calcium intake is much lower in Asians[1,2,11] compared with Caucasians.[4-6] Despite the fact that obese people (BMI >30 kg/m^2) make up only 3–4% of Japanese adults,[11] dieting is quite popular among Japanese people, especially among young women. A recent study showed that 54% of women and 37% of men in Japan have tried to lose body weight.[11] In order to maintain a proper amount of lean mass and BMD, reasonably moderate and healthful dieting should be suggested to these young people.

Our data on Asian young adults indicate that dairy foods together with adequate intake of vitamin D will help not only to decrease body fat mass, but also to increase lean body mass, a finding that has not been investigated previously in slender young Asian women. On the basis of this study, we suggest that enhanced intake of dairy products or calcium and vitamin D may be warranted in Japanese subjects. Furthermore, increased calcium and vitamin D intake may also contribute to a reduction in bone fracture rate and prevention of obesity and disorders associated with the metabolic syndrome[17] in both young and older adults. Further investigation is needed to determine an optimal intake of calcium and vitamin D for each subject and to clarify the mechanisms related to their effect on fat and lean mass.

Acknowledgements This study was supported by Japan Dairy Association.

The authors thank our clue members of Research Laboratory, Tsuji Academy, T. Aoe and H. Ikeda for expert technical assistance. We thank T. Katanosaka for DXA measurements, and all student participants in Tsuji Academy for their continuous effort on dieting program. We also thank Howard S. Barden at GE Lunar for helpful editorial suggestions.

References

1. Hirota T et al. Effect of diet and lifestyle on bone mass in Asian young women. *Am J Clin Nutr*. 1992;55:1168-1173.
2. Hirota T et al. Improvement of nutrition stimulates bone mineral gain in Japanese school children and adolescents. *Osteoporosis Int*. 2005;16:1057-1064.
3. Gulliver P, Horwath CC. Assessing women's perceived benefits, barriers, and stage of change for meeting milk product consumption recommendations. *J Am Diet Assoc*. 2001;101:1354-1357.
4. Davies KM et al. Calcium intake and body weight. *J Clin Endocrinol Metab*. 2000;85:4635-4638.
5. Lin YC et al. Dairy calcium is related to changes in body composition during a two-year exercise intervention in young women. *J Am Coll Nutr*. 2000;19:754-760.
6. Zemel MB et al. Calcium and dairy acceleration of weight and fat loss during energy restriction in obese adults. *Obes Res*. 2004;12:582-590.
7. Zemel MB et al. Effects of calcium and dairy on body composition and weight loss in African-American adults. *Obes Res*. 2005;13:1218-1225.
8. Shapses SA et al. Effect of calcium supplementation on weight and fat loss in women. *J Clin Endocrinol Metab*. 2004; 89:632-637.
9. Trowman R et al. A systematic review of the effects of calcium supplementation on body weight. *Br J Nutr*. 2006;95: 1033-1038.
10. Riedt CS et al. Overweight postmenopausal women lose bone with moderate weight reduction and 1 g/day calcium intake. *J Bone Miner Res*. 2005;20:455-463.
11. Ministry of Health, Labor and Welfare, The national nutrition survey in Japan, 2005. Tokyo: Daiichi Press; 2008.

12. Shi H et al. 1α, 25-Dihydroxyvitamin D3 modulates human adipocyte metabolism via nongenomic action. *FASEB J*. 2001; 15:2751-2753.

13. Arunabh S et al. Body fat content and 25-hydroxyvitamin D levels in healthy women. *J Clin Endocrinol Metab*. 2003;88: 157-161.

14. Parikh SJ et al. The relationship between obesity and serum 1, 25-dihydroxy vitamin D concentrations in healthy adults. *J Clin Endocrinol Metab*. 2004;89:1196-1199.

15. Glerup H et al. Hypovitaminosis D myopathy without biochemical signs of osteomalacic bone involvement. *Calcif Tissue Int*. 2000;66:419-424.

16. Pfeifer M et al. Vitamin D and muscle function. *Osteoporosis Int*. 2002;13:187-194.

17. Bischoff-Ferrari HA et al. Estimation of optimal serum concentrations of 25-hydroxyvitamin D for multiple health outcomes. *Am J Clin Nutr*. 2006;84:18-28.

Trace Elements and Bone

Franz Jakob, Lothar Seefried, Christa Kitz, August Stich,
Barbara Sponholz, Peter Raab, and Regina Ebert

11.1 Introduction

The basic elements, carbon (C), oxygen (O), hydrogen (H), and nitrogen (N) and the abundant elements, calcium (Ca) and phosphate (P), represent 98% of the dry mass of an organism, while 0.5% of the dry mass consists of about 40 trace elements. The present definition of trace elements determines that their concentrations in the organism are below 50 mg/kg. We know from fifteen of these that they are essential trace elements, e.g., arsenic (Ar), copper (Cu), chromium (Cr), cobalt (Co), iron (Fe), fluoride (F), iodine (I), manganese (Mn), molybdenum (Mo), nickel (Ni), selenium (Se), silicon (Si), tin (Sn), vanadium (V), and zinc (Zn), while we do not have sufficient knowledge on elements such as cadmium (Cd), lithium (Li), bromine (Br), and others. Historically, the importance of trace elements was first shown in the nineteenth century for zinc in microorganisms (*Aspergillus niger*, Raulin 1869), and later on, for the relevance of iron in hematopoiesis and anemia, which was described by Osler, Stockman, and Cloetta (for citations see[1]).

Trace elements are often a part of the active centers of enzymes, e.g., copper, zinc, and manganese in superoxide dismutases and selenium in various selenium-dependent enzymes like thioredoxin reductases and glutathione peroxidases.[2] Not only are such trace element-dependent proteins active in the balancing the reactive oxygen species but also in reducing critical cysteins that are involved in protein folding and DNA binding of transcription factors (e.g., estrogen and vitamin D receptors and nuclear factor kappa B NFκB). In consequence, trace elements influence a series of essential processes of life, in health and disease, such as signaling cascades, protection of proteins and DNA from oxidative damage and its consequences such as DNA instability, degenerative diseases and cancer, aging and inflammation processes, reproduction, pregnancy, and lactation, to mention just a few.[2,3]

Micronutrient deficiencies including trace element deficiencies contribute significantly to worldwide disease and mortality burden as recently reviewed for vitamin A, iodine, iron, and zinc by Boy et al.[3] Deficiencies of these compounds cause problems such as growth stunting, blindness, susceptibility to infections such as prevalence of diarrhea and pneumonia, and childhood mortality and this causes worldwide awareness. In contrast, the impact of nutritional trace element deficiencies on the worldwide risk and burden of musculoskeletal diseases is largely unknown. In the European Union, the nutritional situation in, for example, elderly people is presently regarded as sufficient according to present standards, but little is known about other parts of the world and especially about children and adolescents. However taking only zinc as an example, the impact of this trace element on cell biology, growth, infection, aging, senescence and degenerative diseases like Alzheimers disease is impressive. Particularly in case of degenerative diseases, zinc serum levels might not necessarily correlate with intracellular changes because of variable function and expression of zinc transporter molecules.[4,5] Thus it may be anticipated that more research is needed as to the role of trace elements in disease and also in bone biology, especially with respect to their interaction with calcium and phosphate metabolism and the regulators of the parathyroid hormone/vitamin D/calcium endocrine system. We will, in this minireview, focus on the putative roles of

F. Jakob (✉)
Orthopedic Department, Orthopedic Center for Musculoskeletal
Research, University of Wuerzburg, Wuerzburg, Germany
e-mail: f-jakob.klh@uni-wuerzburg.de

P. Burckhardt et al. (eds.), *Nutritional Influences on Bone Health*,
DOI: 10.1007/978-1-84882-978-7_11, © Springer-Verlag London Limited 2010

zinc and selenium and on their putative nutritive and geological interactions with calcium under extreme conditions in some regions of the world (e.g., Nigeria, Gambia, Bangladesh), where calcium deficient rickets are an outstanding problem with a high individual and population-relevant burden of disease.

11.2 Trace Elements and Bone

Bone is a complex tissue, which is formed and resorbed by tightly coupled actions of mesenchymal stem cell-derived osteoblasts/osteocytes and monocyte-derived osteoclasts. The process is influenced by many hormone and growth factor-driven signaling cascades, mechanical loading, and by the nutritional supply of minerals and trace elements.[6] Rickets/osteomalacia and osteoporosis are the most important diseases because of vitamin D and calcium deficiency and bone loss/altered bone quality as a result of multifaceted influences of genetics, aging, lifestyle, and environment.

11.2.1 Zinc in Cell Biology and Bone

Zinc is important for several essential processes in cell biology. Relevant examples are zinc finger-dependent transcription factors of the families of steroid hormone receptors and a superfamily of zinc finger proteins, many of which have not yet been functionally analyzed.[7,8] Zinc atoms in these proteins are surrounded by several cysteins, which form finger-like structures to bind to receptor and conformation-specific DNA response elements resulting in transcription modulation (Fig. 11.1). Besides the fact that the receptors for estrogens, androgens, glucocorticoids, and vitamin D are important players in osteoblast biology and bone formation/remodeling,[6] recent data on other zinc finger proteins demonstrate that some of the yet unknown functions of zinc finger transcription factors may also be involved in bone metabolism. The zinc finger protein Schnurri was reported to be relevant for bone remodeling since KO mice were osteopenic due to both osteoblastic and osteoclastic defects.[9] The zinc finger and BTB domain containing 40 gene ZBTB40 was one of the loci associated with osteoporosis in a large cohort study published in 2008.[10]

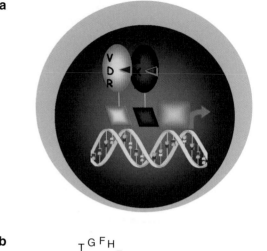

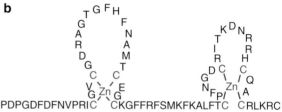

Fig. 11.1 Schematic diagram of the vitamin D receptor/RXR receptor heterodimer binding to DNA (**a**) and of the Zinc finger structure of the vitamin D receptor DNA binding domain (**b**) (according to Ebert et al[23])

A second important field where the trace element zinc is involved is the extracellular matrix metabolism as exerted by proteases, which are also very important in bone biology and metabolism.[11] Zinc-dependent metalloproteases are even developed as small molecule targets for the treatment of MMP-related diseases such as arthritis and cancer. Metalloproteases possess zinc-binding domains that are involved in the efficiency of proteolysis.[12] A HEXXHXXGXXH/D zinc-binding consensus sequence shows three histidines as zinc ligands and glutamic acid as the catalytic base, which is of relevance in the functions of ADAMS proteases and MMPs, as has been shown by structural studies using bacterial serralysins. The zinc metalloprotease Ste24 (Zmpste24) processes Lamin A/C, a key gene involved in premature aging, which was also recently shown to be involved in osteogenic differentiation processes.[13,14]

Zinc and its intracellular homeostasis are being extensively discussed as a putative pathomechanism of degeneration especially in neurodegenerative diseases. Moreover, accumulation of cells with critical telomere shortening has been found to be associated with the alteration of intracellular zinc homeostasis.[15] Since aging is one of the most prominent risk factors of osteoporosis, the role of zinc in osteoporosis pathogenesis as a supporter of segmental aging is likely to be meaningful.

There are some hints to suggest that these data translate into clinical issues. Zinc levels in the serum are one of several reliable means of assessing the zinc status in an individual. Both in animal models and in humans, low zinc intake and zinc deficiency have been reported to be associated with osteopenia and osteoporosis and the incidence of fractures.[16,17] Low levels of zinc (and magnesium) in the serum were associated with osteopenia and fracture risk.[18,19] Mutation close to the zinc-binding domain of the MMP2 gene disrupted MMP2 activity in patients with the multicentric osteolysis and arthritis syndrome, which besides the osteolyses also displayed marked osteoporosis.

Thus robust data are in favor of zinc deficiency being a risk factor for skeletal impairment in development and in adult life, although this has been challenged by recent data in rats consuming a marginally zinc deficient diet.[20] It may, however, be even more stimulating to initiate research on such nutritional issues of worldwide relevance with respect to musculoskeletal diseases.

11.2.2 Selenium in Cell Biology and Bone

Selenium is a trace element, which is being incorporated into the 21st amino acid selenocysteine by a multistep procedure involving a panel of specific proteins and a 3′ hairpin structure in the respective mRNA species, the SECIS element. In the presence of the latter, the opal stop codon TGA encodes for selenocystein, which is incorporated into the growing polypeptide chain. Translation of selenoproteins is dependent on the presence of selenium, and deficiency creates truncated proteins because of translational stop at the opal stop codon. Selenoproteins are involved in many essential processes of life; in several cases, knockout of the protein leads to intrauterine death. Selenoproteins are involved in hormone synthesis (thyroid hormones, deiodinases), reactive oxygen species balance (glutathione peroxidases), sperm production, and fertility,[2,21] but not all selenoproteins have yet been functionally characterized. The human and the prokaryotic selenoproteomes have been identified, but not yet fully characterized.[22]

Selenoproteins are expressed in cells of mesodermal/mesenchymal origin including mesenchymal stem cells and their offspring, which form bone, cartilage, tendons, and other mesenchymal tissues as well as in monocyte/macrophage-derived osteoclasts.[2,23,24] Selenium is known to modulate a specific form of osteoarthritis, the Kashin Beck disease.[25] Selenium-deficient rats display osteopenia and calciuria.[26] Despite many clinical and epidemiological studies on "antioxidants" including selenium and others and their effects on bone loss and osteoporosis, no conclusive data have yet been delivered to establish a causal relationship between antioxidant activity and osteoporosis and to supplement the long list of etiological factors in this respect.[27–29]

11.2.3 Other Trace Elements and Bone

Of the numerous effects, either direct or indirect, of various trace elements on bone, some important ones are listed in Table 11.1. Iodine as an essential constituent of thyroid hormones is of course extremely relevant with respect to osteoporosis and fragility fractures in both hypo- and hyperthyroidism. Others like nickel and cobalt are more important with respect to implant allergies in joint endoprostheses. We have chosen the above discussed ones for their actuality and putative relevance and the reader might refer to the original literature as cited in a minireview of ours for additional information.[30]

11.3 Calcium Deficiency as a Cause of Rickets in Nigeria: Is There a Role for Trace Elements?

Since more than three decades, there are reports about rickets in children in the regions of the world where people sustain abundant sun light exposure, e.g., in Africa (Gambia and Nigeria) and in Asia (Bangladesh) ([31–35];). Generally, there may be several factors influencing this disease, but a main causal factor seems to be calcium deficiency. Recent observations indicate that the incidence of rickets in several regions of Nigeria is

Table. 11.1 Role of some trace elements in bone metabolism (according to Ebert et al[30])

Trace elements	Recommended daily intake	Relevance for bone	Negative influences on bone
Iron	10–15 mg	Unknown	Secondary osteoporosis in hemochromatosis
Fluoride	3.1–3.8 mg	Second line osteoporosis therapy	When overdosed, mechanically incompetent bone
Iodine	200 µg	Thyroid hormones	Fragility fractures in hyper-/hypothyroidism
Cobalt	3 µg	Implant surfaces, part of vitamin B12	Allergy, genomic toxicity
Copper	1–1.5 mg	May be protective in estrogen deficiency, part of SOD1 and Cytochrome C	Developmental problems in deficiency
Lithium	Unknown	Influences wnt-signaling	High fracture risk if discontinued in depression
Manganese	2–5 mg	Enhances BMD in animals	No known ones
Nickel	25–30 µg	Implant surfaces	Allergy, inhibits AP
Selenium	30–70 µg	Antioxidative	Osteopenia in deficiency
Vanadium	Unknown	Implants, stimulates osteoblast differentiation	Inhibition of mineralization in high doses
Zinc	7–10 mg	Part of enzymes and TF, enhances AP	Enhanced senescence in deficiency, zinc finger and BTB domain containing 40 gene (ZBTB40) locus associated with osteoporosis

increasing.[32] More than 30% of children in the region of Kaduna in Nigeria suffer from rickets due to extremely low calcium intake (approximately 200 mg/day). However, in addition to calcium deficiency, other confounding factors such as genetics may contribute to the precipitation of the disease even though common polymorphisms of the vitamin D receptor gene do not seem to be significantly associated with the affected vs. unaffected siblings ([36] and our unpublished results). Geological circumstances certainly contribute very strongly to the incidence of rickets, since there are tribes and villages where people are prone to rickets in comparably close vicinity to others which show considerably lower incidence. Heavy rainfall (>1,300 mm/year) may rapidly wash out calcium from the soil consisting of granitoid rocks with a high content of silicic acid. Very similar conditions might also lead to trace element deficiency, but this remains to be shown. The information about other minerals and trace elements in the soil and in nutrients in the regions with calcium deficient rickets is scarce, but our preliminary results indicate that not only calcium deficiency but also

trace element deficiency (e.g., selenium deficiency) in soil and water might play a role and that the latter might interact with respect to calcium balance and bone metabolism (Fig. 11.2).

11.4 Trace Element Deficiencies and Interactions Between Minerals and Trace Elements

Geological interactions between minerals and trace elements and resulting geomedical problems are well recognized phenomena in veterinary medicine with respect to agriculture or grazing land and livestock reproduction and productivity.[37,38] There is however, little or no scientific interest and clinical information in humans on geomedical problems in general, demineralization processes in our organic and inorganic environment, and the interaction of minerals and trace elements in general, and even less with respect to

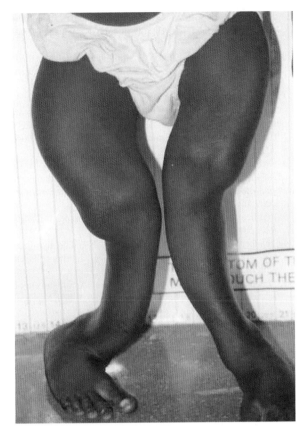

Fig. 11.2 Clinical symptoms of rickets due to calcium deficiency in a Nigerian child from the Kaduna region

calcium and phosphorus metabolism. Committees on nutrition problems around the world have been founded and both scientific and political activities are rising.[39,40] However, due to our rapidly increasing knowledge and similarly rapidly changing environmental circumstances, there is still a lot of work ahead to enhance the awareness and to broaden activities beyond the important and deserving great efforts on e.g., fortification of salt with iodine and sugar with vitamin A.

There are only few studies on the association of serum levels of trace elements with rickets, osteomalacia, osteopenia, and osteoporosis.[19] Here the authors found low serum levels of magnesium and zinc, but not copper in patients with osteoporosis compared to controls. Selenium-deficient rats show calciuria as discussed above.[26] Hence, under conditions of extremely low calcium intake, additional selenium deficiency might impair natural calcium sparing mechanisms to optimize calcium balance. In case of critically affected regions as discussed above, for e.g., Nigeria, this may have considerable impact on not only musculoskeletal but also other diseases such as infections, growth, and development. It might be helpful to study such interactions under these extreme conditions for both the critically affected and the rest of the world.

References

1. Sandstead HH, Klevay LM. History of nutrition symposium: trace element nutrition and human health. *J Nutr*. 2000;130: 483S-484S.
2. Kohrle J, Jakob F, Contempre B, Dumont JE. Selenium, the thyroid, and the endocrine system. *Endocr Rev*. 2005;26: 944-984.
3. Boy E, Mannar V, Pandav C, et al. Achievements, challenges, and promising new approaches in vitamin and mineral deficiency control. *Nutr Rev*. 2009;67(suppl 1):S24-S30.
4. Hess SY, Lonnerdal B, Hotz C, Rivera JA, Brown KH. Recent advances in knowledge of zinc nutrition and human health. *Food Nutr Bull*. 2009;30:S5-S11.
5. Fairweather-Tait SJ, Harvey LJ, Ford D. Does ageing affect zinc homeostasis and dietary requirements? *Exp Gerontol*. 2008;43:382-388.
6. Soltanoff CS, Yang S, Chen W, Li YP. Signaling networks that control the lineage commitment and differentiation of bone cells. *Crit Rev Eukaryot Gene Expr*. 2009;19:1-46.
7. Ganss B, Jheon A. Zinc finger transcription factors in skeletal development. *Crit Rev Oral Biol Med*. 2004;15:282-297.
8. McEwan IJ. Nuclear receptors: one big family. *Methods Mol Biol*. 2009;505:3-18.
9. Saita Y, Takagi T, Kitahara K, et al. Lack of Schnurri-2 expression associates with reduced bone remodeling and osteopenia. *J Biol Chem*. 2007;282:12907-12915.
10. Styrkarsdottir U, Halldorsson BV, Gretarsdottir S, et al. Multiple genetic loci for bone mineral density and fractures. *N Engl J Med*. 2008;358:2355-2365.
11. Krane SM, Inada M. Matrix metalloproteinases and bone. *Bone*. 2008;43:7-18.
12. Tallant C, Marrero A, Gomis-Ruth FX. Matrix metalloproteinases: fold and function of their catalytic domains. *Biochim Biophys Acta*. 2009;1803:20-28.
13. Liu B, Zhou Z. Lamin A/C, laminopathies and premature ageing. *Histol Histopathol*. 2008;23:747-763.
14. Rauner M, Sipos W, Goettsch C, et al. Inhibition of lamin A/C attenuates osteoblast differentiation and enhances RANKL-dependent osteoclastogenesis. *J Bone Miner Res*. 2009;24:78-86.
15. Cipriano C, Tesei S, Malavolta M, et al. Accumulation of cells with short telomeres is associated with impaired zinc homeostasis and inflammation in old hypertensive participants. *J Gerontol A Biol Sci Med Sci*. 2009;64:745-751.
16. Eberle J, Schmidmayer S, Erben RG, Stangassinger M, Roth HP. Skeletal effects of zinc deficiency in growing rats. *J Trace Elem Med Biol*. 1999;13:21-26.

17. Elmstahl S, Gullberg B, Janzon L, Johnell O, Elmstahl B. Increased incidence of fractures in middle-aged and elderly men with low intakes of phosphorus and zinc. *Osteoporos Int*. 1998;8:333-340.

18. Hyun TH, Barrett-Connor E, Milne DB. Zinc intakes and plasma concentrations in men with osteoporosis: the Rancho Bernardo Study. *Am J Clin Nutr*. 2004;80:715-721.

19. Mutlu M, Argun M, Kilic E, Saraymen R, Yazar S. Magnesium, zinc and copper status in osteoporotic, osteopenic and normal post-menopausal women. *J Int Med Res*. 2007;35:692-695.

20. Erben RG, Lausmann K, Roschger P, et al. Long-term marginal zinc supply is not detrimental to the skeleton of aged female rats. *J Nutr*. 2009;139:703-709.

21. Ursini F, Heim S, Kiess M, et al. Dual function of the selenoprotein PHGPx during sperm maturation. *Science*. 1999;285:1393-1396.

22. Kryukov GV, Castellano S, Novoselov SV, et al. Characterization of mammalian selenoproteomes. *Science*. 2003;300: 1439-1443.

23. Ebert R, Ulmer M, Zeck S, et al. Selenium supplementation restores the antioxidative capacity and prevents cell damage in bone marrow stromal cells in vitro. *Stem Cells*. 2006;24: 1226-1235.

24. Jakob F, Becker K, Paar E, Ebert-Duemig R, Schutze N. Expression and regulation of thioredoxin reductases and other selenoproteins in bone. *Methods Enzymol*. 2002;347:168-179.

25. Moreno-Reyes R, Mathieu F, Boelaert M, et al. Selenium and iodine supplementation of rural Tibetan children affected by Kashin-Beck osteoarthropathy. *Am J Clin Nutr*. 2003;78: 137-144.

26. Moreno-Reyes R, Egrise D, Neve J, Pasteels JL, Schoutens A. Selenium deficiency-induced growth retardation is associated with an impaired bone metabolism and osteopenia. *J Bone Miner Res*. 2001;16:1556-1563.

27. Banfi G, Iorio EL, Corsi MM. Oxidative stress, free radicals and bone remodeling. *Clin Chem Lab Med*. 2008;46:1550-1555.

28. Raisz LG. Pathogenesis of osteoporosis: concepts, conflicts, and prospects. *J Clin Invest*. 2005;115:3318-3325.

29. Sheweita SA, Khoshhal KI. Calcium metabolism and oxidative stress in bone fractures: role of antioxidants. *Curr Drug Metab*. 2007;8:519-525.

30. Ebert R, Seefried L, Jakob F. Spurenelemente und Knochengesundheit. (Trace elements and bone health). *Osteologie*. 2008;17:60-66.

31. Craviari T, Pettifor JM, Thacher TD, Meisner C, Arnaud J, Fischer PR. Rickets: an overview and future directions, with special reference to Bangladesh. A summary of the Rickets Convergence Group meeting, Dhaka, 26-27 January 2006. *J Health Popul Nutr*. 2008;26:112-121.

32. Kitz C, Stich A, Ebert R, Jakob F, Raab P, Sponholtz B. Rachitis in Nigeria - Spielen neben extremem Kalziummangel auch genetische Faktoren eine Rolle? *FTR Tropenmedizin*. 2009;16:76-80.

33. Prentice A. Vitamin D deficiency: a global perspective. *Nutr Rev*. 2008;66:S153-S164.

34. Thacher TD, Aliu O, Griffin IJ, et al. Meals and dephytinization affect calcium and zinc absorption in Nigerian children with rickets. *J Nutr*. 2009;139:926-932.

35. Thacher TD, Fischer PR, Pettifor JM, et al. A comparison of calcium, vitamin D, or both for nutritional rickets in Nigerian children. *N Engl J Med*. 1999;341:563-568.

36. Fischer PR, Thacher TD, Pettifor JM, Jorde LB, Eccleshall TR, Feldman D. Vitamin D receptor polymorphisms and nutritional rickets in Nigerian children. *J Bone Miner Res*. 2000;15:2206-2210.

37. Hostetler CE, Kincaid RL, Mirando MA. The role of essential trace elements in embryonic and fetal development in livestock. *Vet J*. 2003;166:125-139.

38. Steinnes E. Soils and geomedicine. *Environ Geochem Health*. 2009;31:523-535.

39. Underwood BA. The Interdepartmental Committee on Nutrition for National Defense surveys: lasting impacts. *J Nutr*. 2005;135(5):1276-1280.

40. Underwood BA. Scientific research: essential, but is it enough to combat world food insecurities? *J Nutr*. 2003; 133(5 suppl 1):1434S-1437S.

Phosphorus and Bone

12

Christel Lamberg-Allardt, Heini Karp, and Virpi Kemi

Abbreviations

BMC	Bone mineral content
BMD	Bone mineral density
Ca	Calcium
DXA	Dual X-ray absorptiometry
FGF23	Fibroblast growth factor 23
Npt2a	Type 2a sodium-phosphate cotransporter
P	Phosphorus
Pi	Inorganic phosphorus
pQCT	Peripheral computerized tomography
PTH	Parathyroid hormone
S-B-ALP	Serum bone-specific alkaline phosphatase activity, marker of bone formation
S-Ca	Serum calcium concentration
S-ICTP	Serum carboxy-terminal telopeptide of type I collagen concentration, marker of bone resorption
S-OC	Serum osteocalcin concentration, marker of bone formation and bone turnover
S-P	Serum Pi concentration
S-PICP	Serum carboxy-terminal propeptide of type I collagen concentration, marker of bone formation
S-PTH	Serum parathyroid hormone concentration
U-DPD	Urinary deoxypyridinoline excretion, marker of bone resorption
U-NTX	Urinary N-terminaltelopeptide of collagen type I excretion, marker of bone resorption
μCT	Micro computerized tomography
(Npt2c)	Type 2c sodium-phosphate cotransporter
$1,25(OH)_2D$	1,25-Dihydroxy-vitamin D

12.1 Introduction

Dietary phosphorus intake, from natural sources and food additives, is high in many Western countries, whereas calcium intake may be low. Phosphorus is readily absorbed from the intestine and the main regulatory site is the kidney. Elevated serum phosphorus concentration increases S-PTH concentration, which in turn increases bone resorption. Animal studies have shown that high phosphorus intake is deleterious to the skeleton. Findings from human studies indicate that a high intake of phosphorus, especially in conjunction with low calcium intake, is harmful to the skeleton. More studies are still needed to confirm these findings.

12.2 Phosphorus Homeostasis

Phosphorus (P) is one of the most abundant minerals in the human body. The total phosphorus content in a 70 kg man is approximately 700 g, 85% of it is in bone tissue and teeth mostly as hydroxyapatite, 14% is in soft tissues, and 1% in the extracellular space. Phosphorus as inorganic phosphate (Pi) has numerous roles in the biological processes such as in cellular metabolism, in cell signaling, as coenzymes, in nucleotide metabolism, in energy metabolism, in membrane function, and in bone mineralization.

Phosphorus homeostasis is mainly determined by the dietary intake, intestinal absorption, and renal tubular reabsorption of phosphorus. The main regulation of P homeostasis happens in the kidney, although the

C. Lamberg-Allardt (✉)
Department of Food and Environmental Sciences,
Calcium Research Unit, University of Helsinki, Helsinki, Finland
e-mail: christel.lamberg-allardt@helsinki.fi

P. Burckhardt et al. (eds.), *Nutritional Influences on Bone Health*,
DOI: 10.1007/978-1-84882-978-7_12, © Springer-Verlag London Limited 2010

movement of Pi from the extracellular fluid space into bone and into cells is also important in determining serum Pi (S-P) concentrations. Intestinal absorption of P is very efficient and about 60–80% is absorbed from bioavailable sources. The kidney filters Pi at the glomerulus, and reabsorbs a large percentage of filtered Pi in the proximal tubule. An increase in intestinal absorption of Pi results in an increase in renal Pi excretion, whereas a decreased absorption results in higher renal Pi reabsorption. The reabsorption in the kidneys is mediated by the type 2a sodium-phosphate cotransporter (Npt2a) and the type 2c sodium-phosphate cotransporter (Npt2c) in the proximal tubular cells. PTH modulates the Npt2a in the apical membrane, but PTH does not play a role in regulating Npt2c expression. An increase in S-P increases the serum PTH concentration (S-PTH) which in turn decreases renal P reabsorption. Fibroblast growth factor 23 (FGF23) is a recently found regulator of Pi as well as vitamin D metabolism. It is synthesized in the osteocytes in response to hyperphosphatemia. FGF23 increases renal P excretion, through the downregulation of both Npt2a and Npt2c. Hence, FGF23 and PTH work in the same direction. In humans, dietary phosphorus supplementation increases S-FGF23, whereas phosphorus restriction decreases S-FGF23 (for review see ref[1]).

Phosphorus homeostasis is closely linked to calcium (Ca) metabolism, which is tightly regulated to maintain serum calcium (S-Ca) at adequate levels. The main regulators of calcium homeostasis are PTH and $1,25(OH)_2D$. In response to a low S-Ca concentration, S-PTH increases, which results in an increased reabsorption of calcium in the kidney as well as a rise in bone resorption and release of Ca and P. Furthermore, PTH increases the production of $1,25(OH)_2D$ in the kidney, which results in increased intestinal Ca and Pi absorption. All these events result in a higher serum calcium concentration, but S-Pi is not affected as PTH decreases the reabsorption of Pi.

Phosphorus and vitamin D metabolism are also closely related. Oral P increases serum concentrations of $1,25(OH)_2D$ (S-$1,25(OH)_2D$) in humans.[2] An elevated S-P stimulates the synthesis of $1,25(OH)_2D$ in the kidney, whereas $1,25(OH)_2D$ induces the release of P from bone during bone resorption and facilitates the intestinal absorption of P. Moreover, FGF23 inhibits the 1a-hydroxylase in the kidney and induces the expression of 24-hydroxylase, thus suppressing the synthesis of $1,25(OH)_2D$ and increasing that of 24,25-dihydroxy-vitamin D.[3]

12.3 Parathyroid Hormone and Bone

PTH is secreted by the parathyroids and its main function is to regulate the level of S-Ca. PTH secretion is regulated primarily by S-Ca through the extracellular calcium receptor. Extracellular calcium is sensed at the surface of the parathyroid cell, and this leads to the suppression of PTH secretion. Low serum calcium results in an increase in S-PTH secretion. $1,25(OH)_2D$ suppresses PTH secretion through the inhibition of the transcription of the PTH gene. Thus, both calcium and $1,25(OH)_2D$ suppress the expression of the PTH gene. Furthermore, both inhibit parathyroid cell proliferation. The relationship between serum calcium and PTH is a sigmoidal one, allowing a response in PTH at very small changes in S-Ca through the extracellular calcium sensing receptor.

PTH has dual effects on bone; long-term continuous exposure as seen in hyperparathyroidism enhances bone resorption, whereas intermittent treatment increases bone formation. In the calcium homeostasis context, PTH increases bone resorption, when S-Ca is low. In primary hyperparathyroidism, S-Ca is increased as a result of accelerated bone resorption. One of the main reasons for secondary hyperparathyroidism is vitamin D insufficiency or deficiency. The elevated S-PTH is a result of lower intestinal calcium absorption, and the increased S-PTH results in increased bone resorption. In contrast, when PTH is administered intermittently, it has an anabolic effect on bone: it stimulates bone formation and suppresses bone resorption.

12.4 Serum Phosphorus Has Direct Effects on Parathyroid Hormone Secretion

The effect of S-P on PTH secretion has been thought to be mediated through changes in S-Ca. There are, nevertheless, a number of studies showing a direct effect of P on PTH secretion independent of changes in serum calcium.

It has been shown in rat experiments that PTH secretion and gene expression is decreased by low phosphate levels[4] and increased by high phosphate levels.[5] In vitro studies have demonstrated that high phosphate levels stimulate PTH secretion in rats.[6] S-P acts directly on PTH secretion and gene expression in human parathyroid tissue in vitro.[7] S-P seems to regulate the PTH secretion by promoting the stability of PTH mRNA.[8] Recently, Martin et al[9] studied the acute regulation of PTH by dietary phosphate in uremic rats in various experimental settings. Their findings indicated that oral Pi increases PTH release in vivo rapidly; this response may be from S-P and an additional signal arising from the gastrointestinal tract.

12.5 Does Phosphorus Have Direct Effects on Bone Cells?

Extracellular phosphorus has direct effects on both osteoclasts and osteoblasts besides those mediated through PTH, $1,25(OH)_2D$, and FGF23. High Pi concentration in culture media inhibits osteoclast formation and also bone resorption by mature osteoclasts,[10] and this seems to be mediated both by upregulating OPG expression and by direct action on osteoclast precursor cells.[11] Moreover, an increase in extracellular Pi inhibits osteoclastic activity, at least in part, by the direct induction of apoptosis of osteoclasts.[11] Increased extracellular Pi increased apoptosis on osteoblast-like cells.[12] Extracellular Pi affects gene expression and cell viability in preosteoblasts and osteoblasts derived from human mesenchymal stem cells (Pekkinen et al, Effect of extracellular phosphate on mRNA expression in mesenchymal and osteoblastic cells, Unpublished).

12.6 Hypophosphatemia as a Result of Low Phosphorus Intake

Chronic Pi insufficiency results in impaired bone mineralization, rickets, and osteomalacia. The clinical consequences besides the skeletal ones affect, for example, the nervous system, muscle tissue, and the kidney. Low dietary phosphorus intake is rare and intestinal absorption of phosphorus is very effective. Vitamin D deficiency or resistance decreases phosphorus absorption.

Renal regulation of Pi excretion is the most important step in P homeostasis and is very efficient. Thus hypophosphatemia due to low intestinal absorption is rare, and it is only when P deprivation has continued for a long time, i.e., diarrhea, that there is a risk for hypophosphatemia.

12.7 Dietary Phosphorus Intake

The American daily dietary recommended intake for P[13] is 700 mg for adults, whereas, it is 600 mg in the European Nordic Countries.[14] In all Western countries, the phosphorus intake is high, often two- to threefold in comparison to the recommended intake. For the typical American diet, young and middle-aged men consume about 1,600 mg P/day, while aged women consume about 1,000 mg/day.[15] The daily P intake in Finland is about 1,200 mg for women and 1,800 for men.[16]

Estimates of dietary phosphorus in food composition tables reflect mostly the natural phosphorus (NP) content of foods. A true estimate of the dietary content of phosphorus, however, requires consideration of two major sources – natural phosphorus and phosphorus added to foods during processing as food additives.

Meat, milk products, and grain products are high in phosphorus and contribute the largest amounts to the total dietary phosphorus intake in an average diet. The bioavailability of P differs among food sources. The biological availability of the various forms of phosphorus in foods must be considered in assessing the phosphorus content of the diet. There is limited information relative to the availability of phosphorus in individual food items; however, some forms of organic phosphorus, such as phytin, are known to be incompletely hydrolyzed and absorbed. In contrast, inorganic phosphate salts such as those used in food processing are readily hydrolyzed in the gastrointestinal tract. Hence, the contribution of phosphate food additives to the serum phosphorus pool is greater than their contribution to diet phosphorus.[17]

The use of food additives containing phosphorus in food industry is widespread. In 1990, phosphorus-containing food additives contributed an estimated 470 mg/day to the daily adult phosphorus intake in the United States.[15] Estimation of phosphorus intakes is difficult because the amounts of phosphate additives used in industrially prepared foods are not well known.[15] In fact, depending on individual food choices, phosphorus intake could be increased by as much as 1,000 mg/day by simply increasing the percentage of processed foods in the diet.[18]

12.8 High Phosphorus Intake and Health

Elevated Pi concentrations contribute significantly to the pathogenesis of secondary hyperparathyroidism seen in patients with chronic renal failure. The decreased renal excretion of P is obviously the reason for the increased S-P concentration, but it can be regulated by decreased P intake. This results in renal osteodystophy, ectopic calcification, and increased coronary and vascular disease risk. Vascular mineralization is an important complication in renal disease. Regulation of dietary P intake is a significant problem in the management of renal disease.

During the last years, serum phosphorus concentrations has gained interest in relation to cardiovascular disease in population studies. Dhinga et al[19] showed that S-P and S-Ca levels were related to the incidence of cardiovascular disease, and recently, S-P was found to be related to coronary atherosclerosis in young adults.[20] The S-P levels were within the normal reference range in these studies. Consequently, a high P intake may play a role in the regulation of S-P in healthy subjects.

12.9 Effect of High Phosphorus Intake on Skeletal Properties in Animal Studies

Long-term animal studies have shown that a high phosphorus intake has deleterious effects on the skeleton. For instance, in a 12 month and a 42 week study in dogs, a diet containing 1.2% P and 0.12% Ca resulted in lower skeletal ash content.[21,22] We have recently studied the effect of increasing doses of P on the skeleton in 30 1-month-old male rats in an 8-week study.[23] The rats were divided into three groups: one receiving normal rat feed (Ca:P ratio 1:1, control group), the second receiving twice as much P (Ca:P 1:2), and the third

receiving thrice as much P(Ca:P 1:3) as the first group. At the beginning and the end of the study period, the right femurs were measured using DXA. Double labeling with tetracycline injection was performed 12 and 2 days before death. After death, hind legs were cut loose. Left femurs were processed for histomorphometry. Right femurs were measured with pQCT. Mechanical testing was performed on the right femoral neck and tibial shaft. Six right tibias were analyzed with μCT. We found that high P intake impaired the growth of the animal, limited bone longitudinal growth, and restricted increase in femur BMC and BMD. Osteoclast number, osteoblast perimeter, and mineral apposition rate were increased, and trabecular area and width were decreased. P decreased femur midshaft total bone BMD, cortical bone BMD, and mean cortical thickness. High-phosphate diet reduced femoral neck and tibial shaft ultimate strength and tibia stiffness and toughness. In addition, serum PTH increased. Thus, in conclusion, high dietary phosphate intake reduced growth, skeletal material, and structural properties and decreased bone strength in growing male rats. Moreover, adequate calcium could not overcome this.

12.10 Could a High Phosphorus Intake Be Harmful to the Skeleton in Healthy Subjects?

A diet high in phosphorus may evidently result in an increase in S-PTH secretion and affect bone metabolism also in humans. Thus, in the long run, high dietary phosphorus intake could lead to secondary hyperparathyroidism, increased bone resorption, and poorer bone quality, especially if the dietary calcium intake is inadequate.

There are some early studies in which the effect of high P intake on PTH and bone markers has been studied for periods between 5 days and 8 weeks. Thirteen 19–36 years old subjects (8 women, 5 men) received 2 g of oral phosphate daily for 5 days.[24] S-P rose by 26% while S-Ca decreased. S-PTH concentrations increased by 50%. A persistent phosphaturia and a 69% fall in urinary calcium were observed. $1,25(OH)_2D$ and urinary hydroxyproline excretion, a marker of bone resorption, did not change significantly. The S-OC rose by 41% by day 2 and remained elevated throughout the study period. S-OC has been considered to be a marker of bone formation, but could also be considered a marker of bone turnover. Consequently, these results would indicate that P increased bone turnover. However, the authors interpreted the results to support the possibility that brief periods of phosphate administration may be useful in the therapy of disorders associated with low bone turnover, such as osteoporosis.

Calvo et al[25] studied if the high phosphorus, moderately low calcium intake typical of U.S. teenagers and young adults alters parathyroid function. They studied 8 men and 8 women, aged 18–25 years, after 8 days of ingesting a control diet that had calcium (820 mg) and phosphorus (930 mg) contents near the recommended daily intakes, and a test diet with calcium and phosphorus contents (1,660 mg phosphorus, 420 mg calcium) typical of US intakes. Both the diets were based on common grocery store foods. The 24-h mean S-PTH levels increased in men by 11% and in women by 22% during the test diet. In both sexes, the test diet significantly increased S-P, plasma $1,25(OH)_2D$, and urinary hydroxyproline excretion. Thus, short-term ingestion of a diet with typical calcium and phosphorus intake resulted in elevated serum PTH levels, and changes in mineral metabolism in young adults. Furthermore, there was an increase in bone resorption.

To determine if the elevation in PTH levels and action persisted with chronic intake of the typical diet, Calvo et al[26] studied the 24-h mineral and hormone responses of fifteen 18–25-year-old women to either high P, low Ca, or basal diets. Each subject served as her own control, first consuming a basal diet (800 mg Ca, 900 mg P) for 28 days; 10 women were then switched to the high P, low Ca test diet (400 mg Ca, 1,700 mg P) for 28 days, while the remaining 5 women in the control group continued eating the basal diet. On days 28 and 56, all subjects were studied for 24 h, with blood drawn every 4 h. S-PTH increased significantly (36%) after 4 weeks of consuming the test diet, whereas there was no change in the control group.

The studies by Calvo et al[25,26] did not indeed show that it was high P per se that induced the effect on S-PTH. Their study diets were also low in Ca and the effect could have been due to the low Ca intake and could possibly be corrected by an increase in Ca intake. The fact, however, remains that their study diets were typical for a Western diet. Consequently, Barger-Lux and Heaney[27] studied 28 healthy premenopausal women before and after manipulating Ca intake. None of the subjects had high-P diets. Women with low Ca intakes at entry were restricted to about 200 mg/day (low Ca), and those with higher self-selected intakes were supplemented to about 2,800 mg/day (high Ca). After 8 weeks, the low-Ca women had higher S-PTH and urine hydroxyproline excretion than the women on the high-Ca diet. Their findings showed that Ca restriction can evoke a persistent PTH response in the absence of a high P intake.

The effect of phosphate supplements on Ca homeostasis and bone turnover was studied in men.[28] The first part of the study was a randomized, controlled, cross-over trial of 1,000 mg/day P given for 1 week. Ten men (19–32 years) had a standard diet of about 800 mg/day each of Ca and P, which was achieved by providing them with evening meals and instructions on what to eat during the day. Blood samples were taken 3 h after breakfast and 24-h urine was collected. The tablets were taken in divided doses over meals. They found an increase in S-PTH, but no effect on the bone markers, S-OC and U-NTX excretion. In the second part of the study, the subjects, 12 healthy men (19–38 years) were given 0, 1,000, 1,500, and 2,000 mg/day phosphate, each given for 1 week, with a similar diet of 1,000 mg/day each of calcium and phosphate. Though there were differences in S-Ca and S-P between the highest and the lowest P diet, they did not find any difference in S-PTH or U-DPD secretion. The authors conclude that phosphate supplementation of the diet did not affect bone turnover in young men. However, the study may have been underpowered to detect changes in the bone markers; the diet was not controlled and the blood samples were not taken after an overnight fast, which could increase the variation.

All the studies showed that increased or high P intake elevates S-PTH concentrations when calcium intake is low. Some studies also showed that bone turnover was increased, as indicated by changes in serum osteocalcin concentration, and some also an effect on bone resorption. However, the bone markers used in these investigations were not very specific and sensitive to be used in this type of studies. The bone markers have developed extremely during the last decades, they are more sensitive, and we have a better knowledge of what they reflect in bone metabolism. The power of the studies may have also been too low to detect differences in the bone markers.

12.11 Studies on the Acute Effect of a High Phosphorus Intake on the Skeleton in Humans

We have studied the effect of high P intake in controlled short-term settings. Kärkkäinen and Lamberg-Allardt[29] studied the effects of a single oral Pi dose as well as those of three consecutive oral phosphate doses on calcium and bone metabolism. In the first part of the study (P1 study), 10 female volunteers were given orally 1,500 mg of Pi in water, as a single dose, or plain water in a randomized order at two different sessions. In the second part of the study (P2 study), 10 female volunteers were given orally 1,500 mg of Pi, as three separate 500 mg doses in water, or plain water in a randomized order. Calcium and bone metabolism was monitored for 24 h. The S-P increased, the S-iCa concentration declined significantly only in the P1 study, the urinary calcium excretion decreased, and the S-PTH concentration rose during the phosphate session as compared with the control session. Of the three markers of bone formation studied, S-PICP declined in the P1 study, and B-ALP activity declined in both parts of the study in after phosphate administration, whereas there was no significant change in S-OC in either of the studies. The markers of bone resorption, S-ICTP and U-DPD, were unaffected by the phosphate load in

both the studies. In conclusion, acute ingestion of phosphate leads to an increase in S-P, a decrease in S-iCa, and an increase in intact PTH secretion. The results indicated that these events may lead to an acute inactivation of the early phases of bone formation. In this setting, there was no indication of enhanced bone resorption despite the increase in PTH secretion.

The effect of increasing doses of P was studied in another acute setting.[30] We studied the short-term effects of four P doses on Ca and bone metabolism in 14 healthy women, 20–28 years of age, who were randomized to four controlled study days; thus each subject served as her own control. P supplement doses of 0 (placebo), 250, 750, or 1,500 mg were taken, divided into three doses during the study day. The meals served

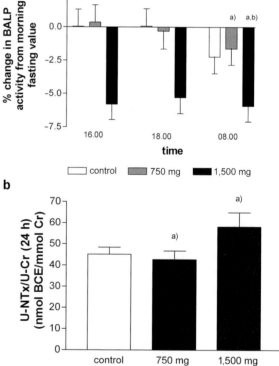

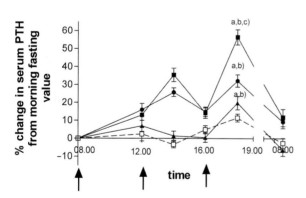

Fig. 12.1 Effect of phosphorus doses on S-PTH concentration. Change in S-PTH during the study days: control day (*open square*), 250 mg P dose (*filled triangle*), 750 mg P dose (*filled circle*) and 1,500 mg P dose (*filled square*). Values are means with their standard errors depicted by vertical bars. *a:* $p < 0.05$ (by ANOVA, repeated measures design). *b, c:* Mean values were significantly different from those of the control day (by contrast analysis): *b:* $p < 0.05$; *c:* $p < 0.001$. *Upward arrow:* P administration times (Kemi et al[30])

Fig. 12.2 Effect of phosphorus doses on bone markers (**a**), change in S-B-ALP activity during the study days (*open square*, control day; *shaded open square* 750 mg P dose; *filled square*, 1,500 mg P dose). (**b**), The 24 h urinary excretion of N-terminal telopeptide of collagen type I corrected for creatinine excretion (U-NTx/U-Cr) during the study days. Values are means with their standard errors depicted by vertical bars. *a:* $p < 0.05$ (by ANOVA, repeated measures design). *b:* Mean value was significantly different from that of the control day (by contrast analysis): $p < 0.05$. *BCE* bone collagen equivalents (Kemi et al[30])

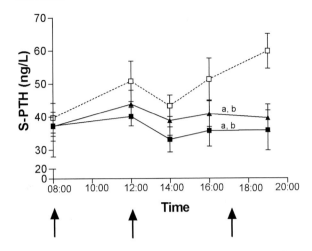

Fig. 12.3 Effect of calcium doses on S-PTH concentration. Change in S-PTH during experiment days: control day (Ca intake 480 mg/day, *open square*), 600 mg Ca dose (Ca intake 1,080 mg/day, *filled triangle*) and 1,200 mg Ca dose (Ca intake 1,680 mg/day, *filled square*). Values are means with their standard errors indicated by vertical bars. *a*: $p < 0.05$ by ANOVA, repeated measure design. Mean values were significantly different from those of the control day (by contrast analysis): *b*: $p < 0.05$. *Upward arrow*: Ca administration times (Kemi et al[31])

were exactly the same during each study day and provided 495 mg P and 250 mg Ca. The P doses affected the serum S-PTH in a dose-dependent manner (Fig. 12.1). There was a decrease in serum ionized Ca concentration only in the highest P dose. The marker of bone formation, B-ALP, decreased and the bone resorption marker U-NTX, increased in response to the P doses (Fig. 12.2). This controlled dose–response study showed that P has a dose-dependent effect on S-PTH and increases PTH secretion significantly when Ca intake is low. In conclusion, acutely high P intake adversely affects bone metabolism by decreasing bone formation and increasing bone resorption, as indicated by the bone metabolism markers.

Could an increase in calcium intake counteract the effects of increased phosphorus intake on the bone markers, that is, is the effect of P only due to a low calcium intake, as indicated by Barger-Lux and Heaney[27]? The effect of increasing doses of calcium on the markers of calcium and bone metabolism when the diet was high in S-P was studied in another acute study.[31] Each of the twelve healthy female subjects aged 21–40 years attended three 24-h study sessions, which were randomized with regard to a Ca dose of 0 (control day), 600, or 1,200 mg, and each subject

served as her own control. The meals on each study day provided 1,850 mg P and 480 mg Ca. S-PTH concentration decreased (Fig. 12.3) and serum ionized Ca concentration increased with increasing Ca doses. The bone formation marker, S-B-ALP, did not differ significantly between sessions (Fig. 12.4), indicating that Ca could not counteract the effect of P. By contrast, the bone resorption marker, U-NTX, decreased significantly with both Ca doses (Fig. 12.4). When P intake was above current recommendations, increased Ca intake was beneficial for bone, as indicated by decreased S-PTH concentration and the marker of bone resorption. However, not even a high-Ca intake

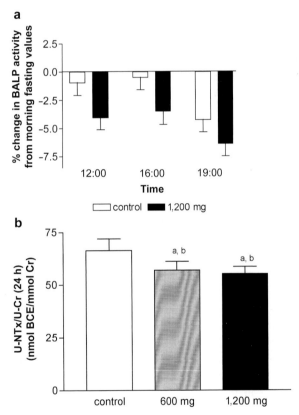

Fig. 12.4 Effect of calcium doses on bone markers. Change in S-B-ALP activity from morning fasting values (**a**) and the 24-h urinary excretion of N-terminal telopeptide of collagen type I corrected for creatinine excretion (NTx:Cr) (**b**) during experiment days: control day (*open square*), 600 mg Ca dose (*shaded open square*) and 1,200 mg Ca dose (*filled square*). Values are means with their standard errors indicated by vertical bars. *a*: $p < 0.05$ by ANOVA, repeated measure design. Mean values were significantly different from those of the control day (by contrast analysis), *b*: $p < 0.05$. *BCE* bone collagen equivalents (Kemi et al[31])

could change the effect of P intake on the bone formation marker.

In the above-mentioned studies, the effect of P was studied using phosphate salts. Karp et al[32] focused on the effect of different P-containing foods (meat, cereals, cheese) on the markers of calcium and bone metabolism in a similar setting. Sixteen healthy women aged 20–30 years were randomized to five controlled 24-h study sessions, each subject serving as her own control. At the control session, calcium intake was about 250 mg and phosphorus intake about 500 mg. During the other four sessions, phosphorus intake was about 1,500, 1,000 mg of which was obtained from meat, cheese, whole grains, or a phosphate supplement, respectively. The foods served were exactly the same during the phosphorus sessions and the control session; only phosphorus sources varied. Only the phosphate supplement increased S-PTH concentration compared with the control session. Relative to the control session, meat increased the markers of both bone formation and bone resorption. Cheese decreased S-PTH and bone resorption due to the high-Ca content of cheese. These data suggest that the metabolic response differ among P-containing foods.

12.12 Habitual P Intake and Calcium and Bone Metabolism

The effect of habitual phosphorus intake on S-PTH was studied in a cross-sectional study.[33] The objective of the study was to investigate whether NP and food additive containing foods (AP) in habitual diets differ in their effects on the markers of calcium metabolism. One hundred and forty women were studied. P intake was estimated based on 4 day food diaries. S-PTH was measured from serum samples, which were collected in the morning after an overnight fast. The authors focused on the consumption of milk and cheese as natural P sources and cheese containing food additives (e.g., spreadable cheese) as sources of food additives. The subjects were divided into groups according to their NP- and AP-containing food consumption and into quartiles according to their total P intake. Higher habitual total dietary P intakes were associated with higher mean S-PTH and lower mean S-iCa concentrations. We observed in the habitual diets of a randomly selected subgroup of women that

AP might affect bone more negatively than other P sources, as indicated by higher mean S-PTH concentrations among participants consuming AP-containing foods. The effects of NP from milk and cheese, excluding processed cheese, on S-PTH were the opposite of those of AP-containing foods, probably due to a higher Ca content in these foods. This may be important as the consumption of processed foods has increased during the last decades, which in turn has increased P intake from AP. The intakes of AP and total P have been shown to rise due to the increasing consumption of fast, snack, and convenience foods. High dietary P intake may no longer be a problem only in patients with impaired renal function, but it may also affect healthy individuals whose diet contains excessive P derived from AP. As the foods we examined represent only one type of NP and AP sources, the effects of other foods, e.g., meat or baked products, might be different, because dairy products are the only foodstuffs containing large amounts of both P and Ca.

12.13 Is the Dietary Calcium/Phosphorus Ratio Important?

The imbalance between phosphorus intake and calcium intake results in a low Ca:P ratio in many Western communities. The overall trend in food consumption in Europe[34,35] as well as in the USA[15,36] is to drink less milk and more phosphoric acid-containing soft drinks. In fact, it was reported that consumption of cola beverages may predict a higher risk of fracture in girls[37] and result in the development of higher S-PTH concentration and hypocalcaemia in postmenopausal women.[38] These types of dietary habits may lead to lower dietary Ca:P ratios that were recently observed in many countries.[16,39–41] Furthermore, recent evidence from Poland revealed that for 10% of young girls and boys, the dietary Ca:P ratio was lower than 0.25.[40] These results support the previous findings among young women in the USA.[26] The recommended optimal Ca:P ratio in the diet is 1.0 on a molar basis,[16,28] which corresponds to 1.3 on a mg basis. Criticism[42] was raised against the American dietary reference intakes.[13] The report excluded several studies whose results supported the importance of the role played by the dietary Ca:P ratio in bone health.

The effect of different Ca:P ratios has not gained much attention and has not been studied to a larger extent. Ca:P ratio only reflects the balance between Ca and P intakes regardless of what the absolute intakes are. Kemi et al[43] focused on the effect of low Ca:P in habitual diets on S-PTH and other markers of calcium metabolism in healthy women with adequate calcium intake. In this cross-sectional analysis of 147 healthy women aged 31–43 years, fasting blood samples and three separate 24-h urinary samples were collected. Participants kept a 4-day food record and were divided into quartiles according to their dietary Ca:P ratios. The first quartile with Ca:P molar ratio ≤0.50 differed significantly from the second (Ca:P molar ratio 0.51–0.57), third (Ca:P molar ratio 0.58–0.64), and fourth (Ca:P molar ratio ≥0.65) quartiles by interfering with Ca metabolism. It is noteworthy that dietary Ca intake among our participants was mostly adequate or high (mean Ca intake 1,056 mg/day). Even in the first quartile, the mean Ca intake was nearly 750 mg/day. This intake reflects the high dairy product consumption of the participants. Nevertheless, none of the participants achieved the suggested Ca:P molar ratio of 1 in their diets. This is mainly due to the excessive P content in their habitual diets, rather than low dietary Ca intake. In the first quartile, mean S-PTH concentration and mean urinary Ca (U-Ca) excretion were higher than in all other quartiles. The higher 24-h U-Ca excretion in the first quartile was unexpected, since the mean dietary Ca intake and Ca:P ratio in the first quartile were the lowest and the mean S-PTH concentration in this quartile was the highest, and thus a low U-Ca would be expected. In normal physiological conditions, elevated S-PTH leads to decreased U-Ca excretion. In primary hyperparathyroidism, an increase in U-Ca excretion is, however, often seen. The U-Ca finding suggests that low dietary Ca:P ratios in habitual diets somehow interfere with Ca homeostasis. An increase in S-PTH due to a low Ca:P ratio would be expected to increase bone resorption, and some of the extra Ca, which has been released from bone, to be excreted in urine. Elevated U-Ca excretion might therefore reflect an increase in bone resorption. Unfortunately, we were not able to measure the bone markers. Because low habitual dietary Ca:P ratios are common in Western diets, more attention should be focused on decreasing excessively high dietary P intake and increasing low Ca intakes to the recommended level.

12.14 Conclusions

Does high phosphorus intake have harmful effects on bone? The results from animal studies point in that direction. Human studies have also shown that a high dietary phosphate intake has negative effects on bone; it increases S-PTH and bone resorption. Most human studies have been performed using high P and low Ca diets. Low Ca may indeed have the same effects on S-PTH as high P. However, the animal studies have been done with normal Ca intakes, and some human studies have shown that high-Ca intake does not counteract the effect of P on bone completely. The Ca:P ratio is low in most Western diets. Increasing the Ca:P ratio when P intake is already high could bring the Ca intake to levels much higher than the recommended dietary intake. The intake of P is increasing due to the use of food additives. The bioavailability of Pi from these is much more effective than that from natural sources, which make them more harmful. No definite conclusions can be made on the effect of high P on the skeleton at this stage. More studies are needed addressing the effect of high P and low Ca:P ratio from both natural and artificial sources on skeletal variables and fractures in population-based as well as controlled long-term intervention studies.

References

1. Sommer S, Berndt T, Craig T, Kumar R. The phosphatonins and the regulation of phosphate transport and vitamin D metabolism. *J Steroid Biochem Mol Biol*. 2007;103:497-503.
2. Portale AA, Halloran BP, Morris RC Jr. Physiologic regulation of the serum concentration of 1, 25-dihydroxyvitamin D by phosphorus in normal men. *J Clin Invest*. 1989;83:1494-1499.
3. Shimada T, Hasegawa H, Yamazaki Y, et al. FGF-23 is a potent regulator of vitamin D metabolism and phosphate homeostasis. *J Bone Miner Res*. 2004;19:429-435.
4. Kilav R, Silver I, Naveh-Many T. Parathyroid hormone gene expression inhypophosphatemic rats. *J Clin Invest*. 1995;96:327-333.
5. Hernandez A, Concepción MT, Rodriguez M, Salido E, Torres A. High phosphate diet increases prepro PTH mRNA independent of calcium and calcitriol in normal rats. *Kidney Int*. 1996;50:1872-1878.
6. Nielsen PK, Feldt-Rasmussen U, Olgaard K. A direct effect in vitro of phosphate on PTH release from bovine parathyroid tissue slices but not from dispersed parathyroid cells. *Nephrol Dial Transplant*. 1996;11:1762-1768.
7. Almaden Y, Hernandez A, Torregrosa V, et al. High phosphate level directly stimulates parathyroid hormone

secretion and synthesis by human parathyroid tissue in vitro. *Am Soc Nephrol*. 1998;9:1845-1852.

8. Moallem E, Kilav R, Silver J, Naveh-Many T. RNA-protein binding and post-transcriptional regulation of parathyroid hormone gene expression by calcium and phosphate. *J Biol Chem*. 1998;273:5253-5259.

9. Martin DR, Ritter CS, Slatopolsky E, Brown AJ. Acute regulation of parathyroid hormone by dietary phosphate. *Am J Physiol Endocrinol Metab*. 2005;289:E729-E734.

10. Yates AJ, Oreffo RO, Mayor K, Mundy GR. Inhibition of bone resorption by inorganic phosphate is mediated by both reduced osteoclast formation and decreased activity of mature osteoclasts. *J Bone Miner Res*. 1991;6:473-478.

11. Kanatani M, Sugimoto T, Kano J, Kanzawa M, Chihara K. Effect of high phosphate concentration on osteoclast differentiation as well as bone-resorbing activity. *J Cell Physiol*. 2003;196:180-189.

12. Meleti Z, Shapiro IM, Adams CS. Inorganic phosphate induces apoptosis of osteoblast-like cells in culture. *Bone* 2000;27:359-366.

13. Institute of Medicine, National Research Council, Standing Committee on the Scientific Evaluation of Dietary Reference Intakes, Food and Nutrition Board. *Dietary Reference Intakes: Calcium Phosphorus, Magnesium, Vitamin D, and Fluoride*. Washington, DC: National Academy Press;1997

14. Nordic Councils of Ministeries. *Nordic Nutrition Recommendations*, 4th ed. Nord, 2004:13, Scanprint, Århus, Denmark, 2005.

15. Calvo MS, Park YK. Changing phosphorus content of the US diet: potential for adverse effects on bone. *J Nutr*. 1996;126:S1168-S1180.

16. Männistö S, Ovaskainen M-L, Valsta L. *The National FINDIET 2002 Study. Kansanterveyslaitoksen julkaisuja (Publications of the National Institute fot Health) B3/2003*. Helsinki, Finland: Hakapaino OY; 2003.

17. Bell RR, Draper HH, Tzeng DYM, Shin HK, Schmidt GR. Physiological responses of human adults to foods containing phosphate additives. *J Nutr*. 1977;107:42-50.

18. Uribarri J, Calvo MS. Hidden sources of phosphorus in the typical American diet; does it matter in nephrology. *Semin Dial*. 2003;16:186-188.

19. Dhingra R, Sullivan LM, Fox CS, et al. Relations of serum phosphorus and calcium levels to the incidence of cardiovascular disease in the community. *Arch Intern Med*. 2007;167: 879-885.

20. Foley CAJ, Herzog CA, Ishani A, Kalra PA. Serum phosphorus levels associate with coronary atherosclerosis in young adults. *J Am Soc Nephrol*. 2009;20:397-404.

21. Saville PD, Krook L, Gustafsson P, Marshall JL, Figarola F. Nutritional secondary hyperparathyroidism in a dog. Morphologic and radioisotope studies with treatment. *Cornell Vet*. 1969;59:155-167.

22. Krook L, Lutwak L, Henrikson PA, et al. Reversibility of nutritional osteoporosis: physicochemical data on bones from an experimental study in dogs. *J Nutr*. 1971;101:233-246.

23. Huttunen MM, Tillman I, Viljakainen HT, et al. High dietary phosphorus reduces bone strength in the growing rat skeleton. *J Bone Mineral Res*. 2007;22:83-92.

24. Silverberg SJ, Shane E, Clemens TL, et al. The effect of oral phosphate administration on major indices of skeletal metabolism in normal subjects. *J Bone Miner Res*. 1986;1:383-388.

25. Calvo MS, Kumar R, Heath H III. Elevated secretion and action of serum parathyroid hormone in young adults consuming high phosphorus, low calcium diets assembled from common foods. *J Clin Endocrinol Metab*. 1988;66: 823-829.

26. Calvo MS, Kumar R, Heath H. Persistently elevated parathyroid hormone secretion and action in young women after four weeks of ingesting high phosphorus, low calcium diets. *J Clin Endocrin Metab*. 1990;70:1334-1340.

27. Barger-Lux MJ, Heaney RP. Effects of calcium restriction on metabolic characteristics of premenopausal women. *J Clin Endocr Metab*. 1993;76:103-107.

28. Whybro A, Jagger H, Barker M, Eastell R. Phosphate supplementation in young men: lack of effect on calcium homeostasis and bone turnover. *Eur J Clin Nutr*. 1998;52:29-33.

29. Kärkkäinen M, Lamberg-Allardt C. An acute intake of phosphate increases parathyroid hormone secretion and inhibits bone formation in young women. *J Bone Miner Res*. 1996; 11:1905-1912.

30. Kemi V, Kärkkäinen M, Lamberg-Allardt C. Low dietary calcium-to-phosphorus ratios negatively affects calcium and bone metabolism in a dose-dependent manner in healthy young females. *Br J Nutr*. 2006;96:545-552.

31. Kemi VE, Kärkkäinen MUM, Karp HJ, Laitinen K, Lamberg-Allardt CJE. Increased calcium intake does not completely counteract the adverse effects of high phosphorus intake on bone: a dose-response study in healthy females. *Br J Nutr*. 2008;99:832-839.

32. Karp H, Vaihia KP, Kärkkäinen MUM, Niemistö M, Lamberg-Allardt CJE. The acute effects of different phosphate sources on calcium and bone metabolism in young women. *Calcified Tissue Int*. 2007;80:251-258.

33. Kemi V, Rita H, Kärkkäinen M, et al. Habitual high phosphorus intakes and foods with phosphate additives negatively affect serum parathyroid hormone concentration: a cross-sectional study on healthy pre-menopausal women. *Public Health Nutr*. 2009;16:1-8.

34. Urho U-M, Hasunen K. Yläasteen kouluruokailu 1998. *Sosiaali- ja terveysministeriön selvityksiä* 1995:5. Helsinki: Edita; 1999.

35. Comité de Nutrición de la Asociación Española de Pediatría. Consumption of fruit juices and beverages by Spanish children and teenagers: health implications of their poor use and abuse. An Pediatr (Barc) 2003;58:584-593.

36. Harnack L, Stang J, Story M. Soft drink consumption among US children and adolescents: nutritional consequences. *J Am Diet Assoc*. 1999;99:436-441.

37. Wyshak G. Teenaged girls, carbonated beverage consumption, and bone fractures. *Arch Pediatr Adolesc*. 2000;154:610-613.

38. Fernando GR, Martha RM, Evangelina R. Consumption of soft drinks with phosphoric acid as a riskfactor for the development of hypocalcemia in postmenopausal women. *J Clin Epidemiol*. 1999;52:1007-1010.

39. Brot C, Jorgensen N, Madsen OR, Jensen LB, Sorensen OH. Relationships between bone mineral density, serum vitamin D metabolites and calcium:phosphorus intake in healthy perimenopausal women. *J Intern Med*. 1999;245:509-516.

40. Chwojnowska Z, Charzewska J, Chabros E, Wajszczyk B, Rogalska-Niedswieds M, Jarosz B. Contents of calcium and phosphorus in the diet of youth from Warsaw elementary schools. *Rocz Panstw Zakl Hig*. 2002;53:157-165.

41. Takeda E, Sakamoto K, Yokota K, et al. Phosphorus supply per capita from food in Japan between 1960 and 1995 (abstract). *J Nutr Sci Vitaminol.* 2002;48:102.

42. Sax L. The Institute of Medicine's 'Dietary reference intake' for phosphorus: a critical perspective. *J Am Coll Nutr.* 2001;20:271-278.

43. Kemi VE, Kärkkäinen MUM, Rita HJ, Laaksonen MML, Outila TA, Lamberg-Allardt CJE. Low calcium-to-phosphorus ratio in habitual diets affects serum parathyroid hormone concentration and calcium metabolism in healthy women with adequate calcium intake. *Br J Nutr* 2010;103: 561-568.

13

Seasonal Differences in Mineral Homeostasis and Bone Metabolism in Response to Oral Phosphate Loading in Older Northern Chinese Adults

B. Zhou, L. Yan, X. Wang, I. Schoenmakers, G.R. Goldberg, and A. Prentice

13.1 Introduction

Vitamin D deficiency in older people has been recognized as an important factor influencing skeletal integrity. This is because it induces secondary hyperparathyroidism which in turn promotes an increase in bone remodeling rate and bone loss.[1,2] However, we have previously shown that vitamin D status of older people in China is very low in winter (40–50% <25 nmol 25-hydroxyvitamin D (25(OH)D)/L), and plasma parathyroid hormone (PTH) is elevated, but the incidence of osteoporotic fracture is low in this population.[3–6] Resistance to the bone resorbing effects and racial differences in PTH dynamics have been reported.[7] We therefore explored ethnic differences in bone and mineral metabolism as challenged by 5 days of oral phosphate (P) loading to stimulate PTH secretion in older British, Chinese, and Gambian adults in summer and winter.[8] In summary, ethnic differences in bone and mineral metabolism were found, in particular, in the rate of renal clearance of phosphate, which was more rapid in the Chinese subjects than in their British and Gambian counterparts. No evidence was found for resistance to the resorbing effects of PTH. Seasonal differences in vitamin D status and bone and mineral metabolisms as challenged by P-loading were found only in the Chinese subjects and are reported here.

13.2 Methods

13.2.1 Subjects

The study was conducted at Shenyang Medical College, Shenyang, China. Thirty healthy adults (15 men, 15 women) aged 60–75 years were recruited. Exclusion criteria were any pathological disorder or medication known to affect mineral or bone metabolism. All the subjects were ambulatory with normal renal function (fasting plasma creatinine <115 μmol/L). To allow for the possible effects of season, subjects were studied once in February–April and once in July–September. Two subjects (1 male, 1 female) were not available in the summer. Ethical approval was given by the Academic Committee of Shenyang Medical College. Informed written consent was obtained from all the subjects.

13.2.2 PTH Stimulation Test

Subjects took a 1 g dose of elemental P (Phosphate-Sandoz, HK Pharma, UK) dissolved in 200 mL water, twice daily (0700–0900 and 1,900–2,100 h) for 5 consecutive days. The stimulation test was preceded within 5 days by a control day in which only 200 mL water was given (day 0). On days 0, 1, 4, and 5, subjects attended the research center between 0700 and 0900 h after an overnight fast. Blood and urine samples were collected on arrival (0 h) and 2 hours (2 h) after consuming the water or morning P dose. Subjects remained sedentary during the 2 h and drank 500 mL water to

I. Schoenmakers (✉)
MRC Human Nutrition Research, Elsie Widdowson
Laboratory, Fulbourn Road, Cambridge CB1 9NL, UK
e-mail: inez.schoenmakers@mrc-hnr.cam.ac.uk

P. Burckhardt et al. (eds.), *Nutritional Influences on Bone Health*,
DOI: 10.1007/978-1-84882-978-7_13, © Springer-Verlag London Limited 2010

standardize the fluid intake, but no other food or liquid was consumed. Subjects were requested to keep to their usual diet the week before and during each stimulation test.

13.2.3 Sample Collections and Laboratory Analyses

Blood samples were collected into tubes containing EDTA or lithium-heparin. Blood ionized Ca (iCa) was measured (ABL77, Radiometer Medical, USA) within 10 min. Plasma was separated from cells within 30 min in a refrigerated centrifuge, and stored at $-80°C$. Urine samples were collected immediately after blood collection. Acidified (HCl, 10 mL/L) and nonacidified aliquots were stored at $-20°C$. Plasma P and urinary P and creatinine (uP and uCr) were measured by colorimetric methods (7170A Hitachi automatic analyzer, Japan). Within and between-assay coefficients of variation (CV) were <2.0 and <4.0% respectively. PTH, osteocalcin (OC), and C-telopeptide of type 1 collagen (CTX) were measured on an automatic analyzer (Elecsys 2010, Roche Diagnostics, USA). Between-assay CVs were 4.7, 3.1, and 4.3% respectively. Plasma 25-OHD and 1,25-dihydroxyvitamin D (1,25 $(OH)_2D$) were measured by radioimmunoassay (DiaSorin, Stillwater, MN and IDS, Tyne and Wear, UK respectively). Within and between-assay CV were 4.1 and 6.1% for 25-OHD, and 7.5 and 9.0% for 1,25$(OH)_2D$. Concentration of uP was expressed as a ratio relative to urinary Cr (uP/Cr).

13.2.4 Data-Handling and Analysis

Statistical analysis was performed using the Linear Model facility in Data Desk 6.1.1 (Data Description, Ithaca, NY). To permit the exploration of proportion relationships, variables were converted to natural logarithms whereby differences$\times 100$ correspond closely to percentage differences [(difference/mean)$\times 100$].[9] All percent differences presented were obtained this way. The change by 2 h (%) was defined as the change in a variable from 0 (before P dose) to 2 h after, on the same day. The response on day 0 was used to control for any change that was independent of the effect of administered P. Change by day 5 (%) was defined as the difference in fasting values between baseline (mean of 0 h on days 0 and 1) and 0 h on day 5. The significance of change from baseline by 2 h and day 5 and seasonal differences in these changes were examined by Student's paired t-test. Because there was no significant season-gender interaction, data were pooled for men and women. p Values ≤ 0.05 were considered significant.

13.3 Results

Baseline mean ($\pm$ SE) 25-OHD (nmol/L) was lower in winter (33.2 ± 2.5) than in summer ($58.8 \pm 2.9, p < 0.01$), but there was no significant seasonal difference in 1,25$(OH)_2D$ (pmol/L), (108.2 in winter and 118.3 in summer).

13.3.1 Change by 2 h Post P-Loading

On all measurement days in winter, significant increases were found in P (34, 31, 34% on day 1, 4, and 5, respectively), PTH (29, 20, 17%), OC (10, 12, 9%), and CTX (9, 12, 15%). There was a significant decrease in the plasma concentration of iCa (3, 3, 2%) on all days and 1,25 $(OH)_2D$ (9, 11, 5%) on day 1 and 5.

In summer, 2 h changes in P (+14, +5, +12% on day 1, 4, and 5, respectively), PTH (+6, +7, +13%), OC (+5, +5, +1%), CTX (0, +1, +4%), iCa (0% on all days), and 1,25 $(OH)_2D$ (−0, +4, +1%) were nonsignificant, but were in the same direction as in winter, except for 1,25 $(OH)_2D$. The % change in uP/Cr in winter (116, 69, 65%) and summer (87, 50, 57%) were significant on all measurement days. There were significant seasonal differences in the 2-h percentage change for all analytes, except for uP/Cr.

13.3.2 Change by 5 Days

The 5-day change from baseline (fasting) was nonsignificant for P, iCa, and OC in both the seasons. uP/Cr increased significantly in winter (92%) and summer (70%), and CTX (12 and 19%, respectively) and 1,25

(OH)$_2$D (25 and 20%) decreased in both the seasons. PTH increased significantly only in winter (22%). The % change in winter was significantly greater than in summer for uP/Cr and PTH ($p < 0.05$), but there were no seasonal differences for P, iCa, OC, and 1,25 (OH)$_2$D.

13.4 Discussion and Conclusion

As expected, oral P-loading induced perturbations in Ca and P homeostasis, consequently inducing changes in PTH secretion and bone metabolism. Although the pattern of change was similar for all analytes except 1,25 (OH)$_2$D, greater changes were found in winter than in summer, especially at 2 h after P-loading. Vitamin D status was significantly lower in winter than in summer evidenced by the lower plasma concentration of 25-OHD. These findings suggest that vitamin D status may modulate the hormonal response to maintain normo-calcaemia after P loading. The long-term implications of seasonal differences in vitamin D status for bone health in this and other populations should be further investigated.

Acknowledgment The study was partly supported by a grant from the Nestlé Foundation. We thank Dr. Lianying Guo and Mr. Zhuo Zhang for their valuable assistance and all the subjects for their participation.

References

1. Szulc P, Munoz F, Marchand F, Chapuy MC, Delmas PD. Role of vitamin D and parathyroid hormone in the regulation of bone turnover and bone mass in men: the MINOS study. *Calcif Tissue Int.* 2003;73:520-530.
2. Kuchuk NO, van Schoor NM, Pluijm SM, Chines A, Lips P. Vitamin D status, parathyroid function, bone turnover, and BMD in postmenopausal women with osteoporosis: global perspective. *J Bone Miner Res.* 2009;24:693-701.
3. Yan L, Zhou B, Prentice A, et al. An epidemiological study of hip fracture in Shenyang, P R China. *Bone.* 1999;24: 151-155.
4. Yan L, Prentice A, Zhang H, et al. Vitamin D status and parathyroid hormone concentrations in Chinese women and men from north-east of the People's Republic of China. *Eur J Clin Nutr.* 2000;54:68-72.
5. Yan L, Zhou B, Wang X, et al. Older people in China and the United Kingdom differ in the relationships among parathyroid hormone, vitamin D, and bone mineral status. *Bone.* 2003;33:620-627.
6. Wang Y, Tao Y, Hyman ME, et al. Osteoporosis in China. *Osteoporosis Int.* 2009;20:1651-1662. doi:10.1007/s00198-009-0925-y.
7. Cosman F, Morgan DC, Nieves JW, et al. Resistance to bone resorbing effects of PTH in black women. *J Bone Miner Res.* 1997;12:958-966.
8. Yan L, Schoenmakers I, Zhou B, et al. Ethnic differences in parathyroid hormone secretion and mineral metabolism in response to oral phosphate administration. *Bone.* 2009;45(2): 238-245.
9. Cole TJ. Sympercents: symmetric percentage differences on the 100 loge scale simplify the presentation of log transformed data. *Stat Med.* 2000;19:3109-3125.

Diabetes Mellitus and Osteoporosis

14

Lorenz C. Hofbauer and Christine Hamann

14.1 Introduction

Diabetes mellitus (DM) is an emerging health problem for industrialized societies with substantial morbidity and mortality and an established risk factor for osteoporosis and fragility fractures.[1] The skeletal alterations in patients with DM are due to insulin deficiency or resistance and hyperglycemia, alterations of the bone marrow microenvironment and bone matrix quality, and impaired neuromuscular–skeletal interactions.[2,3]

A large prospective analysis of 32,089 postmenopausal women in the Iowa Women's Health Study revealed that women with type 1 diabetes mellitus (T1DM) had a 12-times higher risk of having self-reported hip fractures than women without T1DM.[4] Of note, women with type 2 diabetes mellitus (T2DM) also displayed a 1.7-fold higher risk for reporting hip fractures compared to women without T2DM.[4] The higher incidence of falls due to long-standing T2DM was viewed as a potential explanation for the higher fracture risk in T2DM despite the higher bone mineral density (BMD).[1]

In this chapter, we review the risk factors that are associated with low BMD and osteoporotic fractures in patients with DM, discuss the principal mechanisms, and provide recommendations regarding prevention and management.

L.C. Hofbauer (✉)
Department of Medicine III, Division of Endocrinology, Diabetes, and Bone Diseases, University of Dresden Medical Center, Fetscherstrasse 74, 01307 Dresden, Germany
e-mail: lorenz.hofbauer@uniklinikum-dresden.de

14.2 Osteoporosis in Type 1 Diabetes Mellitus

14.2.1 Major Findings

The skeletal findings in T1DM depend upon the age of the patients and the duration of the disease. Two small studies of children with T1DM showed decreased BMD values with Z scores of −1.1 and −0.4 in the lumbar spine, respectively.[5,6] However, two large pediatric studies[7,8] have shown no adverse effect of T1DM on BMD and no correlation between BMD and the duration of disease or glycemic control. In young adults with stable T1DM, most studies point towards a negative effect of T1DM on BMD. Two studies of patients in their forties with long-standing T1DM (20–33 years) detected no significant BMD differences at the spine and the hip[9] or the distal radius.[10] Other studies of patients with T1DM demonstrated lower BMD values at the lumbar spine[11,12] and femoral neck.[11–14] Interestingly, most studies reported no association between BMD and glycemic control.

14.2.2 Predictors of Poor Bone Health

The presence and severity of diabetic complications such as retinopathy,[15–17] peripheral neuropathy,[18] nephropathy,[16,19,20] and peripheral vascular disease[21] rather than long duration predict low BMD in patients with T1DM. Retinopathy of diabetes mellitus *per se* as well as peripheral neuropathy may impair bone health through reduced mobility and an increased propensity

P. Burckhardt et al. (eds.), *Nutritional Influences on Bone Health*,
DOI: 10.1007/978-1-84882-978-7_14, © Springer-Verlag London Limited 2010

of falls. Male gender is a risk factor for low BMD in T1DM, as no women, but 14% of men with T1DM had osteoporosis.[12] Oral contraceptives were positively correlated with the BMD at the spine,[21] whereas cigarette smoking was associated with lower BMD in either gender with T1DM.[16]

14.2.3 Pathogenesis

Lack of the bone-anabolic factor insulin has long been implicated in the development of low BMD and osteoporotic fractures.[22] Because T1DM frequently develops in young people, it is likely that it impairs bone accrual and final peak bone mass. This is supported by an animal model of streptozotocin-induced diabetic mice.[23] In this context, intensive insulin therapy had a favorable effect on bone metabolism over the course of 7 years as compared to conventional insulin therapy.[17] Of interest, amylin is another osteotropic peptide produced by pancreatic β cells which when administered to a rat model of T1DM maintained bone mass, inhibited biochemical markers of bone resorption, and elevated those of bone formation.[24]

14.2.4 Therapeutic Implications

T1DM is a risk factor for osteoporotic fractures.[4] A detailed history and physical examination is aimed at identifying concurrent diseases, low body weight, malnutrition, and lactose intolerance, and, in particular, the extent of retinopathy, neuropathy, nephropathy, and vascular disease. In addition, the risk of falls and fall-provoking circumstances (impaired vision; unstable joints; medications such as sedatives, impaired before vision opiates, or antidepressants) should be evaluated and optimized. BMD should be assessed at the lumbar spine and the hip using DXA, especially in men who carry an increased risk for osteoporosis.[9,12] A healthy life style with increased physical activity and cessation of cigarette smoking[16] should be encouraged. Oral contraceptives are protective for bone health in women with T1DM.[21]

14.3 Osteoporosis in Type 2 Diabetes Mellitus

14.3.1 Major Findings

Based on DXA and fracture data, the Rotterdam study which included 792 elderly patients with T2DM and 5,863 nondiabetic controls indicated that the presence of T2DM on treatment was associated with a 1.3-fold higher fracture risk, although BMD at the femoral neck and the lumbar spine was higher.[25] Increased BMD values in T2DM were confirmed by other investigators who reported a 4–5% higher BMD at the hip of 566 patients (243 women, 323 men)[26] and 11 and 8% higher BMD values at the femoral neck and the spine, respectively, in an all-female cohort[27] compared to healthy controls. Gender differences may play an important role, as spinal BMD was 8% lower in men with T2DM and normal renal function compared to nondiabetic controls, but no such differences were found in women with T2DM,[28] indicating that men are particularly at risk of diabetic osteopenia. Confirmatory findings come from a recent Austrian bone ultrasound study comparing elderly nursing home patients with T2DM with nondiabetic controls.[29] Adjusted for various confounders, calcaneal stiffness scores as well as radial and phalangeal speed of sound scores were higher in diabetic as compared to nondiabetic patients. Longitudinal analysis of these subjects for 2 years showed that hip fracture and nonvertebral fracture rates were comparable between the two groups, suggesting that patients with T2DM do not benefit from the higher BMD, possibly because of the increased risk of falls.[29]

14.3.2 Predictors of Poor Bone Health

According to most studies, obesity confers relative protection against bone loss with positive correlations between BMD and BMI in patients with T2DM[10,28] and a negative association between BMI and the presence of osteoporosis in patients with T2DM.[30] Since both weight-bearing and nonweight-bearing skeletal sites have a higher BMD with increasing BMI, these changes cannot be explained by mechanical loading as a result of higher body weight. Instead, adipocyte-derived cytokines or "adipokines" such as leptin, resistin, and adiponectin may mediate enhanced BMD of obesity as discussed below.

Postmenopausal women with T2DM ($n = 1,682$) from the Iowa Women's Health Study, while having a higher BMI and, thus, presumably a higher mean BMD, had a 1.7-fold higher risk for self-reported hip fractures than nondiabetic women ($n = 30,377$).[4] These findings were essentially confirmed by the Rotterdam study that patients with T2DM have an increased fracture risk despite a higher BMD.[25] After adjustment for multiple confounders, including the frequency of falls, the relative risk for nonvertebral fractures was 1.33, for hip fractures 1.34, and for wrist fractures 1.40 in patients with T2DM compared to nondiabetic individuals.[25] Thus, factors other than BMD and the propensity to falls affect fracture risk.

In the prospective questionnaire-based Study of Osteoporotic Fractures ($n = 9,249$ women), 629 women (6.8%) had diabetes (530 noninsulin-treated diabetes and 99 insulin-treated DM).[31] Interestingly, women with DM on insulin treatment had the highest incidence of falls (age adjusted odds ratio: 2.78), while those without insulin treatment had an incidence of falls (age adjusted odds ratio: 1.68) that was between the insulin treatment group and the nondiabetic group. Most likely, hypoglycemic episodes under insulin therapy may have contributed to the increased risk for falls or insulin therapy was initiated because DM was more severe. Risk factors for self-reported falls in patients with T2DM include advanced age, peripheral neuropathy, impaired balance, and a history of coronary heart disease or arthritis.[31]

14.3.3 Pathogenesis

The hallmarks of T2DM include peripheral insulin resistance with a variable degree of hyperinsulinemia and impaired insulin secretion following metabolic challenge by glucose. Chronic hyperglycemia has several adverse effects on bone metabolism. One in vitro study demonstrated that glucose dose-dependently enhanced the activity of avian osteoclasts.[32] Moreover, hyperglycemia may promote the accumulation of nonenzymatic glycosylation of various bone matrix proteins such as type I collagen, thus contributing to impaired bone quality.[33] Rats which spontaneously developed diabetes (WBN/Kob rat) accumulated glycation-induced nonenzymatic cross-links (pentosidine) with disease progression in their bones, while the amount of enzymatic cross-links, including pyridinoline and deoxypyridinoline decreased.[34] Importantly, a high skeletal content of pentosidine rendered the bones biomechanically less competent on three-point bending compared to nondiabetic controls despite similar BMD values,[34] indicating that nonenzymatic glycosylation may impair bone quality (Fig. 14.1).

Other indirect skeletal complications of hyperglycemia include hypercalciuria due to glycosuria and alterations of the PTH/vitamin D system. Improvement of glycemic control in 78 poorly controlled patients with T2DM reduced urinary excretion of calcium and phosphate as well as serum $1,25(OH)_2D_3$ levels and increased serum phosphate levels, but had no effect on serum calcium or PTH levels.[35]

Of note, area under the glucose curve during oral glucose tolerance testing and total insulin concentrations were inversely correlated with the serum concentration of 25-hydroxyvitamin D_3 in patients with T2DM, of whom one third were 25-hydroxyvitamin D_3 depleted.[36] Two studies indicated that serum levels of leptin[37] and that of adiponectin[38] are positively and negatively correlated with BMD, respectively.

14.3.4 Therapeutic Implications

While patients with T2DM were included in most osteoporosis treatment studies, specific evidence-based recommendations are not available for the prevention and treatment of osteoporosis in T2DM. BMD-based osteoporotic fracture risk may be underestimated in patients with T2DM because bone quality may be impaired and the risk of falls is higher. As a general recommendation, adequate glycemic control delays vascular complications and may limit the degree of nonenzymatic glycosylation of collagen, a determinant of poor bone quality.

Fig. 14.1 Potential mechanisms contributing to low bone mass, poor bone quality, and fragility fractures in patients with diabetes mellitus

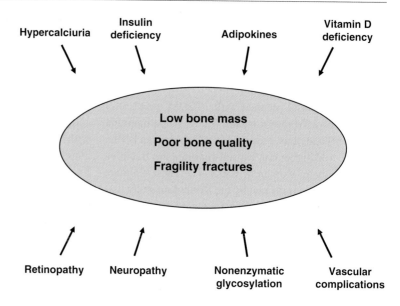

The risk and frequency of falls, the degree of frailty, and the presence of established risk factors for falls (impaired balance, coronary heart disease, peripheral neuropathy)[31] should be assessed. An individualized approach to reduce the risk of falls and fractures should combine some or all of the following components: regular exercise program to improve muscle strength, balance, and proprioception, withdrawal of psychotropic medications, visual assessment, professional environmental hazard assessment and modification, and the use of hip protectors.[39] Adequate vitamin D and calcium supplementation reduced the risk of falls by 49% in elderly nondiabetic women.[40] This has not been shown in patients with T2DM. The insulin sensitizers thiazolidinediones should not be used in patients with T2DM and a high risk of, or established osteoporosis.[41]

14.4 Summary

Both DM and osteoporosis are pandemic diseases with an increasing prevalence in the future. Patients with T1DM are a high-risk population for osteoporotic fractures. Apart from the short period of insulin deficiency which is associated with impaired bone formation, diabetic complications such as peripheral neuropathy, nephropathy, and peripheral vascular disease are predictors of osteoporotic fractures. Thus, prevention and treatment of

these complications by intensive insulin therapy, screening for low BMD, and a high index of suspicion is recommended in patients with T1DM.

Despite higher mean BMD values, patients with T2DM have an increased fracture risk which is only partially attributable to an increased risk of falls. This suggests that normal BMD values may be misleading. As in T1DM, adequate glycemic control as well as early detection and treatment of diabetic complications are meaningful recommendations to protect skeletal health in patients with T2DM. A comprehensive and individualized practical approach combining regular exercise, vitamin D supplementation, critical review, concurrent medications, visual assessment, environmental hazard assessment, and the use of hip protectors may be useful to reduce the risk of osteoporotic fractures. Thiazolidinediones should be avoided in patients with T2DM and osteoporosis, while bisphosphonates appear to be efficacious and safe drugs in T2DM.

References

1. Schwartz AV. Diabetes mellitus: does it affect bone? *Calcif Tissue Int.* 2003;73:515-519.
2. Inzerillo AM, Epstein S. Osteoporosis and diabetes mellitus. *Rev Endocr Metab Disord.* 2004;5:261-268.
3. Leidig-Bruckner G, Ziegler R. Diabetes mellitus - a risk for osteoporosis? *Exp Clin Endocrinol Diabetes.* 2001;109:493-514.

4. Nicodemus KK, Folsom AR; Iowa Women's Health Study. Type 1 and type 2 diabetes and incident hip fractures in postmenopausal women. *Diabetes Care*. 2001;24:1192-1197.

5. Gunczler P, Lanes R, Paz-Martinez V, et al. Decreased lumbar spine bone mass and low bone turnover in children and adolescents with insulin dependent diabetes mellitus followed longitudinally. *J Pediatr Endocrinol Metab*. 1998;11: 413-419.

6. Valerio G, del Puente A, Esposito-del Puente A, Buono P, Mozzillo E, Francese A. The lumbar bone mineral density is affected by long-term poor metabolic control in adolescents with type 1 diabetes mellitus. *Horm Res*. 2002;58:266-272.

7. Pascual J, Argente J, Lopez MB, et al. Bone mineral density in children and adolescents with diabetes mellitus type 1 of recent onset. *Calcif Tissue Int*. 1998;62:31-35.

8. Liu EY, Wactawski-Wende J, Donahue RP, Dmochowski J, Hovey KM, Quattrin T. Does low bone mineral density start in post-teenage years in women with type 1 diabetes? *Diabetes Care*. 2003;26:2365-2369.

9. Ingberg CM, Palmer M, Aman J, Arvidsson B, Schvarcz E, Berne C. Body composition and bone mineral density in longstanding type 1 diabetes. *J Intern Med*. 2004;255:392-398.

10. Bridges MJ, Moochhala SH, Barbour J, Kelly CA. Influence of diabetes on peripheral bone mineral density in men: a controlled study. *Acta Diabetol*. 2005;42:82-86.

11. Lopez-Ibarra PJ, Pastor MM, Escobar-Jimenez F, et al. Bone mineral density at time of clinical diagnosis of adult-onset type 1 diabetes mellitus. *Endocr Pract*. 2001;7:346-351.

12. Kemink SA, Hermus AR, Swinkels LM, Lutterman JA, Smals AG. Osteopenia in insulin-dependent diabetes mellitus; prevalence and aspects of pathophysiology. *J Endocrinol Invest*. 2000;23:295-303.

13. Tuominen JT, Impivaara O, Puukka P, Ronnemaa T. Bone mineral density in patients with type 1 and type 2 diabetes. *Diabetes Care*. 1999;22:1196-1200.

14. Hampson G, Evans C, Petitt RJ, et al. Bone mineral density, collagen type 1 α 1 genotypes and bone turnover in premenopausal women with diabetes mellitus. *Diabetologia*. 1998;41:1314-1320.

15. Rozadilla A, Nolla JM, Montana E, et al. Bone mineral density in patients with type 1 diabetes mellitus. *Joint Bone Spine*. 2000;67:215-218.

16. Munoz-Torres M, Jodar E, Escobar-Jimenez F, Lopez-Ibarra PJ, Luna JD. Bone mineral density measured by dual X-ray absorptiometry in Spanish patients with insulin-dependent diabetes mellitus. *Calcif Tissue Int*. 1996;58:316-319.

17. Campos Pastor MM, Lopez-Ibarra PJ, Escobar-Jimenez F, Serrano Pardo MD, Garcia-Cervigon AG. Intensive insulin therapy and bone mineral density in type 1 diabetes mellitus: a prospective study. *Osteoporos Int*. 2000;11:455-459.

18. Rix M, Andreassen H, Eskildsen P. Impact of peripheral neuropathy on bone density in patients with type 1 diabetes. *Diabetes Care*. 1999;22:827-831.

19. Clausen P, Feldt-Rasmussen B, Jacobsen P, et al. Microalbuminuria as an early indicator of osteopenia in male insulin-dependent diabetic patients. *Diabet Med*. 1997;14: 1038-1043.

20. Olmos JM, Perez-Castrillon JL, Garcia MT, Garrido JC, Amado JA, Gonzalez-Macias J. Bone densitometry and biochemical bone remodeling markers in type 1 diabetes mellitus. *Bone Miner*. 1994;26:1-8.

21. Lunt H, Florkowski CM, Cundy T, et al. A population-based study of bone mineral density in women with longstanding type 1 (insulin dependent) diabetes. *Diabetes Res Clin Pract*. 1998;40:31-38.

22. Thrailkill KM, Lumpkin CK Jr, Bunn RC, Kemp SF, Fowlkes JL. Is insulin an anabolic agent in bone? Dissecting the diabetic bone for clues. *Am J Physiol Endocrinol Metab*. 2005; 289:E735-E745.

23. Einhorn TA, Boskey AL, Gundberg CM, Vigorita VJ, Devlin VJ, Beyer MM. The mineral and mechanical properties of bone in chronic experimental diabetes. *J Orthop Res*. 1988; 6:317-323.

24. Horcajada-Molteni MN, Chanteranne B, Lebecque P, et al. Amylin and bone metabolism in streptozotocin-induced diabetic rats. *J Bone Miner Res*. 2001;16:958-965.

25. de Liefde II, van der Klift M, de Laet CE, van Daele PL, Hofman A, Pols HA. Bone mineral density and fracture risk in type-2 diabetes mellitus: the Rotterdam Study. *Osteoporos Int*. 2005;16:1713-1720.

26. Strotmeyer ES, Cauley JA, Schwartz AV, et al.; Health ABC Study. Diabetes is associated independently of body composition with BMD and bone volume in older white and black men and women: the Health, Aging, and Body Composition Study. *J Bone Miner Res*. 2004;19:1084-1091.

27. Gerdhem P, Isaksson A, Akesson K, Obrant KJ. Increased bone density and decreased bone turnover, but no evident alteration of fracture susceptibility in elderly women with diabetes mellitus. *Osteoporos Int*. 2005;16:1506-1512.

28. Wakasugi M, Wakao R, Tawata M, Gan N, Koizumi K, Onaya T. Bone mineral density measured by dual energy x-ray absorptiometry in patients with non-insulin-dependent diabetes mellitus. *Bone*. 1993;14:29-33.

29. Dobnig H, Piswanger-Sölkner JC, Roth M, et al. Type 2 diabetes mellitus in nursing home patients: effects on bone turnover, bone mass, and fracture risk. *J Clin Endocrinol Metab*. 2006;91:3355-3363.

30. Perez-Castrillon JL, De Luis D, Martin-Escudero JC, Asensio T, del Amo R, Izaola O. Non-insulin-dependent diabetes, bone mineral density, and cardiovascular risk factors. *J Diabetes Complications*. 2004;18:317-321.

31. Schwartz AV, Hillier TA, Sellmeyer DE, et al. Older women with diabetes have a higher risk of falls: a prospective study. *Diabetes Care*. 2002;25:1749-1754.

32. Williams JP, Blair HC, McDonald JM, et al. Regulation of osteoclastic bone resorption by glucose. *Biochem Biophys Res Commun*. 1997;235:646-651.

33. Vashishth D, Gibson GJ, Khoury JI, Schaffler MB, Kimura J, Fyhrie DP. Influence of nonenzymatic glycation on biomechanical properties of cortical bone. *Bone*. 2001;28: 195-201.

34. Saito M, Fujii K, Mori Y, Marumo K. Role of collagen enzymatic and glycation induced cross-links as a determinant of bone quality in spontaneously diabetic WBN/Kob rats. *Osteoporos Int*. 2006;17:1514-1523.

35. Okazaki R, Totsuka Y, Hamano K, et al. Metabolic improvement of poorly controlled noninsulin-dependent diabetes mellitus decreases bone turnover. *J Clin Endocrinol Metab*. 1997;82:2915-2920.

36. Baynes KC, Boucher BJ, Feskens EJ, Kromhout D. Vitamin D, glucose tolerance and insulinaemia in elderly men. *Diabetologia*. 1997;40:344-347.

37. Thomas T, Burguera B, Melton LJ III, et al. Role of serum leptin, insulin, and estrogen levels as potential mediators of the relationship between fat mass and bone mineral density in men versus women. *Bone.* 2001;29:114-120.

38. Lenchik L, Register TC, Hsu FC, et al. Adiponectin as a novel determinant of bone mineral density and visceral fat. *Bone.* 2003;33:646-651.

39. Kannus P, Sievannen H, Palvanen M, Jarvinen T, Parkkari J. Prevention of falls and consequent injuries in elderly people. *Lancet.* 2005;366:1885-1893.

40. Bischoff HA, Stahelin HB, Dick W, et al. Effects of vitamin D and calcium supplementation on falls: a randomized controlled trial. *J Bone Miner Res.* 2003;18:343-351.

41. Schwartz AV, Sellmeyer DE, Vittinghoff E, et al. Thiazolidinedione use and bone loss in older diabetic adults. *J Clin Endocrinol Metab.* 2006;91:3349-3354.

Vitamin D and Muscle

15

Heike Bischoff-Ferrari and Bess Dawson-Hughes

15.1 Introduction

Vitamin D modulates fracture risk in two ways: by decreasing falls and increasing bone density. Two 2009 metaanalyses of double-blind randomized controlled trials came to the conclusion that vitamin D reduces the risk of falls by 19%, the risk of hip fracture by 18%, and the risk of any nonvertebral fracture by 20%; however, this benefit was dose-dependent. Fall prevention was only observed in trial of at least 700 IU vitamin D per day, and fracture prevention required a received dose (treatment dose*adherence) of more than 400 IU vitamin D per day. Antifall efficacy started with achieved 25-hydroxyvitamin D levels of at least 60 nmol/L (24 ng/mL) and antifracture efficacy started with achieved 25-hydroxyvitamin D levels of at least 75 nmol/L (30 ng/mL) and both end points improved further with higher achieved 25-hydroxyvitamin D levels.

Based on these evidence-based data derived from the general older population, vitamin D supplementation should be at least 700–1,000 IU/day and taken with good adherence to cover the needs for both fall and fracture prevention. Ideally, the target range for 25-hydroxyvitamin D should be at least 75 nmol/L, which may need more than 700–1,000 IU vitamin D in individuals with severe vitamin D deficiency or those overweight.

15.1.1 Target Both Muscle and Bone

Critical for the understanding and prevention of fractures, especially at older age, is their close relationship with muscle weakness[1] and falling.[2,3] Over 90% of fractures occur after a fall, and fall rates increase with age[4] and poor muscle strength or function.[4] Mechanistically, the circumstances[5] and the direction[6] of a fall determine the type of fracture, whereas bone density and factors that attenuate a fall, such as better strength or better padding, critically determine whether a fracture will take place when the person lands on a certain bone.[7] Moreover, falling may affect bone density through increased immobility from self-restriction of activities.[8] It is well known that falls may lead to psychological trauma known as fear of falling.[9] After their first fall, about 30% of people develop fear of falling resulting in self-restriction of activities and decreased quality of life.[8]

Notably, bisphosphonate treatment alone may not reduce fractures among individuals of 80 years of age and older in the presence of nonskeletal risk factors for fractures, such as muscle weakness and falling, despite an improvement in bone metabolism.[10]

15.1.2 Vitamin D: Its Role in Muscle Health

In humans, four lines of evidence support a role of vitamin D in muscle health. First, proximal muscle weakness is a prominent feature of the clinical syndrome of vitamin D deficiency.[11] Vitamin D deficiency myopathy includes proximal muscle weakness, diffuse muscle pain, and gait impairments such as waddling

H. Bischoff-Ferrari (✉)
Department of Rheumatology and Institute of Physical Medicine, Centre on Aging and Mobility, University Hospital Zurich, Gloria Strasse 25, 8091 Zurich, Switzerland
e-mail: heikeabischoff@aol.com

P. Burckhardt et al. (eds.), *Nutritional Influences on Bone Health*,
DOI: 10.1007/978-1-84882-978-7_15, © Springer-Verlag London Limited 2010

way of walking.[12] Second, VDR is expressed in human muscle tissue,[13] and VDR activation may promote de novo protein synthesis in muscle.[14] Suggesting a role of vitamin D in muscle development, mice lacking the VDR show a skeletal muscle phenotype with smaller and variable muscle fibers and persistence of immature muscle gene expression during adult life.[15,16] These abnormalities persist after correction of systemic calcium metabolism by a rescue diet.[16]

Third, several observational studies suggest a positive association between 25-hydroxyvitamin D and muscle strength or lower extremity function in older people.[17,18] Finally, in several double-blind randomized controlled trials, vitamin D supplementation increased muscle strength and balance[19,20] and reduced the risk of falling in community-dwelling individuals,[20–22] as well as in institutionalized individuals.[19,23] Notably, a study by Glerup and colleagues suggests that vitamin D deficiency may cause muscular impairment even before adverse effects on bone occur.[11]

15.1.3 Importance of 25-Hydroxyvitamin D Status and Dose of Vitamin D with Respect to Function, Strength, and Risk of Falling

A dose–response relationship between vitamin D status and muscle health was examined in NHANES III (The Third National Health and Nutrition Examination Survey) including 4,100 ambulatory adults of 60 years of age and older. Muscle function measured as the 8-foot walk test and the repeated sit-to-stand test was poorest in subjects with the lowest 25-hydroxyvitamin D (below 20 nmol/L) levels. Similar results were found in a Dutch cohort of older individuals.[17] Notably, while from the smaller Dutch cohort a threshold of 50 nmol/L has been suggested for optimal function,[17] a threshold beyond which function would not further improve was not identified in the larger NHANES III survey, even beyond the upper end of the reference range (> 100 nmol/L).[18] In NHANES III, a similar benefit of higher 25-hydroxyvitamin D status was documented by gender, level of physical activity, and level of calcium intake.

These associations between higher 25-hydroxyvitamin D status and better function observed in epidemiologic

studies in the US and Europe were confirmed by three recent double-blind RCTs with 800 IU vitamin D3 plus calcium compared to calcium alone resulting in a 4–11% gain in lower extremity strength or function,[19,20] and in an up to 28% improvement in body sway[20,22] in older adults of 65+ years of age, within 2–12 month of treatment.

A dose-dependent benefit of vitamin D in regard to fall prevention was suggested by a 2004 metaanalysis[24] and a recent multidose double-blind RCT among 124 nursing home residents receiving 200, 400, 600, or 800 IU vitamin D compared to placebo over a 5-month period.[23] Participants in the 800 IU group had a 72% lower rate of falls than those taking placebo or a lower dose of vitamin D (rate ratio=0.28; 95% confidence interval=0.11–0.75).[23] Including this trial, *a most recent metaanalysis of 8 high-quality double-blind RCTs* ($n=2,426$) found significant heterogeneity by dose (low-dose: <700 IU/day vs. higher dose: 700–1,000 IU/day; p-value 0.02) and achieved 25-hydroxyvitamin D level (<60 nmol/L vs. ≥60 nmol/L; p-value = 0.005).[25] *Higher dose supplemental vitamin D* reduced fall risk by 19% (pooled relative risk (RR)=0.81; 95% CI, 0.71–0.92; $n=1,921$ from seven trials), but a lower dose did not (pooled RR = 1.10, 95% CI, 0.89–1.35 from two trials); also, achieved serum 25-hydroxyvitamin D concentrations less than 60 nmol/L did not reduce the risk of falling (pooled RR = 1.35, 95% CI, 0.98–1.84). Notably, at the higher dose of 700–1,000 IU vitamin D, this metaanalysis documented a 38% reduction in the risk of falling with treatment duration of 2–5 months and a sustained significant effect of 17% fall reduction with treatment duration of 12–36 months. Thus benefits of vitamin D on fall prevention are rapid and sustained, provided a high enough dose.

15.1.4 Dose-Dependent Benefit of Vitamin D for Any Nonvertebral Fractures and Fractures of the Hip

Consistent with the 2009 metaanalysis of vitamin D and fall prevention, a 2009 metaanalysis of 12 double-blind RCTs for nonvertebral fractures ($n=42,279$) and 8 RCTs for hip fractures ($n=40,886$) found that antifracture efficacy of vitamin D is dose-dependent and increases significantly with a higher achieved level of

Table 15.1 Nonvertebral fracture reduction with vitamin D based on evidence from double-blind RCTs

Subgroups by received dose of vitamin D	Fracture (%)	Reduction
Pooled analysis from three trials with low-dose vitamin D (340–380 IU/day)	+2	Ø
Pooled analysis from nine trials with higher dose vitamin D (482–770 IU/day)	−20	Sig.
Pooled subgroup analysis from trials with higher dose vitamin D (482–770 IE/Tag)		
Vitamin D2	−10	Ø
Vitamin D3	−23	Sig.
Age 65–74	−33	Sig.
Age 75+	−17	Sig.
Institutionalized 65+	−15	Sig.
Community-dwelling 65+	−29	Sig.
Vitamin D plus calcium	−21	Sig.
Vitamin D main effects	−21	Sig.

Adapted from Bischoff-Ferrari et al. Copyright (2009), American Medical Association[26]

25-hydroxyvitamin D in the treatment group starting at 75 nmol/L.[26] No fracture reduction was observed for a received dose of 400 IU or less per day, while a higher received dose of 482–770 IU supplemental vitamin D per day reduced nonvertebral fractures by 20% (pooled RR = 0.80; 95% CI, 0.72–0.89; n = 33,265 from nine trials) and hip fractures by 18% (pooled RR = 0.82; 95% CI, 0.69–0.97; n = 31,872 from five trials). Notably, subgroup analyses for the prevention of nonvertebral fractures with the higher received dose suggested a benefit in all subgroups of the older population, and possibly better fracture reduction with D3 compared to D2, while additional calcium did not further improve antifracture efficacy (see Table 15.1).

15.1.5 Adding Calcium to Vitamin D

The observed calcium-independent benefit of vitamin D on nonvertebral fracture prevention at a vitamin D dose greater than 400 IU/day may be explained by a calcium-sparing effect of vitamin D,[27,28] which is supported by two recent epidemiologic studies suggesting that both PTH suppression[28] and hip bone density[29] may only depend on a higher calcium intake if serum 25-hydroxyvitamin D levels are very low.

Thus as calcium absorption is improved with higher serum 25-hysdroxyvitamin D levels,[28,30] future studies may need to evaluate whether current calcium intake recommendations with higher doses of vitamin D beyond 2,000 IU/day are safe or require downward adjustment.[30] If dietary calcium is a threshold nutrient, as suggested by Dr. Heaney,[31] then the threshold for optimal calcium absorption may be at a lower calcium intake when vitamin D supplementation is adequate.

15.1.6 Are Current Recommended Intakes for Vitamin D Sufficient for Optimal Musculoskeletal Health?

The recommended adequate intake of vitamin D as defined by the Institute of Medicine in 1997 is 200 IU/day for adults up to 50 years of age, 400 IU/day for adults between 51 and 70 years of age, and 600 IU/day for those aged 70 years and over. These recommendations are insufficient to meet the requirements of optimal fall and nonvertebral fracture prevention. The current intake recommendation for older persons (600 IU/day) may bring most individuals to 50–60 nmol/L, but not to a threshold of at least 75 nmol/L[32] where fall and fracture prevention occurs.

Studies suggest that 700–1,000 IU of vitamin D per day may bring 50% of younger and older adults up to 75–100 nmol/L.[33-35] Thus to bring most older adults to the desirable range of at least 75 nmol/L, vitamin D doses higher than 700–1,000 IU would be needed. According to studies in younger adults, intakes of as high as 4,000–10,000 IU are safe,[36,37] and 4,000 IU may bring 88% of healthy young men and women to at least 75 nmol/L.[37] Heaney and colleagues, in a study of healthy men, estimated that 1,000 IU cholecalciferol per day are needed during winter months in Nebraska to maintain a late summer starting level of 70 nmol/L, while baseline levels between 20 and 40 nmol/L may require a daily dose of 2,200 IU vitamin D to reach and maintain 80 nmol/L.[31,36] These results indicate that individuals with a lower starting level may need a higher dose of vitamin D to achieve desirable levels, while relatively lower doses may be sufficient in individuals who start at higher baseline levels.

Based on a dose–response calculation proposed by Dr. Heaney of about 1.0 nmol per 40 IU at the lower end of the distribution and 0.6 nmol per 40 IU at the upper end,[31] 2,000 IU vitamin D per day may bring a large majority of the US population into the range of 80 nmol/L or higher. Thus, high 25-hydroxyvitamin D levels observed in healthy outdoor workers are 135 nmol/L in farmers and 163 nmol/L[38] in lifeguards. As a first sign of toxicity, only serum 25(OH)D levels of above 220 nmol/L have been associated with hypercalcemia.[39]

Most vulnerable to low vitamin D levels are older individual,[40,41] individuals living in northern latitudes with prolonged winters,[42,43] obese individuals,[44] and individuals of all ages with dark skin pigmentation living in northern latitudes.[32,45,46]

15.1.7 In Summary

Based on the evidence from randomized controlled trials, vitamin D supplementation reduces both falls and nonvertebral fractures, including those at the hip. However, this benefit is dose-dependent. According to two 2009 metaanalyses of double-blind RCTs, no fall reduction was observed for a dose of less than 700 IU/day, while a higher dose of 700–1,000 IU supplemental vitamin D per day reduced falls by 19%.[25] Similarly, no fracture reduction was observed for a received dose of 400 IU or less per day, while a higher received dose of 482–770 IU supplemental vitamin D per day reduced nonvertebral fractures by 20% and hip fractures by 18%. The antifracture effect was present in all subgroups of the older population and was most pronounced among those community-dwelling (−29%) and those of 65–74 years of age (−33%).

With respect to desirable 25-hydroxyvitamin D levels, fall prevention and nonvertebral fracture prevention increased significantly with higher achieved 25-hydroxyvitamin D levels in the 2009 metaanalyses. Fall prevention occurred with 25-hydroxyvitamin D levels of 60 nmol/L up to 95,[25] while 75–112 nmol/L were required for nonvertebral fracture prevention.[26] Given the absence of data beyond this beneficial range, these recent metaanalyses do not preclude the possibility that higher doses or higher achieved 25-hydroxyvitamin D concentrations would have been even more efficient in reducing falls and nonvertebral fractures.

References

1. Cummings SR, Nevitt MC, Browner WS, et al. Risk factors for hip fracture in white women. Study of Osteoporotic Fractures Research Group. *N Engl J Med.* 1995;332:767-773.
2. Prevention CoDCa. Fatalities and injuries from falls among older adults–United States, 1993-2003 and 2001-2005. *Morb Mortal Wkly Rep.* 2006;55:1221-1224.
3. Schwartz AV, Nevitt MC, Brown BW Jr, Kelsey JL. Increased falling as a risk factor for fracture among older women: the study of osteoporotic fractures. *Am J Epidemiol.* 2005;161:180-185.
4. Tinetti ME. Risk factors for falls among elderly persons living in the community. *N Engl J Med.* 1988;319:1701-1707.
5. Cummings SR, Nevitt MC. Non-skeletal determinants of fractures: the potential importance of the mechanics of falls. Study of Osteoporotic Fractures Research Group. *Osteoporos Int.* 1994;4 suppl 1:67-70.
6. Nguyen ND, Frost SA, Center JR, Eisman JA, Nguyen TV. Development of a nomogram for individualizing hip fracture risk in men and women. *Osteoporos Int.* 2007;17:17.
7. Nevitt MC, Cummings SR. Type of fall and risk of hip and wrist fractures: the study of osteoporotic fractures. The Study of Osteoporotic Fractures Research Group. *J Am Geriatr Soc.* 1993;41:1226-1234.
8. Vellas BJ, Wayne SJ, Romero LJ, Baumgartner RN, Garry PJ. Fear of falling and restriction of mobility in elderly fallers. *Age Ageing.* 1997;26:189-193.
9. Arfken CL, Lach HW, Birge SJ, Miller JP. The prevalence and correlates of fear of falling in elderly persons living in the community. *Am J Public Health.* 1994;84:565-570.
10. McClung MR, Geusens P, Miller PD, et al. Effect of risedronate on the risk of hip fracture in elderly women. Hip Intervention Program Study Group. *N Engl J Med.* 2001;344:333-340.
11. Glerup H, Mikkelsen K, Poulsen L, et al. Hypovitaminosis D myopathy without biochemical signs of osteomalacic bone involvement. *Calcif Tissue Int.* 2000;66:419-424.
12. Schott GD, Wills MR. Muscle weakness in osteomalacia. *Lancet.* 1976;1:626-629.
13. Bischoff-Ferrari HA, Borchers M, Gudat F, Durmuller U, Stahelin HB, Dick W. Vitamin D receptor expression in human muscle tissue decreases with age. *J Bone Miner Res.* 2004;19:265-269.
14. Sorensen OH, Lund B, Saltin B, et al. Myopathy in bone loss of ageing: improvement by treatment with 1 alpha-hydroxycholecalciferol and calcium. *Clin Sci (Colch).* 1979;56:157-161.
15. Bouillon R, Bischoff-Ferrari H, Willett W. Vitamin D and health: perspectives from mice and man. *J Bone Miner Res.* 2008;28:28.
16. Endo I, Inoue D, Mitsui T, et al. Deletion of vitamin D receptor gene in mice results in abnormal skeletal muscle development with deregulated expression of myoregulatory transcription factors. Endocrinology 2003;144:5138-5144. Epub 2003 Aug 13.
17. Wicherts IS, van Schoor NM, Boeke AJ, et al. Vitamin D status predicts physical performance and its decline in older persons. *J Clin Endocrinol Metab.* 2007;6:6.
18. Bischoff-Ferrari HA, Dietrich T, Orav EJ, et al. Higher 25-hydroxyvitamin D concentrations are associated with better lower-extremity function in both active and inactive persons aged ≥60 y. *Am J Clin Nutr.* 2004;80:752-758.

19. Bischoff HA, Stahelin HB, Dick W, et al. Effects of vitamin D and calcium supplementation on falls: a randomized controlled trial. *J Bone Miner Res.* 2003;18:343-351.

20. Pfeifer M, Begerow B, Minne HW, Suppan K, Fahrleitner-Pammer A, Dobnig H. Effects of a long-term vitamin D and calcium supplementation on falls and parameters of muscle function in community-dwelling older individuals. *Osteoporos Int.* 2008;16:16.

21. Bischoff-Ferrari HA, Orav EJ, Dawson-Hughes B. Effect of cholecalciferol plus calcium on falling in ambulatory older men and women: a 3-year randomized controlled trial. *Arch Intern Med.* 2006;166:424-430.

22. Pfeifer M, Begerow B, Minne HW, Abrams C, Nachtigall D, Hansen C. Effects of a short-term vitamin D and calcium supplementation on body sway and secondary hyperparathyroidism in elderly women. *J Bone Miner Res.* 2000;15:1113-1118.

23. Broe KE, Chen TC, Weinberg J, Bischoff-Ferrari HA, Holick MF, Kiel DP. A higher dose of vitamin d reduces the risk of falls in nursing home residents: a randomized, multiple-dose study. *J Am Geriatr Soc.* 2007;55:234-239.

24. Bischoff-Ferrari HA, Dawson-Hughes B, Willett CW, et al. Effect of vitamin D on falls: a meta-analysis. *JAMA.* 2004;291:1999-2006.

25. Bischoff-Ferrari HA, Dawson-Hughes B, Staehelin HB, et al. Fall prevention with supplemental and active forms of vitamin D: a meta-analysis of randomized controlled trials. *Br Med J.* 2009;339:b3692.

26. Bischoff-Ferrari HA, Willett WC, Wong JB, et al. Prevention of nonverterbal fractures with oral vitamin D and dose dependency: a meta-analysis of randomized controlled trials. *Arch Intern Med.* 2009;169:551-561.

27. Heaney RP, Barger-Lux MJ, Dowell MS, Chen TC, Holick MF. Calcium absorptive effects of vitamin D and its major metabolites. *J Clin Endocrinol Metab.* 1997;82:4111-4116.

28. Steingrimsdottir L, Gunnarsson O, Indridason OS, Franzson L, Sigurdsson G. Relationship between serum parathyroid hormone levels, vitamin D sufficiency, and calcium intake. *JAMA.* 2005;294:2336-2341.

29. Bischoff-Ferrari HA, Kiel DP, Dawson-Hughes B, et al. Dietary calcium and serum 25-hydroxyvitamin D status in relation to BMD among U.S. adults. *J Bone Miner Res.* 2009;24:935-942.

30. Heaney RP, Dowell MS, Hale CA, Bendich A. Calcium absorption varies within the reference range for serum 25-hydroxyvitamin D. *J Am Coll Nutr.* 2003;22:142-146.

31. Heaney RP. The Vitamin D requirement in health and disease. *J Steroid Biochem Mol Biol.* 2005;15:15.

32. Bischoff-Ferrari HA, Dietrich T, Orav EJ, Dawson-Hughes B. Positive association between 25-hydroxy vitamin d levels and bone mineral density: a population-based study of younger and older adults. *Am J Med.* 2004;116:634-639.

33. Tangpricha V, Pearce EN, Chen TC, Holick MF. Vitamin D insufficiency among free-living healthy young adults. *Am J Med.* 2002;112:659-662.

34. Barger-Lux MJ, Heaney RP, Dowell S, Chen TC, Holick MF. Vitamin D and its major metabolites: serum levels after graded oral dosing in healthy men. *Osteoporos Int.* 1998;8:222-230.

35. Dawson-Hughes B. Impact of vitamin D and calcium on bone and mineral metabolism in older adults. In: Holick MF, ed. *Biologic Effects of Light 2001.* Boston, MA: Kluwer Academic; 2002:175-183.

36. Heaney RP, Davies KM, Chen TC, Holick MF, Barger-Lux MJ. Human serum 25-hydroxycholecalciferol response to extended oral dosing with cholecalciferol. *Am J Clin Nutr.* 2003;77:204-210.

37. Vieth R, Chan PC, MacFarlane GD. Efficacy and safety of vitamin D3 intake exceeding the lowest observed adverse effect level. *Am J Clin Nutr.* 2001;73:288-294.

38. Haddad JG, Chyu KJ. Competitive protein-binding radioassay for 25-hydroxycholecalciferol. *J Clin Endocrinol Metab.* 1971;33:992-995.

39. Vieth R, Chan PC, MacFarlane GD. Efficacy and safety of vitamin D3 intake exceeding the lowest observed adverse effect level Vitamin D supplementation, 25-hydroxyvitamin D concentrations, and safety. *Am J Clin Nutr.* 2001;73:288-294.

40. McKenna MJ. Differences in vitamin D status between countries in young adults and the elderly. *Am J Med.* 1992;93:69-77.

41. Theiler R, Stahelin HB, Tyndall A, Binder K, Somorjai G, Bischoff HA. Calcidiol, calcitriol and parathyroid hormone serum concentrations in institutionalized and ambulatory elderly in Switzerland. *Int J Vitam Nutr Res.* 1999;69:96-105.

42. Webb AR, Kline L, Holick MF. Influence of season and latitude on the cutaneous synthesis of vitamin D3: exposure to winter sunlight in Boston and Edmonton will not promote vitamin D3 synthesis in human skin. *J Clin Endocrinol Metab.* 1988;67:373-378.

43. Dawson-Hughes B, Harris SS, Dallal GE. Plasma calcidiol, season, and serum parathyroid hormone concentrations in healthy elderly men and women. *Am J Clin Nutr.* 1997;65:67-71.

44. Parikh SJ, Edelman M, Uwaifo GI, et al. The relationship between obesity and serum 1, 25-dihydroxy vitamin D concentrations in healthy adults. *J Clin Endocrinol Metab.* 2004;89:1196-1199.

45. Looker AC, Dawson-Hughes B, Calvo MS, Gunter EW, Sahyoun NR. Serum 25-hydroxyvitamin D status of adolescents and adults in two seasonal subpopulations from NHANES III. *Bone.* 2002;30:771-777.

46. Nesby-O'Dell S, Scanlon KS, Cogswell ME, et al. Hypovitaminosis D prevalence and determinants among African American and white women of reproductive age: third National Health and Nutrition Examination Survey, 1988-1994. *Am J Clin Nutr.* 2002;76:187-192.

Vitamin D and Bone Health

Paul Lips

16

16.1 Introduction

Vitamin D deficiency and insufficiency are widespread among the population, especially in risk groups such as young children, pregnant women, older persons, in particular the homebound and institutionalized, and nonwestern immigrants.[1–3] Consequences are mineralization defects, resulting in rickets or osteomalacia, and secondary hyperparathyroidism resulting in osteoporosis and fractures. Many studies have been done in older persons, but data from the general adult population are lacking. Vitamin D deficiency and insufficiency can be prevented and the potential gain is high. This paper starts with the pathophysiological background and the data coming from molecular biology, in particular the knock-out models. Subsequently, mineralization disorders, as well as risk factors, are discussed. This is followed by the relationship between vitamin D deficiency, osteoporosis, and fractures. The pathophysiology and the prevention of bone loss and fractures will be discussed. Subsequently the implications for public health, vitamin D requirement, and the use of supplements will be discussed.

16.2 Pathophysiological Background

Vitamin D3 is synthesized in the skin under the influence of ultraviolet radiation. Subsequently, it is hydroxylated in the liver to 25-hydroxyvitamin D (25(OH)D) and in

the kidney to 1,25-dihydroxyvitamin D (1,25(OH)2D). The active metabolite, 1,25(OH)2D, stimulates the absorption of calcium from the gut, which is used for the formation of hydroxyl apatite during the process of bone mineralization.[4] However, the mineralization of new organic bone matrix (osteoid tissue) can occur independently of vitamin D. It is a passive process mainly dependent upon the availability of calcium and phosphate. More recently, it has become clear from studies with knock-out mice that 1,25(OH)2D is not needed for bone mineralization.[5] The mouse that lacks the 1-α hydroxylase enzyme cannot synthesize 1,25(OH)2D, but a high calcium and lactose diet can cure the rickets. The vitamin D receptor null mouse can function without genomic vitamin D effect. Longitudinal growth is disturbed in this model and there is no hair growth, but mineralization can be normal when a very high calcium rescue diet is offered. Patients with a nonfunctional vitamin D receptor have decreased longitudinal bone growth, which is clearly visible in families with vitamin D-dependent rickets type 2. These are characterized by rickets, low body height, and baldness.[6]

16.3 Rickets and Osteomalacia

In case of long-standing severe vitamin D deficiency, mineralization defects will develop resulting in rickets in children and osteomalacia in adults. In children, the hypertrophied cartilage zone of the growth plate does not mineralize and cartilage proliferation is prolonged. The growth plate becomes thick, wide, and irregular. This results in wide and thick epiphysial zones. In children as well as in adults, remodeling is abnormal during long-standing severe vitamin D deficiency. After bone resorption, a new bone matrix is formed, the osteoid

P. Lips
Internal Medicine Division, Section of Endocrinology,
VU University Medical Center, De Boelelaan 1117,
Amsterdam 1081 HV, The Netherlands
e-mail: p.lips@vumc.nl

P. Burckhardt et al. (eds.), *Nutritional Influences on Bone Health*,
DOI: 10.1007/978-1-84882-978-7_16, © Springer-Verlag London Limited 2010

tissue, but this does not mineralize leading to osteomalacia.[7] Rickets and osteomalacia are characterized by generalized bone pain and muscle weakness, especially of the proximal muscles. In children with rickets, the bones may be weaker than normal and may show bowing. Rickets and osteomalacia occur with very low serum 25(OH)D levels, usually lower than 12.5 nmol/L (5 ng/mL). A low calcium diet, low dairy intake, and malabsorption, as in coeliac disease, increase the risk of rickets and osteomalacia.

Laboratory findings include low serum calcium and phosphate, low urinary calcium excretion, and elevated serum alkaline phosphatase level. Radiologic findings include unsharp images of the spine and tubular bones, and Looser zones or pseudo fractures. The diagnosis can be confirmed by demonstrating increased osteoid tissue (osteoid seam thickness >15 μm) and absent tetracycline double labels.[7] Rickets and osteomalacia were very rare three or four decades ago, but now occur more frequently due to vitamin D deficiency in risk groups such as older persons and immigrants.

16.4 Bone Loss, Osteoporosis, and Fractures

When vitamin D deficiency is less severe, mineralization may occur almost normally. However, the somewhat lower calcium absorption results in secondary hyperparathyroidism. This leads to high bone turnover and bone loss. This may contribute to the risk of osteoporosis and fractures (Fig. 16.1).

Many epidemiologic studies confirm that mean serum parathyroid hormone (PTH) levels are higher in case of vitamin D deficiency (serum 25(OH)D <25 nmol/L) or insufficiency (serum 25(OH)D between 25 and 50 nmol/L). Serum PTH may be 15–30% higher in patients with vitamin D deficiency or insufficiency compared to vitamin D replete subjects (serum 25(OH)D >50 nmol/L).

In the Longitudinal Aging Study Amsterdam, serum PTH decreased from 5.1 pmol/L when serum 25(OH)D was lower than 25 nmol/L to 3.3 pmol/L when serum 25(OH)D was between 50 and 75 nmol/L.[8] According to a Loess plot, serum PTH decreased further to 3.1 pmol/L when serum 25(OH)D became higher than 75 nmol/L (Fig. 16.2). The latter decrease was marginal and confidence intervals increased. In the same study serum osteocalcin decreased from 2.5 nmol/L when serum 25(OH)D was lower than 25 pmol/L to 2.1 nmol/L when serum 25(OH)D was higher than 40 nmol/L. The bone resorption marker urinary DPD/creatinine decreased from 6.7 nmol/mL with low serum 25(OH)D to 5.5 nmol/mL when serum 25(OH)D was higher than 40 nmol/L. The bone mineral density in the total hip, femoral trochanter, and total body increased with serum 25(OH)D to about 50 nmol/L. The increases of BMD were significant in the lower part of the curve only (Fig. 16.2). Very similar

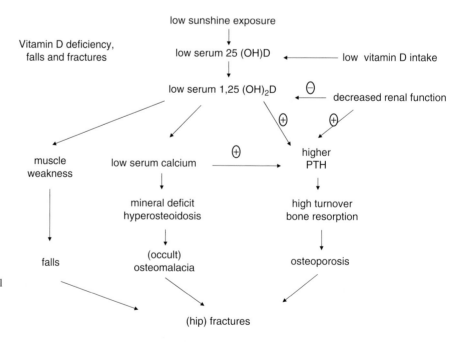

Fig. 16.1 Pathophysiological pathways from vitamin D deficiency to falls and fractures

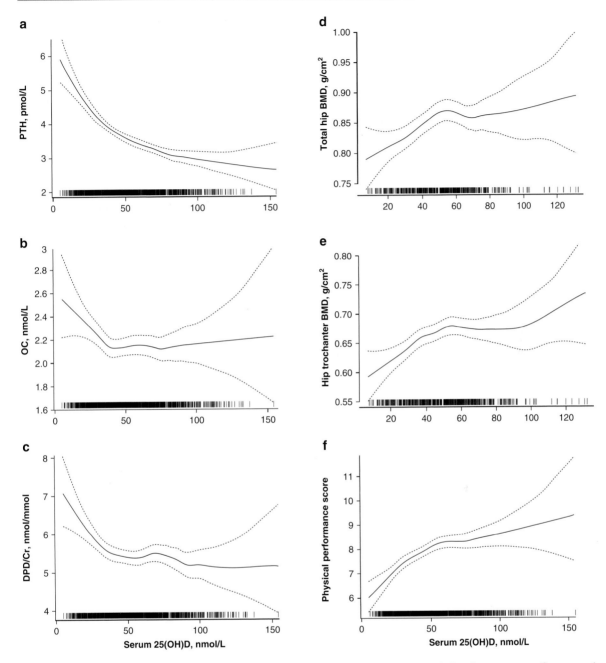

Fig. 16.2 Relationship between serum 25(OH)D and serum PTH (**a**), bone turnover markers osteocalcin (OC) (**b**), deoxypyridino-line/creatinine (DPD/Cr) (**c**), bone mineral density in total hip (**d**) and trochanter (**e**), and physical performance score (**f**), presented as LOESS plots. Reproduced with permission from Kuchuk et al.[8] *Copyright 2009, The Endocrine Society*

cross-sectional data have come from the baseline results of a very large clinical trial on the selective estrogen receptor modulator bazedoxifen.[9] Results of the NHANES-III study showed that with increasing serum 25(OH)D, bone mineral density of the hip increased up to serum 25(OH)D of about 90 nmol/L.[10]

The risk for falls and fractures was also studied in LASA. An interaction with age was observed with significant results between 65 and 75 years and no significance over 75 years of age.[11] Persons with serum 25(OH)D lower than 30 nmol/L had a relative risk of about three compared to persons with serum 25(OH)D higher than 30 nmol/L. A similar threshold was observed regarding the risk of falls.[12] A study from Australia in patients with severe vitamin D deficiency showed a plateau for serum 1,25(OH)2D, calcium absorption, and bone markers at a serum 25(OH)D of 25 nmol/L.[13]

Many randomized placebo-controlled clinical trials have been performed with bone mineral density and fracture incidence as outcomes. In the Amsterdam Vitamin D Study, the BMD of the femoral neck increased 2.2% after 2-year supplementation with 400 IU of vitamin D3 and an increase of serum 25(OH)D from 22 to 60 nmol/L.[14] The BMD increase in most trials was less than that could be predicted from cross-sectional epidemiological data. The results of clinical trials with fracture incidence as outcome have been equivocal. Most trials have combined vitamin D and calcium vs. double placebo such as the classical trial from Lyon.[15] A trial with 100,000 IU of vitamin D per 4 months without calcium showed a decrease of fractures in the United Kingdom.[16] The other trials used combinations of 400 or 800 IU of vitamin D in combination with calcium.[17–21] Several excellent metaanalyses have been done showing small differences.[22–25] Two French studies using vitamin D 800 IU/day and calcium 1,200 mg/day vs. double placebo in nursing home residents have a major impact on the results of these metaanalyses as both trials were significantly positive and showed a fracture reduction of 20%.[15,26] A metaanalysis of Bischoff-Ferrari showed that trials with 800 IU/day tended to be more often significant than trials with 400 IU/day.[22] The metaanalysis of Tang included a sensitivity analysis showing that the results were significantly better in the age groups of 80 years and older compared to younger age groups, in institutionalized elderly compared with older persons in the community, when compliance was higher than 80% compared with lower compliance, a vitamin D dose of 800 IU or higher compared with a dose lower than 800 IU, a low baseline dietary calcium intake compared with a normal baseline intake, and with a calcium supplement of 1,200 mg/day or higher compared with lower than 1,200 mg.[25] The latter results confirm the high impact of the two trials from Lyon where the nursing home residents had a very low baseline calcium intake.[15,26] It can be learned from the individual trials and the metaanalyses that results of vitamin D and calcium supplementation highly depend on the setting and the baseline situation. In general, a reduction of fracture incidence of about 10% can be obtained with calcium and vitamin D supplementation.

16.5 Implications for Public Health

Cross-sectional epidemiological studies show relationships between serum 25(OH)D and serum PTH, bone turnover markers, bone mineral density, and fall and fracture risk. The required serum 25(OH)D levels or thresholds were different for these outcomes being higher than 75 nmol/L for serum PTH, 25–40 nmol/L for bone turnover parameters, between 50 and 90 nmol/L for bone mineral density, and 30 nmol/L for fracture risk.[8,10,13] Cross-sectional epidemiological studies show a higher impact of vitamin D status on bone mineral density than clinical trials, but there is clearly a lack of data on bone mineral density from randomized clinical trials. Almost all data refer to populations of older persons, and data for adults between 20 and 65 years of age are scarce. The establishment of the required serum 25(OH)D level has a major impact on required vitamin D intake or vitamin D supplementation dose. When the required serum 25(OH)D level is increased from 30 to 50 nmol/L, all older persons should take a vitamin D supplement. When the required serum 25(OH)D is increased from 50 to 75 nmol/L, then almost all adults should take vitamin D supplements for most of the year or throughout the year. When vitamin supplementation is recommended, it can mean life-long supplementation and the side effects of supplementation use for many years are not known. In the Women's Health Initiative Study, vitamin D supplementation led to an increase of renal stones.[21] However, it is not known whether some persons are more sensitive to side effects of vitamin D than others. A parallel to possible side effects of calcium supplementation with regard to the cardiovascular system should be drawn.[27] Nevertheless, it is of utmost importance to improve vitamin D status in large parts of the population, particularly in risk groups such as young children, persons with pigmented skin and little sunshine exposure, pregnant women, and older persons especially the institutionalized. According to this, recent recommendations of the Dutch Health Council[28] are made (Table 16.1). Food fortification should also be stimulated. The effect of such programs should be investigated.

Table 16.1 Dutch Health Council: new recommendations for vitamin D

Daily 10 μg (400 IU) extra for
Children up to 4 years
Women 4–50 years, men 4–70 years with dark skin and little sunshine exposure
Women up to 50 years with veil
Pregnant women, breast feeding
Women >50 years and men >70 years

Daily 20 μg (800 IU) extra for
Patients with osteoporosis
Residents of care or nursing homes
Women >50 years, men >70 years with dark skin and little sunshine exposure
Women >50 years with veil

16.6 Conclusions

Vitamin D deficiency and insufficiency are widespread in the population, particularly in risk groups. Rickets and osteomalacia may occur when serum 25(OH)D is lower than 12.5 nmol/L. High bone turnover, bone loss, osteoporosis, and fractures may occur in case of vitamin D deficiency or insufficiency; in general, when serum 25(OH)D is lower than 50 nmol/L. The risk is higher when calcium intake is low. Cross-sectional epidemiological data show different thresholds regarding PTH, markers of bone turnover, bone mineral density, and fracture risk. Randomized clinical trials show equivocal results and are more positive in older institutionalized persons, with a vitamin D dose of 800 IU/day or higher, combined with calcium. An increase of the required serum 25(OH)D level has a major impact on the proportion of the population that should use vitamin D supplements, either only in winter or all year long. The side effects of long-term vitamin D supplementation are insufficiently known. There is generally a lack of data on the consequences of vitamin D insufficiency in the adult population and on the long-term effects and side effects of vitamin D supplementation.

References

1. Van der Meer IM, Karamali NS, Boeke AJ, et al. High prevalence of vitamin D deficiency in pregnant non-Western women in The Hague, Netherlands. *Am J Clin Nutr.* 2006;84: 350-353.
2. Van der Meer IM, Boeke AJ, Lips P, et al. Fatty fish and supplements are the greatest modifiable contributors to hydroxyvitamin D concentration in a multi-ethnic population. *Clin Endocrinol.* 2008;68:466-472.
3. Lips P. Vitamin D deficiency and secondary hyperparathyroidism in the elderly: consequences for bone loss and fractures and therapeutic implications. *Endocrine Rev.* 2001;22:477-501.
4. Lips P. Vitamin D physiology. *Prog Biophys Mol Biol.* 2006;92:4-8.
5. Bouillon R, Carmeliet G, Verlinden L, et al. Vitamin D and human health: Lessons from vitamin D receptor null mice. *Endocrine Rev.* 2008;29:726-776.
6. Liberman UA, Samuel R, Halabe A, et al. End-organ resistance to 1, 25-dihydroxycholecalciferol. *Lancet.* 1980;1: 504-506.
7. Lips P, van Schoor NM, Bravenboer N. Vitamin D-related disorders. In: *Primer on the Metabolic Bone Diseases and Disorders of Mineral Metabolism.* 7th edn. USA: American Society for Bone and Mineral Research; 2008:329-335 [chapter 71].
8. Kuchuk NO, Pluijm SM, van Schoor NM, Looman CW, Smit JH, Lips P. Relationships of serum 25-hydroxyvitamin D to bone mineral density and serum parathyroid hormone and markers of bone turnover in older persons. *J Clin Endocrinol Metab.* 2009;94:1244-1250.
9. Kuchuk NO, van Schoor NM, Pluijm SM, Chines A, Lips P. Vitamin D status, parathyroid function, bone turnover, and BMD in postmenopausal women with osteoporosis: global perspective. *J Bone Miner Res.* 2009;24:693-701.
10. Bischoff-Ferrari HA, Dietrich T, Orav EJ, Dawson-Hughes B. Positive association between 25-hydroxy vitamin D levels and bone mineral density: a population-based study of younger and older adults. *Am J Med.* 2004;116:634-639.
11. Van Schoor NM, Visser M, Pluijm SMF, Kuchuk N, Smit JH, Lips P. Vitamin D deficiency as a risk factor for osteoporotic fractures. *Bone.* 2008;42:260-266.
12. Snijder MB, van Schoor NM, Pluijm SMF, van Dam RM, Visser M, Lips P. Vitamin D status in relation to one-year risk of recurrent falling in older men and women. *J Clin Endocrinol Metab.* 2006;91:2980-2985.
13. Need AG, O'Loughlin PD, Morris HA, Coates PS, Horowitz M, Nordin BEC. Vitamin D metabolites and calcium absorption in severer vitamin D deficiency. *J Bone Miner Res.* 2008;23:1859-1863.
14. Ooms ME, Roos JC, Bezemer PD, van der Vijgh WJF, Bouter LM, Lips P. Prevention of bone loss by vitamin D supplementation in elderly women: a randomized double-blind trial. *J Clin Endocrin Metab.* 1995;80:1052-1058.
15. Chapuy MC, Arlot ME, Duboeuf F, et al. Vitamin D3 and calcium to prevent hip fractures in the elderly women. *N Engl J Med.* 1992;327:1637-1642.
16. Trivedi DP, Doll R, Khaw KT. Effect of four monthly oral vitamin D3 supplementation on fractures and mortality in men and women living in the community: randomised double blind controlled trial. *BMJ.* 2003;326:469.
17. Dawson-Hughes B, Harris SS, Krall EA, Dallal GE. Effect of calcium and vitamin D supplementation on bone density in men and women 65 years of age and older. *N Engl J Med.* 1997;337:670-676.
18. The RECORD Trial Group. Oral vitamin D3 and calcium for secondary prevention of low-trauma fractures in elderly

people: a randomised placebo-controlled trial. *Lancet.* 2005; 365:1621-1628.

19. Larsen E, Mosekilde L, Foldspang A. Vitamin D and calcium supplementation prevents osteoporotic fractures in elderly community dwelling residents: a pragmatic population-based 3-year intervention study. *J Bone Miner Res.* 2004;19: 370-378.

20. Porthouse J, Cockayne S, King C, et al. Randomised controlled trial of supplementation with calcium and cholecalciferol (vitamin D3) for prevention of fractures in primary care. *BMJ.* 2005;330:1003-1006.

21. Jackson RD, LaCroix AZ, Gass M, et al. Calcium plus vitamin D supplementation and the risk of fractures. *N Engl J Med.* 2006;354:669-683.

22. Bischoff-Ferrari HA, Willett WC, Wong JB, Giovannucci E, Dietrich T, Dawson-Hughes B. Fracture prevention with vitamin D supplementation: a meta-analysis of randomized controlled trials. *JAMA.* 2005;293:2257-2264.

23. Avenell A, Gillespie W, Gillespie L, O'Connell D. Vitamin D and vitamin D analogues for preventing fractures associated with involutional and post-menopausal osteoporosis. *Cochrane Database Syst Rev.* 2005;3:CD000227.

24. Boonen S, Lips P, Bouillon R, Bischoff-Ferrari HA, Vanderschueren D, Haentjens P. Need for additional calcium to reduce the risk of hip fracture with vitamin D supplementation: evidence from a comparative meta-analysis of randomized controlled trials. *J Clin Endocrinol Metab.* 2007; 92:1415-1423.

25. Tang BMP, Eslick GD, Nowson C, Smith C, Bensoussan A. Use of calcium or calcium in combination with vitamin D supplementation to prevent fractures and bone loss in people aged 50 years and older: a meta-analysis. *Lancet.* 2007;370: 657-666.

26. Chapuy M, Pamphile R, Paris E, et al. Combined calcium and vitamin D3 supplementation in elderly women: confirmation of reversal of secondary hyperparathyroidism and hip fracture risk: the Decalyos II study. *Osteoporosis Int.* 2002;13:257-264.

27. Bolland MJ, Barber A, Doughty RN, et al. Vascular events in healthy older women receiving calcium supplementation: randomised controlled trial. *BMJ.* 2008;336:262-266.

28. Gezondheidsraad. *Naar een toereikende inname van vitamine D.* Den Haag: Gezondheidsraad; 2008: publicatienr. 2008/15.

Effects of Vitamin D on Bone Health in Healthy Young Adults

17

Kevin D. Cashman

17.1 Introduction

Osteoporosis is a global health problem that will take on increasing significance as people live longer and the world's population continues to increase in number.[1] For example, currently in the United States (US) alone, ten million individuals already have osteoporosis, and a further 34 million have low bone mass, which make them increasingly susceptible to this disorder.[2] While osteoporosis is characterized by low bone mass and microarchitectural deterioration of bone tissue, fragility fractures are the hallmark of osteoporosis and are particularly common in the spine, hip, and distal forearm, although they can occur throughout the skeleton. These fractures are a significant cause of morbidity and mortality and can have a serious impact on quality of life in patients with osteoporosis. It is estimated that one in eight European Union (EU) citizens over the age of 50 years will fracture their spine this year.[1] Furthermore, because of the increase in incidence rates of osteoporotic fractures with age,[3] the demographic changes and increasing life expectancy predicted for Europe, the US, and elsewhere will have a huge impact on the number of fractures which can be expected to occur.

From an economic perspective, the expenses of hospital care and rehabilitation associated with osteoporotic fractures are a considerable fiscal drain for the health care system, exceeding those of other highly prevalent pathologies of the elderly, such as myocardial infarction.[4] Osteoporosis costs national treasuries over €3,500 million annually in hospital health care alone.[1] Thus

prevention of osteoporosis and its complications is an essential socioeconomic priority. There is an urgent need to develop and/or implement nutritional approaches and policies for the prevention and treatment of osteoporosis, which could – with time – offer a foundation for population-based preventive strategies.

17.2 Risk Factors for Osteoporosis

Low bone mineral mass is the main factor responsible for osteoporotic fracture. Bone mass in later life depends on the peak bone mass achieved during growth and the rate of subsequent age-related bone loss (Fig. 17.1). Accordingly, development of maximal bone mass during growth and reduction of loss of bone later in life are the two main strategies of preventing osteoporosis.[5] While, unquestionably, accrual of bone mass during the growth trajectory in childhood and adolescence is an opportunity in relation to skeletal health, there is

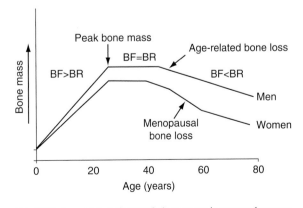

Fig. 17.1 Age-related changes in bone mass in men and women

K.D. Cashman
Department of Food and Nutritional Sciences,
School of Medicine, University College Cork, Cork, Ireland
e-mail: k.cashman@ucc.ie

P. Burckhardt et al. (eds.), *Nutritional Influences on Bone Health*,
DOI: 10.1007/978-1-84882-978-7_17, © Springer-Verlag London Limited 2010

potential for gain in bone mass in young adults for about 10 years after longitudinal bone growth has stopped.[6] Consequently, any factor that influences the development and consolidation of peak bone mass or the loss of bone in adulthood will affect later fracture risk. Several authoritative bodies have stressed on the importance of nutrition, in particular adequate dietary calcium and vitamin D intake/status, as a major contributor to bone health for individuals of all ages.[1,2,6–8]

17.3 Vitamin D Status in Young Adults

Vitamin D, through its active form (1,25-dihydroxyvitamin D), is essential for intestinal calcium absorption and plays a central role in maintaining calcium homeostasis and skeletal integrity.[6] It is well-established that prolonged and severe clinical vitamin D deficiency (represented as serum/plasma 25-hydroxyvitamin D [25(OH)D] concentrations <10–25 nmol/L) leads to rickets in children and osteomalacia in adults.[7] Less severe vitamin D deficiency causes secondary hyperparathyroidism and increases bone turnover and bone loss.[9,10] Currently in the UK, a plasma concentration of 25 nmol/L of 25(OH)D is used as the lower threshold for vitamin D status.[7] There is, however, a lack of consensus on the cut-off values of plasma 25(OH)D that define the lower limit of adequacy/sufficiency, and values between 30 and 80 nmol/L have been suggested.[6,11,12]

It is of concern that a high prevalence of low vitamin D status has been reported in adults from many countries (see reviews[13–16]). In addition, the age profile of those with low vitamin D status is contrary to previously accepted wisdom; for example, younger adults in the UK are more likely to have serum 25(OH)D values below 25 nmol/L than older adults (20.2% vs. 11.7% for men and women aged 19–34 years and 35–64 years, respectively).[17] Data from the third National Health and Nutrition Examination Survey (NHANES III) show that of several age groups (encompassing those aged 12–80+ years), adult males and females (20–39 years) had the highest percentage of wintertime serum 25(OH)D concentrations below 37.5 nmol/L.[18] Relatively low habitual dietary intakes of vitamin D by high proportions of young adults in many countries are likely to have a major role in the observed low wintertime vitamin D status in this age

group.[19–21] For example, nearly 75% of Irish adults fail to reach a dietary intake of vitamin D of 5 µg/day.[20] This is due in particular to the rather limited number of foods that are rich in vitamin D.[20]

17.4 Impact of Low Vitamin D Status on Bone Health in Young Adults

A key question is whether this low vitamin D status impacts bone health in young adults? Positive associations have been reported between serum 25(OH)D (or low parathyroid hormone (PTH), as a secondary measure of vitamin D status) and bone mineral density (BMD) of the forearm, lumbar spine, femoral neck, and hip in healthy young adults.[22–24] Bischoff-Ferrari et al.,[25] using data from NHANES III, have shown that compared to subjects in the lowest quintile of serum 25(OH)D, those in the highest quintile had mean BMD that was 4.1% higher in young White adult (20–49 years) subjects, and that serum 25(OH)D concentrations higher than 100 nmol/L was associated with higher BMD. However, such epidemiological data do not provide evidence of causality.

Unfortunately, data from intervention studies investigating the effect of improving vitamin D status on bone health outcomes, particularly on BMD, in this age group are relatively limited. There are three studies in young adults (18–40 years[26–28]) and two in adults in a wider age bracket (21–70 years),[29,30] which reported the effect of vitamin D supplementation on BMD and/or markers of bone turnover. In a double-blind, randomized controlled intervention study by Barnes et al.,[26] 18–27-year-old adult men and women (*n* 15) who received daily supplementation with 15 µg vitamin D₃ (and 1,500 mg calcium/day) had a significant increase in mean serum 25(OH)D over the 8 weeks of winter (from 47.9 to 86.5 nmol/L from January to March, respectively). However, there was no significant change in markers of bone turnover (serum bone-specific alkaline phosphatase (BAP) or carboxyterminal cross-linked telopeptide of type I collagen (CTx)) or in PTH over the 8 weeks of the study compared to the control group (who received 1,500 mg calcium/day only). We have recently shown that in a double-blind, placebo-controlled, randomized 22-week intervention study, the median serum 25(OH)D concentration in a group of 20–40 year olds (men and women; *n* 53) who received 15 µg vitamin D_3/day over the extended winter period was similar in November (75.9 nmol/L) and March (69.0 nmol/L), suggesting that this level of supplementation largely prevented the seasonal decline in vitamin D status.[27] We also included two further doses of vitamin D_3 (5 and 10 μg/day), which had, as expected, a diminished ability to prevent the seasonal decline in serum 25(OH)D concentration. There was, however, a lack of effect of vitamin D supplementation on markers of bone turnover (serum osteocalcin, bone-specific alkaline phosphatase, CTx or cross-linked N-terminal telopeptides of type I collagen (NTx)), which may have been related to the lack of its effect on serum PTH. While PTH increased (by 11–17%) in the placebo group and all three vitamin D groups throughout winter, there was no significant difference in this increment among groups. Furthermore, the increase was within the normal physiological range. Lips (11) has suggested that mild vitamin D deficiency (serum 25(OH)D in range 25–50 nmol/L) may be associated with increases in serum PTH of <15% with normal/high bone turnover.

It is also noteworthy that in our study there was no increase in markers of bone turnover even in the placebo group from early Autumn to early Spring, despite a significant decrease in serum 25(OH)D and increase in serum PTH, potentially suggesting a lack of seasonal variation in bone turnover.[27] Patel et al.[29] reported the effect of season and vitamin D supplementation on bone metabolism and density in healthy adult women (mean age, 45.3 (range 23–70) years). There was no effect of season on serum PTH, bone markers, or BMD even though serum 25(OH)D was significantly increased. Furthermore, while supplementation with vitamin D_3 increased serum 25(OH)D, there was no effect on serum PTH, bone markers, or BMD. To further test the impact of seasonality, we investigated the effect of supplementation with 15 μg vitamin D_3/day for 4 weeks in a double-blind, placebo-controlled randomized intervention study in a combined cohort of young (18–35 years old) and older (36–63 years old) adults.[28] Subjects were recruited in two waves (late-Autumn and late-Winter, during which vitamin D status would be at its peak and nadir, respectively.[31]) There was no effect of vitamin D supplementation on markers of bone turnover (serum osteocalcin or bone-specific alkaline phosphatase, or urinary NTx) in either wave separately or when combined in the young adults.[28]

In contrast, Viljakainen et al.[30] recently showed that in a 6-month double-blinded vitamin D intervention study in healthy Caucasian Finnish men (aged 21–49 years), there was a seasonal (November to April) decline in serum 25(OH)D and elevation in PTH in the placebo group, but serum BAP was unchanged and, unexpectedly, serum TRACP (a marker of bone resorption) significantly decreased. Supplementation with vitamin D (at 10 and 20 μg/day) inhibited the winter elevation of PTH (20 μg/day only), decreased serum BAP, and tended ($p = 0.09$) to increase cortical BMD of proximal radius with increasing vitamin D.

17.5 Dietary Requirement of Vitamin D to Reach Proposed Thresholds of Serum 25-Hydroxyvitamin D

Bischoff-Ferrari et al.,[25] using data from NHANES III, have shown that a serum 25(OH)D concentration higher than 100 nmol/L was associated with higher BMD in young adult (20–49 years) White subjects. A quasiconsensus of vitamin D experts for a serum 25(OH)D threshold of >70–80 nmol/L has been suggested for optimal bone health for all adults.[32] However, while a secondary analysis is possibly limited by the number of subjects with serum levels that exceeded the threshold, stratifying subjects in our study with serum 25(OH)D levels above or below 80 nmol/L had no effect on the response of serum PTH or bone markers to vitamin D supplementation.[27] Similarly, Patel et al.[29] also showed that there was no significant difference in the response of serum PTH or bone markers to vitamin D supplementation in subjects with low (<60 nmol/L) or high (>80 nmol/L) serum 25(OH)D concentration at baseline.

Considerable variation exists between authoritative dietary recommendations for vitamin D intakes for adults.[6–8,33] The UK Committee on Medical Aspects of Food and Nutrition Policy (COMA) in 1991 chose not to set a reference nutrient intake (RNI) for people aged 4–64 years on the basis that skin synthesis of vitamin D would generally ensure adequacy,[7] a recommendation confirmed in 1998 by the UK COMA subgroup on bone health.[8] In contrast, the US Dietary Reference Intake (DRI) panel for calcium and related nutrients set adequate intakes (AI) for vitamin D in 1997.[6] The US DRI panel concluded that there was insufficient evidence to set estimated average requirements (EAR, the foundation for setting recommended dietary allowances [RDA]) for vitamin D, emphasizing the fact that contributions from sunlight and food are difficult to determine.[6] An AI for vitamin D (5 µg/day for adults aged 18–50 years) was set on the basis of intakes necessary to achieve "normal" ranges of serum 25(OH)D concentrations. However, in establishing the AI, the US DRI panel assumed that there was no cutaneous synthesis of vitamin D through sun exposure.[6] The European dietary recommendation (population reference intake [PRI]) for vitamin D for adults ranges from 0 to 10 µg/day to account for the widely varying latitudes where EU citizens live in (35–70°N).[33]

Recently, we have established based on a randomized controlled intervention study in adults (aged 20–40 years) using supplemental levels (0, 5, 10, and 15 µg/day) of vitamin D₃ throughout winter, established the distribution of dietary requirements for the maintenance of nutritional adequacy of vitamin D during late winter.[34] We placed strong emphasis on using a cut-off for serum 25(OH)D of 25 nmol/L on the basis that concentrations of around 20–27.5 nmol/L are considered to be consistent with vitamin D deficiency and rickets/osteomalacia,[8] and the 25 nmol/L threshold has been used by the various important authorities at least up to now.[6-8,33] The intake required to maintain 97.5% of the young adult population with wintertime serum 25(OH)D concentrations above 25 nmol/L was 8.7 µg/day. However, we have also reported dietary requirements for vitamin D in these young adults using a number of other serum 25(OH)D cut-off values (37.5, 50, and 80 nmol/L) (Table 17.1). In particular, our estimate of the dietary vitamin D requirement needed to maintain serum 25(OH)D concentrations above 80 nmol/L in 97.5% of the sample of 20–40 year olds was 41 µg/day.[34] This is considerably less than the 114 µg/day suggested

by Heaney et al.,[35] who performed an extended vitamin D supplementation study (supplementation range 0–250 µg/day) in adult males (mean age 38.7 years) in Omaha, Nebraska, US (41.2°N) and used pharmacokinetic modeling to estimate the vitamin D intake required to maintain prewinter serum 25(OH)D levels and/or to reach levels of 80 nmol/L during winter. Our data also show that even for the lowest cut-off of serum 25(OH)D (25 nmol/L) and certainly for the more intermediate cut-off of 50 nmol/L serum 25(OH)D, the dietary requirement (8.7 and 28.0 µg/day, respectively) is still higher than that being consumed currently by adult populations.[19-21]

17.6 Conclusion

Low vitamin D status, particularly during wintertime, is common in young adults. The impact of this low vitamin D status on skeletal health in this age group is unclear. Data from intervention studies investigating the effect of improving vitamin D status on bone health outcomes, particularly on BMD, in young adults are relatively limited and the findings are mixed. In light of recent findings that suggest that vitamin D intakes in the region of ~40 µg/day, and may be as high as 100 µg/day, would be required to ensure that nearly all of healthy 20–40 year olds would maintain serum 25(OH)D concentrations above 80 nmol/L,[34,35] there is an urgent need for more data from vitamin D intervention studies, which confirm benefits of these high concentrations in terms of skeletal health.

References

Table 17.1 Estimated dietary requirements for vitamin D at selected percentiles in 215 men and women aged 20–40 years to maintain serum 25(OH)D above selected biochemical cut-off levels during winter[a]

Serum 25(OH)D cut-off	97.5th percentile[a] (µg/day)
>25 nmol/L	8.7 (6.5, 11.1)
>37.5 nmol/L	19.9 (17.2, 23.5)
>50 nmol/L	28.0 (24.2, 32.8)
>80 nmol/L	41.1 (35.4, 48.7)

[a]Results presented as estimate (95% confidence interval)
Data from[34]

1. Commission E. *Report on osteoporosis in the European Community: action for prevention.* Luxembourg: Office for Official Publications for the European Commission; 1998.
2. U.S. Department of Health and Human Services. The 2004 Surgeon General's Report on Bone Health and Osteoporosis. Washington, DC: U.S. Department of Health and Human Services, Office of the Surgeon General; 2004.
3. Compston J. Osteoporosis. In: Campbell G, Compston J, Crisp A, eds. *The Management of Common Metabolic Bone Disorders.* Cambridge, UK: Cambridge University Press; 1993:29-62.
4. Schurch M, Rizzoli R, Mermillod B, Vasey H, Michel J, Bonjour J. A prospective study on socioeconomic aspects of fracture of the proximal femur. *J Bone Miner Res.* 1996; 11:1935-1942.

5. Weaver CM. The growing years and prevention of osteoporosis in later life. *Proc Nutr Soc.* 2000;59:303-306.

6. Institute of Medicine Food and Nutrition Board. *Dietary Reference Intakes: Calcium, Magnesium, Phosphorus, Vitamin D, and Fluoride.* Washington, DC: National Academy Press; 1997.

7. UK Department of Health. Dietary Reference Values for Food Energy and Nutrients for the United Kingdom. Report on Health and Social Subjects (41). London, United Kingdom: Her Majesty's Stationery Office; 1991.

8. UK Department of Health. Nutrition and Bone health: with particular reference to calcium and vitamin D. Report on Health and Social Subjects (49). London, United Kingdom: The Stationary Office, 1998.

9. Lips P. Vitamin D deficiency and secondary hyperparathyroidism in the elderly: consequences for bone loss and fractures and therapeutic implications. *Endocr Rev.* 2001;22:477-501.

10. Parfitt AM, Gallagher JC, Heaney RP, Johnston CC, Neer R, Whedon GD. Vitamin D and bone health in the elderly. *Am J Clin Nutr.* 1982;36:1014-1031.

11. Lips P. Which circulating level of 25-hydroxyvitamin D is appropriate? *J Steroid Biochem Mol Biol.* 2004;89–90:611-614.

12. Chapuy MC, Preziosi P, Maamer M, et al. Prevalence of vitamin D insufficiency in an adult normal population. *Osteoporos Int.* 1997;7:439-443.

13. McKenna MJ. Differences in vitamin D status between countries in young adults and the elderly. *Am J Med.* 1992;93:69-77.

14. van der Wielen RP, Lowik MR, van den Berg H, et al. Serum vitamin D concentrations among elderly people in Europe. *Lancet.* 1995;346(8969):207-210.

15. Lips P, Duong T, Oleksik A, et al. A global study of vitamin D status and parathyroid function in postmenopausal women with osteoporosis: baseline data from the multiple outcomes of raloxifene evaluation clinical trial. *J Clin Endocrinol Metab.* 2001;86:1212-1221.

16. Lips P, Hosking D, Lippuner K, et al. The prevalence of vitamin D inadequacy amongst women with osteoporosis: an international epidemiological investigation. *J Intern Med.* 2006;260:245-254.

17. Ruston D, Hoare J, Henderson L, Gregory J (2004) The National Diet and Nutrition Survey: Adults Aged 19-64 Years – Nutritional Status (anthropometry and blood analytes), Blood Pressure and Physical Activity. London, United Kingdom: The Stationery Office. (ISBN 0 11 621569 0).

18. Looker AC, Dawson-Hughes B, Calvo MS, Gunter EW, Sahyoun NR. Serum 25-hydroxyvitamin D status of adolescents and adults in two seasonal subpopulations from NHANES III. *Bone.* 2002;30:771-777.

19. Henderson L, Irving K, Gregory J, et al. *The National Diet and Nutrition Survey: Adults Aged 19 to 64 Years – Vitamin and Mineral Intake and Urinary Analytes.* London, United Kingdom: The Stationery Office; 2003.

20. Hill TR, O'Brien MM, Cashman KD, Flynn A, Kiely M. Vitamin D intakes in 18-64-y-old Irish adults. *Eur J Clin Nutr.* 2004;58:1509-1517.

21. Moore CE, Murphy MM, Holick MF. Vitamin D intakes by children and adults in the United States differ among ethnic groups. *J Nutr.* 2005;135:2478–2485

22. Lamberg-Allardt CJ, Outila TA, Kärkkainen MU, Rita HJ, Valsta LM. Vitamin D deficiency and bone health in healthy adults in Finland: could this be a concern in other parts of Europe? *J Bone Miner Res.* 2001;11:2066-2073.

23. Välimäki VV, Alfthan H, Lehmuskallio E, et al. Vitamin D status as a determinant of peak bone mass in young Finnish men. *J Clin Endocrinol Metab.* 2004;89:76-80.

24. Roy DK, Berry JL, Pye SR, et al. Vitamin D status and bone mass in UK South Asian women. *Bone.* 2007;40: 200-204.

25. Bischoff-Ferrari HA, Dietrich T, Orav EJ, Dawson-Hughes B. Positive association between 25-hydroxy vitamin D levels and bone mineral density: a population-based study of younger and older adults. *Am J Med.* 2004;116:634-639.

26. Barnes MS, Robson PJ, Bonham MP, Strain JJ, Wallace JM. Effect of vitamin D supplementation on vitamin D status and bone turnover markers in young adults. *Eur J Clin Nutr.* 2006;60:727-733.

27. Seamans KM, Hill TR, Wallace JM, et al. Cholecalciferol supplementation throughout winter does not affect markers of bone turnover in healthy young and elderly adults. *J Nutr.* 2010;140:454-60.

28. Hill TR, Brennan L, O'Connor A, et al. Effect of probiotic and vitamin D supplementation on markers of vitamin D status and bone turnover in healthy adults. *Proc Nutr Soc.* 2009;68 (OCE), E114.

29. Patel R, Collins D, Bullock S, Swaminathan R, Blake GM, Fogelman I. The effect of season and vitamin D supplementation on bone mineral density in healthy women: a double-masked crossover study. *Osteoporos Int.* 2001;12:319-325.

30. Viljakainen HT, Väisänen M, Kemi V, et al. Wintertime vitamin D supplementation inhibits seasonal variation of calcitropic hormones and maintains bone turnover in healthy men. *J Bone Miner Res.* 2009;24:346-352.

31. Webb AR, Kline L, Holick MF. Influence of season and latitude on the cutaneous synthesis of vitamin D3: exposure to winter sunlight in Boston and Edmonton will not promote vitamin D3 synthesis in human skin. *J Clin Endocrinol Metab.* 1988;67:373-378.

32. Dawson-Hughes B, Heaney RP, Holick MF, Lips P, Meunier PJ, Vieth R. Estimates of optimal vitamin D status. *Osteoporos Int.* 2005;16:713-716.

33. Commission of the European Communities. Vitamin D. In: *Nutrient and Energy Intakes of the European Community.* Report of the Scientific Committee for Food (31st series). Brussels, Luxembourg; 1993:132-139.

34. Cashman KD, Hill TR, Lucey AJ, et al. Estimation of the dietary requirement for vitamin D in healthy adults. *Am J Clin Nutr.* 2008;88:1535-1542.

35. Heaney RP, Davies KM, Chen TC, Holick MF, Barger-Lux MJ. Human serum 25-hydroxycholecalciferol response to extended oral dosing with cholecalciferol. *Am J Clin Nutr.* 2003;77: 204-210.

Vitamin D Effects on Bone Structure in Childhood and Aging

18

Kun Zhu and Richard L. Prince

18.1 Introduction

Persistent severe vitamin D deficiency causes rickets in children and osteomalacia in adults, and mild vitamin D deficiency has been reported to be associated with hyperparathyroidism and increased bone turnover. In older people, low vitamin D status may lead to bone loss and fractures.[1]

The serum 25-hydroxyvitamin D [25(OH)D] level is regarded as the best indicator of overall vitamin D status, because it is quantitatively related to the supply of vitamin D over preceding weeks.[2] During puberty, vitamin D requirements relate to both dietary calcium intake and growth velocity. With the increased demand for calcium to meet the mineralization requirement of the rapid expending skeleton, there is an increase in the metabolism of 25(OH)D to 1,25-dihydroxyvitamin D ($1,25(OH)_2D$). There is as yet no consensus on the ideal level of 25(OH)D for maintaining normal calcium metabolism and the achievement of optimal peak bone mass in children and adolescents. In adults, it is generally considered that 25(OH)D should be higher than 50 nmol/L in all postmenopausal women and elderly men for maintaining bone health[3] and many clinicians and researchers favor a higher level of 75 nmol/L.[4] In this chapter, we reviewed the evidence of the effects of vitamin D on bone mass during childhood and aging.

18.2 Vitamin D Effects on Bone Structure During Childhood

18.2.1 Epidemiological Studies on Serum 25(OH)D Levels and Bone Mass During Childhood and Adolescence

Majority of the studies on vitamin D status and bone health during childhood and adolescence were conducted in girls. Only two studies included male subjects and neither of them has shown any association.[5,6] The studies in girls have shown various results, which could be related to the stage of sexual maturation, the rate of linear growth at the time of measurement, and the different growth patterns of different skeletal sites. It seems that the role of vitamin D is more important during pubertal years when there is a greater demand for calcium, as studies in older adolescent girls of 16–20 years of age[7] and prepubertal children and young adults[6] did not find an association between vitamin D status and bone mass.

Studies conducted in adolescent girls of up to 16 years of age have shown a positive association between vitamin D status and bone mass. In a cross-sectional study with 178 healthy Finnish adolescent girls of 14–16 years old, Outila et al. reported that females with serum 25(OH)D concentrations below 40 nmol/L had lower radial BMD (bone mineral density, $p<0.05$) and ulna BMD ($p=0.08$) compared to those with 25(OH)D levels above 40 nmol/L.[8] In another cross-sectional study with 266 12-year-old and 250 15-year-old girls, it was found that girls with high vitamin D status (>74.1 nmol/L) in both age groups had significantly higher forearm BMD as determined by peripheral instantaneous X-ray imager bone densitometer ($p<0.05$).[5] Such association was not

K. Zhu (✉)
Department of Endocrinology and Diabetes,
Sir Charles Gairdner Hospital, Hospital Avenue,
Nedlands, WA 6152, Australia
e-mail: kzhu@meddent.uwa.edu.au

P. Burckhardt et al. (eds.), *Nutritional Influences on Bone Health*,
DOI: 10.1007/978-1-84882-978-7_18, © Springer-Verlag London Limited 2010

observed for heel BMD.[5] This study also included 260 12-year-old and 239 15-year-old boys, and as mentioned earlier, no correlation between vitamin D status and BMD was observed in boys in either age group.[5]

A 3-year prospective study evaluated the association of vitamin D status and bone mineral accretion in 171 healthy Finnish girls aged 9–15 years at baseline. In this longitudinal study, the gain in spinal BMD over 3 years was significantly greater in those with high baseline vitamin D status (12.7, 13.1, and 16.7% for lowest, middle, and highest tertiles, respectively; $p = 0.01$) in the 129 girls with advanced sexual maturation at baseline.[9] However, such effect was not observed for femoral neck BMD ($p = 0.15$).[9] For early pubertal years, in a study with 193 Finnish girls of 10–12 years of age at Tanner stage 1 or 2, it was found that girls with 25(OH)D below 25 nmol/L had significantly lower cortical volumetric BMD of the distal radius ($p < 0.001$) and the tibia shaft ($p = 0.002$) as measured by peripheral quantitative computed tomography (pQCT) compared to those with higher vitamin D status. However, no vitamin D effects on DXA (Dual energy X-ray absorptiometry) total body, femoral neck, and lumbar spine bone mass had been observed.[10]

The average calcium intakes were 700–1,500 mg/day in the above mentioned studies with Caucasian adolescents. Very few studies examined the association between vitamin D status and bone mass in those with low calcium intakes, where vitamin D status is more important for calcium absorption. In a study with 301 Beijing girls aged 15 years old with an average calcium intake of 450 mg/day, it was found that girls with 25(OH)D concentrations above 50 nmol/L had significantly higher BMC at all skeletal sites measured (totally body, distal and proximal forearm) compared to those with 25(OH)D levels below 25 nmol/L ($p < 0.05$), and the effects remained after adjustment for bone and body size, pubertal stage, handgrip muscle strength, physical activity, and dietary vitamin D and calcium intakes.[11]

18.2.2 Effects of Vitamin D Supplementation on Vitamin D Status and Bone Mineral Accretion During Puberty

There are limited data on the effect of vitamin D supplementation on vitamin D status and bone mineral accretion during adolescence. In a 3-year prospective

study, the effects of vitamin D supplementation on vitamin D status were evaluated in 171 peri-pubertal Finnish girls aged 9–15 years. The mean baseline serum 25(OH)D concentration was 34.0 nmol/L. In the first 2 years, girls received 400 IU of vitamin D_2 daily from October to February, and those with calcium intake below 1,000 mg/day also received 500 mg of calcium per day. As improvement in vitamin D status was not observed in wintertime at this supplementation dose, the dose was increase to 800 IU/day in the third year, which significantly increased the serum 25(OH)D concentrations in winter (3,200–5,600 IU supplementation per week: 45.5 nmol/L vs. no supplementation 31.8 nmol/L, $p < 0.001$). The intervention had greater effects in those with baseline 25(OH)D concentrations below 20 nmol/L than those whose 25OHD levels were above 37.5 nmol/L (increase in serum 25(OH)D: 24.2 nmol/L vs. 0.9 nmol/L, $p < 0.001$).[12]

Similar increase in 25(OH)D level was observed with smaller supplementation dose in Chinese girls with low vitamin D status in a 2-year school milk intervention trial. The study subjects were 757 Beijing Chinese girls aged 10 years at baseline, and they were randomized into three groups according to their schools. Subjects either received a carton of 330 mL milk fortified with calcium (providing 560 mg calcium in each carton) on school days ($n = 238$) or the same quantity of milk additionally fortified with 200–320 IU of vitamin D ($n = 260$) or acted as unsupplemented controls ($n = 259$). The mean baseline calcium intake was 436 mg/day. The mean baseline 25(OH)D concentration was 19.4 nmol/L at the end of winter (March and early April), which improved to 47.6 nmol/L in the group that received both calcium and vitamin D fortified milk, but remained unchanged in the other two groups. The group that received milk fortified with both calcium and vitamin D had significantly greater increase in size-adjusted bone mineral content (BMC) than both the control group (2.5%, $p = 0.005$) and the group that received milk fortified with calcium alone (1.4%, $p = 0.05$) after 2 years.[13,14] Both the supplemented groups had significantly greater increases in total body BMD compared to the control group, and the effect in the calcium and vitamin D fortified milk group was greater (calcium fortified milk group: 3.1%, $p = 0.03$; calcium and vitamin D fortified milk group: 5.4%, $p = 0.003$).[14] There were no significant differences between the two supplemented groups as regard the increase in bone size as measured by combined cortical thickness, suggesting that the group that received additional vitamin D might had greater increase in volumetric BMD rather than bone size.[15] However, 3 years after the supplement withdrawal, the effects on bone mass and vitamin D status largely disappeared,[16] indicating that short-term intervention during early pubertal years does not have long-lasting effects on bone mineral accretion in Chinese girls with low habitual calcium intake and low vitamin D status.

18.2.3 Vitamin D Status and Calcium Absorption, PTH, and Bone Turnover During Growth

The primary role of vitamin D during growth is to increase calcium absorption to meet the demands of bone mineralization. However, in Caucasian, Mexican American, and African American children with average calcium intakes ranging between 821 and 1,110 mg/day, no correlations between serum 25(OH)D and fractional calcium absorption were observed in any race.[17,18] Furthermore, in a study with 12 Chinese girls aged 9–17 years with relatively lower calcium intake of 591 mg/day, there was a negative association between 25(OH)D concentrations and fractional calcium absorption.[19] It is not clear whether this was due to more 25(OH)D been converted to $1,25(OH)D_2$ to meet the requirement for calcium during this growth period.

The effects of vitamin D on bone mass could be mediated by reduced level of parathyroid hormone (PTH) and reduced rate of bone turnover. Most studies in Caucasian adolescents found that vitamin D deficiency was associated with an elevation of PTH concentration in blood and a rise in the blood concentration of markers for bone turnover.[5,8,10] However, in a study with 196 Swiss boys and girls aged 11–16 years, the authors reported that there was no correlation between 25(OH)D levels and markers of collagen formation (P1NP) and degradation (serum c-terminal telopeptides, S-CTX).[20] In Chinese adolescent girls aged 15 years, a significant inverse association was found between plasma 25(OH)D and iPTH concentrations ($r=-0.110$, $p<0.05$), and plasma iPTH levels started to rise steeply when 25(OH)D levels fell below 60 nmol/L.[21] Those girls with 25(OH)D levels above 50 nmol/L also had reduced rate of bone turnover as reflected by reduced levels of bone alkaline phosphatase and urinary deoxypyridinoline ($p<0.05$).[11] In the school milk intervention trial with Chinese girls aged 10 years, the group that received calcium and vitamin D fortified milk had significantly lower serum PTH at 12 (-46.2%, $p=0.04$) and 24 months (-16.4%, $p=0.01$) compared to the unsupplemented control group.[15]

However, increase in PTH levels during puberty may not be driven by the same mechanism as in adults,[22] and PTH concentration normally raise during puberty as the rate of remodeling and consolidation is at peak.[23] Therefore, the ideal 25(OH)D level during adolescence cannot be determined as in adults based on the 25(OH)D level that reduces PTH level to a plateau.

18.2.4 Summary

A high prevalence of vitamin D deficiency and insufficiency has been reported in healthy growing children and adolescents in a number of countries.[10,24,25] In Finnish girls aged 10–12 year, serum 25(OH)D concentrations in winter were below 25 nmol/L in 32% of the girls and range between 26 and 40 nmol/L in 46% of them.[10] In Beijing girls aged 15 years old with an average calcium intake of 450 mg/day, it was found that at the end of winter (March and April), 31.2% of the girls had 25(OH)D levels below 25 nmol/L, 57.8% between 25 and 50 nmol/L and only 11% had 25(OH)D levels above 50 nmol/L.[11] Low vitamin D status may result in suboptimal bone mass accretion during growth. Increasing serum 25(OH)D through increasing sunlight exposure and vitamin D intake or taking supplements should be recommended for these children as a cost-effective means of improving bone health, especially during rapid growing period and in those with low calcium intakes.

18.3 Vitamin D Effects on Bone Structure in Aging

18.3.1 Epidemiological Studies on Serum 25(OH)D Levels and Bone Mass in Older Adults

Several cross-sectional epidemiological studies in older people have shown that subjects with low 25(OH)D levels had decreased BMD, with the 25(OH)D threshold ranging from 25–30[1,26] to 75 nmol/L.[27] In the NHANES III, in the analysis with 5,917 older adults aged over 50 years, compared to those in the lowest quintile of 25(OH)D, the highest quintile had higher mean BMD of 4.8% in White ($p < 0.001$), 3.6% in Mexican American ($p = 0.01$), and 2.5% in Black subjects.[27] Similar association was also observed in younger adults aged less than 50 years.[27] In the regression plots, higher serum 25(OH)D levels were associated with higher BMD up to 90–100 nmol/L in all ethnic groups.[27] In another analysis of the NHANES III data collected in 4,958 women and 5,003 men aged above 20 years, total hip BMD increased stepwise with 25(OH)D levels (<50, 50–74, >75 nmol/L, p for trend ≤ 0.001) in both men and women.[28] This study also showed that calcium intake only related to hip BMD in women with 25(OH)D concentrations below 50 nmol/L.[28] However, low vitamin D status might be a reflection of general poor health and lack of physical activity, and casual relation cannot be established from cross-sectional studies. Randomized controlled trials provide the best evidence on the effects of vitamin D on bone health.

18.3.2 Effects of Vitamin D Supplementation on Bone Density in Older People

18.3.2.1 Vitamin D Supplementation Alone

Without adequate calcium intake, vitamin D cannot, in general, correct the raised PTH level and reduce the rate of bone loss. This could explain why some studies of the effects of vitamin D supplementation alone, i.e., in the absence of adequate calcium intake, on BMD have shown little or no effects. A randomized controlled trial of 800 IU vitamin D_3 supplementation with 79 female monozygotic twin pairs aged 47–70 years (mean age 58.7 years) for 24 months showed that there were no significant treatment effects on hip and spinal BMD or calcaneal ultrasound, although the serum 25(OH)D levels increased by 35 nmol/L in the supplemented group.[29] In a 2-year randomized controlled study with 41 men aged 27–77 years with primary osteoporosis and at least one baseline fragility fracture, there were no significant differences between the group

that received calcitriol supplementation of 0.5 μg/day and the group that received 1,000 mg calcium per day in the change in femoral neck and spinal BMD and the incidence of vertebral fractures.[30] In both of the above studies, the baseline serum 25(OH)D levels were in normal range (mean serum 25(OH)D concentrations 70–90 nmol/L).

Vitamin D supplementation alone appears to be more effective in older subjects and those with low vitamin D status or low calcium intakes. In a study in 316 women with a mean age of 73.7 years and 122 men with a mean age of 75.9 years, subjects were randomized to receive placebo, 750 mg calcium, or 600 IU of 25(OH)D over 4 years. Calcium supplementation prevented bone loss, whereas 25(OH)D supplementation was less effective, but showed an effect in those with low calcium intakes.[31] In a 2-year trial in 380 women aged 70 years and older, those subjects who received 400 IU vitamin D_3 per day had significantly increased serum 25(OH)D (increased by 35 nmol/L) and 1,25-$(OH)_2D$ (increased by 7.0 pmol/L) levels and significantly decreased PTH(1–84) secretion (−0.74 pmol/L) after 1 year. The vitamin D group had 1.9% and 2.6% higher BMD at the left and right femoral neck, respectively, compared to the placebo group.[32] In another trial in 15 subjects (13 women and 2 men, mean age of 75 years) with vitamin D insufficiency and primary hyperparathyroidism, after successful treatment of vitamin D insufficiency in all subjects, significant improvement were observed at hip and spinal BMD, even in five subjects with persistent inappropriate production of PTH.[33]

18.3.2.2 Vitamin D and Calcium Supplementation Comparing to Calcium Alone

Several studies have shown that supplementation with both calcium and vitamin D reduced the rate of bone loss compared to placebo.[34,35] However, trials comparing supplementation of calcium plus vitamin D and supplementation of calcium alone have yielded conflicting results. In a 1-year trial in 249 postmenopausal women living at Boston (Latitude 42°) who received 377 mg of calcium and either placebo or 400 IU of vitamin D, it was found that vitamin D supplementation could reduce spinal bone loss in winter significantly (vitamin D −0.54%, Placebo −1.22%, $p = 0.03$).[36] In contrast, in another trial with 280 healthy Black postmenopausal women aged 50–75 years where all women received calcium supplementation to ensure a total calcium intake of 1,200–1,500 mg/day, vitamin D supplementation (800 IU for the first 2 years and 2,000 IU for the third year) showed no effect on bone loss or bone turnover markers.[37]

The effects of vitamin D and calcium and calcium alone had been compared in elderly Australian women with low vitamin D status in a 1-year randomized, double-blind, placebo-controlled trial. The study subjects were 302 elderly women aged 70–90 years with serum 25(OH)D concentrations less than 60 nmol/L.[38] They were randomized to receive either calcium 1,000 mg alone or 1,000 mg calcium plus 1,000 IU vitamin D_2 per day. The average calcium intake at baseline was 1,000 mg/day and 25(OH)D was 44.7 nmol/L. Serum 25(OH)D increased in the vitamin D group by 34%, but not the placebo group after 1 year (59.8 vs. 45.0 nmol/L, $p < 0.001$). Total hip and total body BMD increased significantly during the study with no significant difference between the treatment groups (Hip BMD change: vitamin D +0.5%, control +0.2%; Total body BMD change: vitamin D +0.4%, control +0.4%). Therefore, this short-term 1 year study showed that vitamin D_2 1,000 IU has no extra beneficial effect on bone structure over an additional 1,000 mg of calcium even in patients with low vitamin D status.

18.3.2.3 Long-Term Intervention Study

Most of the vitamin D intervention studies were less than 2 years. The long-term effects of calcium with or without vitamin D on hip BMD were evaluated in a 5-year randomized controlled double-blind trial of 120 community-dwelling Australian women aged 70–80 years.[39] During the 5-year study, subjects received calcium 1,200 mg/day with placebo or 1,000 IU/day vitamin D_2 or double placebo. At year one, hip BMD was preserved in the group that received both calcium and vitamin D (−0.17%) or calcium alone (0.19%), but not the control group (−1.27%). Whereas at years 3 and 5, hip BMD was only maintained in the group that received both calcium and vitamin D (Fig. 18.1). The beneficial effects were mainly in those with baseline 25(OH)D levels below the median (68 nmol/L) (Fig. 18.2).

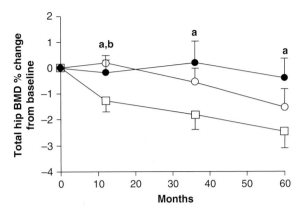

Fig. 18.1 Percent change (mean ± SE) relative to baseline in total hip BMD in a 5-year trial with elderly Australian women. Ca group (*open circle*) Ca + vitamin D group (*filled circle*) Control group (*open square*); (**a**) $p < 0.05$ Ca + vitamin D group Cf Control group; (**b**) $p < 0.05$ Ca group Cf Control group (reproduced from Zhu et al[39])

18.3.3 Vitamin D Effects on Calcium Absorption, PTH, and Bone Turnover in Older Adults

It has been shown that in postmenopausal women, the true fractional absorption rate was significantly higher in those with 25(OH)D concentrations averaging 86 nmol/L than those averaging 50 nmol/L (35.3% vs. 22.5% of the 500 mg calcium load, $p < 0.01$).[40] However, in the 1-year study with elderly Australian women with low vitamin D status who received either 1,000 mg calcium per day alone or 1,000 mg calcium and 1,000 IU vitamin D_2, the increase in 25(OH)D achieved with vitamin D supplementation had no extra effect on active fractional intestinal calcium absorption, which fell equally in both groups (vitamin D −17.4%; control −14.8%) (Fig. 18.3).[38] Similarly, in the 5-year intervention study with elderly Australian women, the calcium absorption rate of both calcium alone and calcium and vitamin D groups, but not the placebo group, reduced significantly at 24 months compared to baseline.[39] Both studies indicated that vitamin D does not enhance intestinal calcium absorption at high calcium intakes in older people.

In the 3-year trial in Black postmenopausal women[37] and the 1-year trial with elderly Australian women with low vitamin D status,[38] vitamin D and calcium supplementation showed no effects on bone turnover markers compared to calcium alone. The later trial also

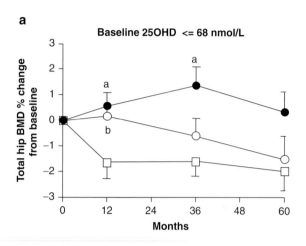

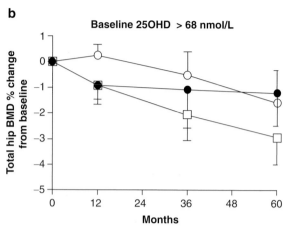

Fig. 18.2 Percent change (mean ± SE) relative to baseline in total hip BMD by baseline vitamin D status in a 5-year trail with elderly Australian women. Ca group (*open circle*) CaD group (*filled circle*) Control group (*open square*); (**a**) $p<0.05$ Ca + vitamin D group Cf Control group; (**b**) $p<0.05$ Ca group Cf Control group; (**c**) $p=0.06$ Ca + vitamin D group Cf Control group (reproduced from Zhu et al[39])

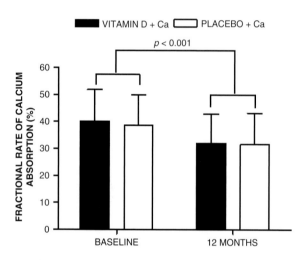

Fig. 18.3 Fractional rate of calcium absorption in a 1-year trial in elderly Australian women with low vitamin D status who received 1,000 mg calcium citrate per day with either 1,000 IU ergocalciferol (vitamin D_2) or identical placebo (control) over 12 months. *Error bars* represent SD (reproduced from Zhu et al[38] with permission of the American Society for Bone and Mineral Research)

did not show an effect on PTH. In the 5-year study with elderly Australian women, at year one, both the groups that received both calcium and vitamin D and calcium alone had lower plasma alkaline phosphatase (calcium: −6.8%, calcium and vitamin D −11.3, $p \leq 0.02$) and urinary DPD/Cr ratio (calcium: −28.7%, calcium and vitamin D −34.5%, $p \leq 0.05$) compared to

the placebo group.[39] However, at 5 years, this suppression was only maintained in the group that received both calcium and vitamin D supplementation, indicating that the long-term beneficial effects on bone density of addition of vitamin D to calcium is probably mediated by a long-term reduction in bone turnover rate. This study also found that the group that received both calcium and vitamin D had significantly low PTH levels compared to the placebo group at 3 and 5 years (27.8% and 31.3%, $p \leq 0.005$) in those subjects with high baseline PTH levels.[39]

18.3.4 Summary

Older people are at increased risk of inadequate vitamin D production in the skin because of reduced sun exposure and the reduced ability of the skin to synthesize vitamin D.[41] The resulting low vitamin D status may have negative effects on the maintenance of bone mass. Considering that vitamin D supplementation could reduce the risk of falling[42] and a meta-analysis that showed that vitamin D supplementation between 700 and 800 IU/day could reduce the risk of hip fracture by 26% and nonvertebral fracture by 23% in ambulatory or institutionalized elderly,[43] calcium and vitamin D supplementation should be recommended to all postmenopausal women and elderly men as first-line treatment for improving bone health and preventing fracture.

18.4 Conclusions

Puberty is a critical period for bone mineral accretion. Cross-sectional, prospective, and intervention studies have shown a positive association between vitamin D status and bone mass in adolescent girls aged up to 16 years. Such association was not observed in studies in prepubertal children, older adolescents, and young adults, indicating that vitamin D is more important during pubertal years when there is greater demand for calcium to meet the mineralization requirement of the growing skeleton. In older adults, a number of cross-sectional studies have shown that higher vitamin D status was related to higher bone mass. Intervention studies with vitamin D alone have only shown effects in older subjects and those with low vitamin D status. Short-term studies comparing supplementation of both calcium and vitamin D and calcium alone have shown conflicting results, which may be related to subjects' calcium intake. A long-term 5-year study has shown that the effects of calcium and vitamin D, but not calcium alone on hip BMD, were maintained at 5 years, which was probably mediated by the long-term reduction in bone turnover rate in the group that received both calcium and vitamin D.

In conclusion, vitamin D deficiency and insufficiently may result in suboptimal bone mineral accretion during growth and increased bone loss in later life. Maintaining adequate vitamin D status through increased sunlight exposure or taking vitamin D supplement should be recommended throughout life for the maintenance of bone health.

References

1. Lips P. Vitamin D deficiency and secondary hyperparathyroidism in the elderly: consequences for bone loss and fractures and therapeutic implications. *Endocr Rev*. 2001;22:477-501.
2. Hollis BW. Assessment of vitamin D nutritional and hormonal status: what to measure and how to do it. *Calcif Tissue Int*. 1996;58:4-5.
3. Norman AW, Bouillon R, Whiting SJ, Vieth R, Lips P. 13th Workshop consensus for vitamin D nutritional guidelines. *J Steroid Biochem Mol Biol*. 2007;103:204-205.
4. Dawson-Hughes B, Heaney RP, Holick MF, Lips P, Meunier PJ, Vieth R. Estimates of optimal vitamin D status. *Osteoporos Int*. 2005;16:713-716.
5. Cashman KD, Hill TR, Cotter AA, et al. Low vitamin D status adversely affects bone health parameters in adolescents. *Am J Clin Nutr*. 2008;87:1039-1044.
6. Oliveri MB, Wittich A, Mautalen C, Chaperon A, Kizlansky A. Peripheral bone mass is not affected by winter vitamin D deficiency in children and young adults from Ushuaia. *Calcif Tissue Int*. 2000;67:220-224.
7. Kristinsson JO, Valdimarsson O, Sigurdsson G, Franzson L, Olafsson I, Steingrimsdottir L. Serum 25-hydroxyvitamin D levels and bone mineral density in 16-20 years-old girls: lack of association. *J Intern Med*. 1998;243:381-388.
8. Outila TA, Karkkainen MU, Lamberg-Allardt CJ. Vitamin D status affects serum parathyroid hormone concentrations during winter in female adolescents: associations with forearm bone mineral density. *Am J Clin Nutr*. 2001;74:206-210.
9. Lehtonen-Veromaa MK, Mottonen TT, Nuotio IO, Irjala KM, Leino AE, Viikari JS. Vitamin D and attainment of peak bone mass among peripubertal Finnish girls: a 3-y prospective study. *Am J Clin Nutr*. 2002;76:1446-1453.
10. Cheng S, Tylavsky F, Kroger H, et al. Association of low 25-hydroxyvitamin D concentrations with elevated parathyroid hormone concentrations and low cortical bone density in early pubertal and prepubertal Finnish girls. *Am J Clin Nutr*. 2003;78:485-492.
11. Foo LH, Zhang Q, Zhu K, et al. Low vitamin D status has an adverse influence on bone mass, bone turnover, and muscle strength in Chinese adolescent girls. *J Nutr*. 2009;139:1002-1007.
12. Lehtonen-Veromaa M, Mottonen T, Nuotio I, Irjala K, Viikari J. The effect of conventional vitamin D(2) supplementation on serum 25(OH)D concentration is weak among peripubertal Finnish girls: a 3-y prospective study. *Eur J Clin Nutr*. 2002;56:431-437.
13. Du X, Zhu K, Trube A, et al. School-milk intervention trial enhances growth and bone mineral accretion in Chinese girls aged 10-12 years in Beijing. *Br J Nutr*. 2004;92:159-168.
14. Du X, Zhu K, Trube A, et al. Effects of school-milk intervention on growth and bone mineral accretion in Chinese girls aged 10-12 years: accounting for cluster ransomisation. *Br J Nutr*. 2005;94:1038-1039.
15. Zhu K, Du X, Cowell CT, et al. Effects of school milk intervention on cortical bone accretion and indicators relevant to bone metabolism in Chinese girls aged 10-12 y in Beijing. *Am J Clin Nutr*. 2005;81:1168-1175.
16. Zhu K, Zhang Q, Foo LH, et al. Growth, bone mass, and vitamin D status of Chinese adolescent girls 3 y after withdrawal of milk supplementation. *Am J Clin Nutr*. 2006;83:714-721.
17. Abrams SA, Copeland KC, Gunn SK, Stuff JE, Clarke LL, Ellis KJ. Calcium absorption and kinetics are similar in 7- and 8-year-old Mexican-American and Caucasian girls despite hormonal differences. *J Nutr*. 1999;129:666-671.
18. Abrams SA, O'Brien KO, Liang LK, Stuff JE. Differences in calcium absorption and kinetics between black and white girls aged 5-16 years. *J Bone Miner Res*. 1995;10:829-833.
19. Lee WT, Jiang J, Hu P, Hu X, Roberts DC, Cheng JC. Use of stable calcium isotopes (42Ca & 44Ca) in evaluation of calcium absorption in Beijing adolescents with low vitamin D status. *Food Nutr Bull*. 2002;23:42-47.
20. Ginty F, Cavadini C, Michaud PA, et al. Effects of usual nutrient intake and vitamin D status on markers of bone turnover in Swiss adolescents. *Eur J Clin Nutr*. 2004;58:1257-1265.
21. Foo LH, Zhang Q, Zhu K, et al. Relationship between vitamin D status, body composition and physical exercise of adolescent girls in Beijing. *Osteoporos Int*. 2009;20:417-425.

22. Guillemant J, Cabrol S, Allemandou A, Peres G, Guillemant S. Vitamin D-dependent seasonal variation of PTH in growing male adolescents. *Bone*. 1995;17:513-516.

23. Cadogan J, Blumsohn A, Barker ME, Eastell R. A longitudinal study of bone gain in pubertal girls: anthropometric and biochemical correlates. *J Bone Miner Res*. 1998;13:1602-1612.

24. Gordon CM, DePeter KC, Feldman HA, Grace E, Emans SJ. Prevalence of vitamin D deficiency among healthy adolescents. *Arch Pediatr Adolesc Med*. 2004;158:531-537.

25. Looker AC, Dawson-Hughes B, Calvo MS, Gunter EW, Sahyoun NR. Serum 25-hydroxyvitamin D status of adolescents and adults in two seasonal subpopulations from NHANES III. *Bone*. 2002;30:771-777.

26. Ooms ME, Lips P, Roos JC, et al. Vitamin D status and sex hormone binding globulin: determinants of bone turnover and bone mineral density in elderly women. *J Bone Miner Res*. 1995;10:1177-1184.

27. Bischoff-Ferrari HA, Dietrich T, Orav EJ, Dawson-Hughes B. Positive association between 25-hydroxy vitamin D levels and bone mineral density: a population-based study of younger and older adults. *Am J Med*. 2004;116:634-639.

28. Bischoff-Ferrari HA, Kiel DP, Dawson-Hughes B, et al. Dietary calcium and serum 25-hydroxyvitamin D status in relation to BMD among U.S. adults. *J Bone Miner Res*. 2009;24:935-942.

29. Hunter D, Major P, Arden N, et al. A randomized controlled trial of vitamin D supplementation on preventing postmenopausal bone loss and modifying bone metabolism using identical twin pairs. *J Bone Miner Res*. 2000;15:2276-2283.

30. Ebeling PR, Wark JD, Yeung S, et al. Effects of calcitriol or calcium on bone mineral density, bone turnover, and fractures in men with primary osteoporosis: a two-year randomized, double blind, double placebo study. *J Clin Endocrinol Metab*. 2001;86:4098-4103.

31. Peacock M, Liu G, Carey M, et al. Effect of calcium or 25OH vitamin D3 dietary supplementation on bone loss at the hip in men and women over the age of 60 [see comments]. *J Clin Endocrinol Metab*. 2000;85:3011-3019.

32. Ooms ME, Roos JC, Bezemer PD, van der Vijgh WJ, Bouter LM, Lips P. Prevention of bone loss by vitamin D supplementation in elderly women: a randomized double-blind trial. *J Clin Endocrinol Metab*. 1995;80:1052-1058.

33. Kantorovich V, Gacad MA, Seeger LL, Adams JS. Bone mineral density increases with vitamin D repletion in patients with coexistent vitamin D insufficiency and primary hyperparathyroidism. *J Clin Endocrinol Metab*. 2000;85:3541-3543.

34. Dawson-Hughes B, Harris SS, Krall EA, Dallal GE. Effect of calcium and vitamin D supplementation on bone density in men and women 65 years of age or older. *N Engl J Med*. 1997;337:670-676.

35. Meier C, Woitge HW, Witte K, Lemmer B, Seibel MJ. Supplementation with oral vitamin D3 and calcium during winter prevents seasonal bone loss: a randomized controlled open-label prospective trial. *J Bone Miner Res*. 2004;19:1221-1230.

36. Dawson-Hughes B, Dallal GE, Krall EA, Harris S, Sokoll LJ, Falconer G. Effect of vitamin D supplementation on wintertime and overall bone loss in healthy postmenopausal women. *Ann Intern Med*. 1991;115:505-512.

37. Aloia JF, Talwar SA, Pollack S, Yeh J. A randomized controlled trial of vitamin D3 supplementation in African American women. *Arch Intern Med*. 2005;165:1618-1623.

38. Zhu K, Bruce D, Austin N, Devine A, Ebeling PR, Prince RL. Randomized controlled trial of the effects of calcium with or without vitamin D on bone structure and bone-related chemistry in elderly women with vitamin D insufficiency. *J Bone Miner Res*. 2008;23:1343-1348.

39. Zhu K, Devine A, Dick IM, Wilson SG, Prince RL. Effects of calcium and vitamin D supplementation on hip bone mineral density and calcium-related analytes in elderly ambulatory Australian women: a five-year randomized controlled trial. *J Clin Endocrinol Metab*. 2008;93:743-749.

40. Heaney RP, Dowell MS, Hale CA, Bendich A. Calcium absorption varies within the reference range for serum 25-hydroxyvitamin D. *J Am Coll Nutr*. 2003;22:142-146.

41. MacLaughlin J, Holick MF. Aging decreases the capacity of human skin to produce vitamin D3. *J Clin Invest*. 1985;76:1536-1538.

42. Bischoff-Ferrari HA, Dawson-Hughes B, Willett WC, et al. Effect of Vitamin D on falls: a meta-analysis. *JAMA*. 2004;291:1999-2006.

43. Bischoff-Ferrari HA, Willett WC, Wong JB, Giovannucci E, Dietrich T, Dawson-Hughes B. Fracture prevention with vitamin D supplementation: a meta-analysis of randomized controlled trials. *JAMA*. 2005;293:2257-2264.

Dietary Patterns and Bone Health

19

Helen M. Macdonald and Antonia C. Hardcastle

19.1 Introduction

This chapter details the different methods used in the study of dietary patterns, covering the advantages and disadvantages of the general approach. It includes methodological considerations with regard to generating dietary patterns and gives examples of where the dietary pattern approach has been used to help further our understanding of diet and disease. Finally, it highlights examples of the application of the dietary pattern approach in more novel situations.

Research into nutrition and bone health is dominated by the nutrients calcium and vitamin D, which is partly historical because of the clear effects these nutrients have in the cure and prevention of rickets. Recently, the research focus has widened to include other nutrients: magnesium, vitamin K, and protein. There has been increased interest in the nutrients associated with fruits and vegetables. The benefits on bone health have been attributed either to their acid-balancing properties or the nutrients they contain, including minerals (calcium, magnesium, potassium, silicon, and boron), vitamins (vitamin C, vitamin K, and folate), and other potential bioactive compounds such as flavonoids and phytoestrogens. However, focusing on nutrients may not be the ideal way to study the effects of diet on disease. People do not eat separate nutrients and most of us eat a mixture of different foods which make up our diet. There are a number of

reasons why the single nutrient or single food approach may be flawed.

First, there is the issue of the accuracy of the food composition database that is used in the analysis of the dietary data for generating nutrient intakes. This can be avoided when food intake is studied. We know that the food matrix can affect the absorption of nutrients, for example, calcium can reduce the absorption of iron. There are also numerous examples of nutrients where the form of the nutrient available "off-the-shelf" may not be the same as the form that is found in food. Folate is produced and sold as folic acid because that is the form of the nutrient that is most stable. However, there are many different forms of folate in foods. Similarly, the mineral silicon is found as silica, which is not bioavailable, or as orthosilicic acid, the form of silicon that can be readily absorbed (Table 19.1). Perhaps, most important is the issue of colinearity of nutrients, which exists because many nutrients have common food sources. For example, dietary intake of potassium may be a marker for magnesium or many other nutrients associated with fruit and vegetable intake.

For these reasons, it is important to consider intakes of foods, not just nutrients. Still, one has to be careful when investigating a single food or food group because this can still give misleading results. If a subject has a higher intake or increases the intake of one type of food, it is likely that intakes of other foods will be different or change (i.e., lowered or decreased) in order to compensate for the difference or change in energy intakes. If there is no compensation, then overall energy intakes will be higher or increase. These problems can be avoided if one examines the diet as a whole. The challenge is to be able to manage the large of amount of data that is generated when analyzing what people eat.

H.M. Macdonald (✉)
Department of Applied Medicine, University of Aberdeen, Foresterhill, Aberdeen, AB25 2ZD, UK
e-mail: h.macdonald@abdn.ac.uk

P. Burckhardt et al. (eds.), *Nutritional Influences on Bone Health*,
DOI: 10.1007/978-1-84882-978-7_19, © Springer-Verlag London Limited 2010

Table 19.1 Examples of the different forms of particular nutrients in food

Nutrient	Nutrient forms available
Folic acid (folate)	Monoglutamyl folate (folic acid) 5-methyltetrahydrofolate 5,10 methylenetetrahydrofolate 5,10 methenyltetrahyrdofolate 10-formyltetrahydrofolate Folates have glutamyl side chains of differing lengths
Vitamin E	Gamma tocopherol (gamma is 7,8-dimethyl) Alpha tocopherol (alpha is 5,7,8-trimethyl) Beta tocopherol (beta is 5,8-dimethyl) Delta tocopherol (delta is 8-methyl) Tocotrienes (available in alpha, beta, gamma and delta forms)
Vitamin K	Phylloquinone (vitamin K1) Menaquinones (vitamin K2) Menadione (synthetic, vitamin K3)
Carotenoids	Alpha carotene (provitamin A) Beta carotene (provitamin A) Beta cryptoxanthin (provitamin A) Lycopene Lutein Zeaxanthin
Silicon	Silica (silicon dioxide), silicates monosilicic acid (orthosilicic acid), $(Si(OH)_4)$
Vitamin D	Cholecalciferol (vitamin D3) Ergocalciferol (vitamin D2) A number of metabolites of vitamin D3 are found in meat

There are many bioactive compounds present in plants and there are different metabolites of vitamins in animal products

19.2 Generate Dietary Patterns (Table 19.2)

19.2.1 Non-computer-Generated Approaches

Dietary patterns can be obtained using an intuitive approach. The investigator decides which groups should be combined (e.g., summing intakes of different types of meat (pork, beef, lamb) for total meat) and how many food groups should be included in the dietary pattern. The dietary patterns themselves are defined by the investigator. The investigator may use national dietary guidelines as the basis of a dietary pattern and score foods according to how much they represent the healthy eating pattern. This approach has been used to show how adhering to dietary recommendations is associated with reduced mortality[1].

19.2.2 Common Computer-Generated Approaches

More recently, specific data reduction techniques have been employed to generate dietary patterns. The two methods most widely used are cluster analysis and factor analysis. They can be found as features of common statistical software packages (e.g., SPSS, SPSS Inc., Chicago, US). The factor analysis technique used in most studies is principal components analysis (PCA),

Table 19.2 Summary of different approaches to generate dietary patterns

Method	Comment
Manually derived	
Intuitive	Investigator defines the dietary pattern
Targeted	Predefined dietary patterns usually based on recommended dietary guidelines
Computer software-derived	
Cluster analysis	Data reduction technique. Subjects are sorted (clustered) based on dietary intakes
Factor analysis	Data reduction technique. Principal components analysis. The aim is to explain the maximum amount of variance in the diet with the minimum number of factors derived from the dietary variables
Reduced rank regression	Similar to principal components analysis, but the aim is to explain the maximum amount of variance in a marker of health or disease with the minimum number of dietary variables
Other	
Partial least squares analysis	Not a data reduction technique, but helps define which components of the diet are most important in relation to a marker of disease outcome

and further details on methodological considerations regarding PCA are given in Sect. 19.2.4 of this chapter.

In cluster analysis, it is the people or cases that are sorted or clustered. For example, people who eat large amounts of fruit and small amounts of meat will cluster differently from people who eat small amounts of fruit and large amounts of meat. The disease trait (e.g., bone mineral density) or disease outcome (e.g., fracture) is then compared between the different dietary clusters. For PCA, the focus is on the dietary data (the independent variable), not the subjects or cases. PCA is concerned with the total variance in the diet, and highly correlated variables are converted to components or factors. The aim of this technique is to explain the maximum amount of variance by the minimum number of factors.

19.2.3 Other Computer-Generated Approaches

Reduced rank regression and partial least squares (PLS) analysis are newer statistical methods that can be used to explore dietary patterns. In reduced rank regression, the diet is regressed on an outcome variable. It is similar to PCA, but whereas for PCA the aim is to generate dietary components that explain the maximum variation in diet, the aim of reduced rank regression is to generate dietary components that explain the maximum amount of variation in a set of biomarkers.

In PLS analysis, the dietary variables (food groups) and outcome measures (the disease traits, e.g., blood pressure, bone mineral density) are combined and the relationships between the food groups and the outcome markers are quantified.

19.2.4 Methodological Considerations in Principal Components Analysis

The objective of PCA is to explain the maximum amount of variation with the minimum number of variables. In case of diet, the statistical analysis packages can produce factors from the complete range of foods

that are recorded for a particular study. However, to help interpret the results, most investigators do not include each individual food that is eaten by each subject. Instead, they group foods according to similarity, and this is done prior to the statistical data reduction. Therefore, there is a subjective element to this method, regarding the initial choice of food groups. Energy intake is considered a confounder when studying the different aspects of the diet, and energy adjustment is routinely done when studying the influence of nutrient intake on health or disease outcome. Using this rationale, most studies investigating dietary patterns have the foods "energy-adjusted," usually by regressing the food on energy intake.[2]

19.3 Choice of Food Groups

Table 19.3 shows typical food groupings that can be made prior to the data reduction step. The choice of groupings may change from study to study, depending on the types of food eaten in the population under investigation, but the main groupings are often comparable. Although it is harder to interpret the output, it is worthwhile rerunning PCA with the ungrouped foods to check that the dietary patterns generated from both approaches are similar. The category of miscellaneous foods is sometimes problematic, because there is a danger that unlike foods may be grouped together inappropriately. Tomato sauce may be combined with mayonnaise or salad dressing, but there could be an argument for tomato products to be included as a fruit and vegetable item. Similarly, nuts and crisps are nutritionally quite different, but often combined as snack item. Even foods that appear to belong to a particular group may better be considered separately, for example, tinned (canned) fruit could be considered as a separate group from total fruit.

19.4 Interpreting the Statistical Output

Scree plots help us to assess whether the data reduction technique has achieved its aim. The scree plot is a graph of the variance explained vs. the number of factors that are generated by the data reduction technique. It is usually characterized by a steep slope at the start, which

Table 19.3 Examples of food groupings prior to data reduction

Foods	Food groups
Lamb, beef, pork	Red meat
Beefburgers, sausages, ham	Processed meat
Chicken	Poultry
Herring, mackerel, salmon	Oily fish
Cod, haddock, plaice	White fish
Eggs	Eggs
Yogurt, milk	Low fat milk and milk products
Cheese, cream	High fat milk products
Weetabix, Rice Krispies, Special K, porridge	Breakfast cereals
Spaghetti, pasta, rice	Rice and pasta
White bread, brown bread, bread rolls	Bread
Apples, oranges, raspberries, mango	Fresh fruit
Canned peaches, pears	Canned fruit
Prunes, sultanas, raisins	Dried fruit
Orange juice, apple juice	Fruit juice
Jacket potatoes, mashed potatoes, chips	Potatoes
Carrots, parsnips, swede	Root vegetables
Broccoli, green beans	Green vegetables
Tomatoes, peppers, cucumber	Salad vegetables
Biscuits, cakes, puddings	Sweets
Chocolates, sweets	Confectionery
Butter, hard margarine, lard	High fat spread
Low fat margarine	Low fat spread
Tea	Tea
Coffee	Coffee
Cola, coke, lemonade	Carbonated beverages
Diet coke, diet lemonade	Diet carbonated beverages
Red wine, white wine	Wine
Beer, lager	Beer
Vodka, gin, whisky, port	Spirits
Crisps and nuts	Savory snacks
Jam, honey, sauces, mayonnaise	Miscellaneous

The list is not exhaustive. Some foods (e.g., bread, pasta and rice) may be split into wholemeal and white

then levels off (Fig. 19.1). This indicates that the first few factors explain most of the variance in the data. If the slope is linear, it suggests that each factor in turn explains a small amount of the variance and there is no advantage over examining the dietary groups individually.

Tables are produced showing the score for each food group with regard to each factor or particular dietary pattern. The score can be negative or positive and cut-offs can be defined for ease of interpretation. Usually, cut-offs of 0.2–0.3 are employed so that scores below these values are not shown in the score table. This makes it easier to see which food groups are the main contributors to each factor or dietary pattern. The cut-off does not remove these data from the analysis, but the absence of the minor-contributing foods helps the investigator to distinguish the type of diet for each factor.

19.5 Studies Involving Dietary Patterns

19.5.1 Dietary Patterns from Different Countries

Although foods eaten around the world can be quite different, the patterns generated often fall into two types, arbitrarily labeled by investigators as – the healthy, prudent, or traditional diet and the unhealthy, "westernized," processed food diet (Table 19.4). Comparison between four different European countries showed that two main dietary patterns – one with high consumption of salad vegetables and the other with high consumption of pork, processed meat, and potatoes – were similar.[3]

19.5.2 Dietary Patterns and Chronic Disease

The dietary pattern approach has been used to define relationships between diet and mortality[4,5] and with many chronic diseases or conditions including heart disease,[6,7] blood pressure,[8] diabetes,[9,10] cancer,[11–14] and with lipid biomarkers.[15] When dietary patterns were examined in the Multi-Ethnic Study of Atherosclerosis (MESA), only processed meat intake was found to be associated with telomere length.[16]

Fig. 19.1 Example of Scree plots generated using principal components analysis (PCA)

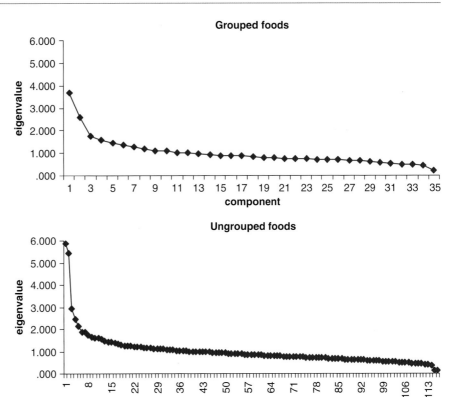

Table 19.4 Typical examples of two dietary patterns

Prudent/healthy diet	Western/unhealthy food diet
Foods with positive factor loadings	Foods with positive factor loadings
Fruit	Processed meat
Vegetables	Red meat
Fish	Fats/oil
Pasta/cereal	Cakes/desserts/confectionery products
Foods with negative factor loadings	
Red meat	
Processed meat products	

19.5.3 Dietary Patterns and Bone Health

At the 2000 ISNAO meeting, we reported the association of food groups with bone loss in perimenopausal and early postmenopausal women.[17]

There are four published studies that have investigated the dietary patterns generated by data reduction techniques in relation to bone health. Tucker et al used cluster analysis in the Framingham study, to generate six key patterns.[18] Men in the fruit, vegetable, and cereal group had higher BMD compared to men in the candy group, and women in the candy group had lower BMD at the radius compared to women in the other dietary groups. Okubo et al used PCA in their study of Japanese farmwomen.[19] They found that a healthy dietary pattern (high intakes of green and yellow vegetables, mushrooms, fish and shellfish, processed fish and fruits) was associated with BMD, whereas there was a trend for a "Western" dietary pattern (high intakes of fats; oil, meat, and processed meat) to be inversely associated with BMD. Also, a recently published study involving Greek women used PCA to identify ten dietary patterns.[20] The dietary pattern that was characterized by high consumption of fish and olive oil and low intakes of red meat was associated with LS BMD and total body BMD.

A prudent dietary pattern (generated by PCA) in late pregnancy was predictive of the child's bone mineral density at the age of 9 years.[21] The prudent diet was characterized by high intakes of fruits, vegetables, wholemeal bread, rice, and pasta, and low intakes of processed food. The same dietary pattern in early pregnancy was not significantly associated with BMD in the child.

In addition, data from the Aberdeen Prospective Osteoporosis Screening study show associations with BMD and bone resorption markers (Hardcastle et al, submitted). A summary of the studies that show an association between dietary patterns and markers of bone health is given in Table 19.5.

Recently, the dietary modification trial of the women's health initiative study (which involved 48,835 postmenopausal women aged 50–79 years) found that an intervention diet requiring lower intakes of fat and increased fruits, vegetables, and grains modestly reduced the risk of multiple falls and slightly lowered hip BMD, but did not affect the risk of osteoporotic fractures.[22]

19.6 Novel Approaches

Most of the work done, so far, on dietary patterns has focused on reducing the information collected for the whole diet in some way and then relating that information to health outcomes. The dietary pattern approach can be widened to include other aspects for the study of diet and disease.

19.6.1 Within Food Groups

Alcohol drinking patterns were associated with risk factors for atherosclerosis in men in France.[23] In the US, beer-drinking in men and wine-drinking in women were associated with improved BMD.[24]

The PLS method can highlight what foods contribute the most to a particular dietary pattern. This technique can be exploited further to study foods within food groups. For example, PLS can be used to examine which fruit or vegetable may be important in the relationship between fruit and vegetable intake and markers of bone health (Hardcastle et al, submitted). Figure 19.2 shows a typical output from PLS analysis. The "variable importance plot" shows that oranges, peppers, green vegetables, salad, tomatoes, onions, grapes, apples, and tomatoes were important in the maintenance of spine BMD in premenopausal and perimenopausal women.

19.7 Timing of Food Intake

The time of day when a food is eaten and the intervals between meals may affect bone metabolism. Calcium taken in the evening appears to suppress bone turnover, whereas this does not happen if supplements are taken in the morning.[25] There is debate as to whether this is beneficial for bone health, because the normal circadian rhythm is for parathyroid hormone to increase overnight and in postmenopausal women, who lose bone at a faster rate, this overnight rise is blunted. Work on rats has shown that food fractionation (dividing the daily food intake into portions) maintains bone mineral content,[26-28] an effect that appeared to be mediated by PTH.[29] The authors suggested that if this situation applied to humans, then "frequent small meals of appropriate composition may help prevent osteoporosis." Clowes and coworkers found that bone turnover makers were suppressed after giving glucose orally and that octreotide, an inhibitor of gastrointestinal hormone production, abolished the bone turnover response to glucose intake, and that PTH secretion increased.[30] They suggested that the change in bone turnover which occurs on feeding is probably mediated by an octreotide-inhibitable endocrine factor.

In the current climate of increasing obesity, there is interest in the timing of food intake in relation to satiety.[31-33] Much of the work involves categorizing macronutrient intakes, for example, according to how much is consumed at fixed times of the day.[34] An alternative approach is to use the data reduction techniques that have been employed in investigating dietary patterns. One can use either the time of day, intermeal interval, or meal number. Preliminary work shows that this approach is promising (Macdonald et al manuscript in preparation), but there are limitations for each of the three methods: (1) The arbitrary cut-off regarding the time of day may mean that lunchtime for one individual is placed in a different category compared to where lunchtimes are placed for other individuals; (2) similar intermeal intervals may apply to different times of day; and (3) depending on the number of meals eaten, the third meal of the day may be midmorning snack for one person, but the evening meal for another. It is likely that a combination of approaches may be required.

Table 19.5 Summary of recent studies involving dietary patterns and bone health

Study	*n*	Subjects	Statistical analysis method	Dietary patterns	Outcome
Tucker et al[18]	907	Older men and women (Framingham study) age 69–96 years, US	Cluster analysis: six patterns from FFQ	(1) Meat, dairy, and bread (2) meat and sweet baked products (3) sweet baked products (4) alcohol (5) candy (6) fruits, vegetables, and cereal	Men with a dietary pattern rich in candy diet had lower BMD than those with a dietary pattern characterized by high intakes of fruits, vegetables and cereal ($p<0.05$) after adjustment for confounders
Okubo et al[19]	291	Premenopausal farmwomen age 40–55 years, Japan	PCA: four patterns from diet history questionnaire	(1) Healthy: vegetables, fruits, fish, and mushrooms (2) traditional Japanese (3) Western: fats and oils, meats and processed meat (4) Beverage and meats	The healthy pattern was associated with BMD ($p<0.05$) and there was a trend for the Western diet to be inversely associated with BMD ($p=0.08$) after adjustment for confounders
Kontogianni et al[20]	220	Adult women mean age 48 ± 12 years (50:50 premeno-pausal and peri-/postmenopausal), Greece	PCA: ten patterns from 3-day food records	(1) Dairy, cereals, red meat, and olive oil (2) vegetables, fruits, and olive oil (3) fish, olive oil (low red meat/products) (4) Poultry and nuts (low red meat/products) (5) alcohol (6) legumes (7) sweets 8) fruit drinks (9) coffee (10) soft drinks	A pattern characterized by high consumption of fish and olive oil and low intake of red meat was positively associated with LS BMD ($p=0.017$) and total body BMC ($p=0.048$). Scores for adherence to the Mediterranean diet were not associated with bone health
Cole et al[21]	198	Pregnant mothers age 17–43 years, UK	PCA: unknown number of patterns from FFQ. Details of one pattern were reported	(1) Prudent diet: fruits and vegetables, wholemeal bread, rice pasta, yogurt, cheese, fish, and milk.	The prudent diet in late pregnancy was associated with BMC and areal BMD of the offspring at the age of 9 years ($p=0.04$ after adjustment for confounders)
Hardcastle et al	3226	Postmenopausal women, age 50–59 years, UK	PCA: five patterns from FFQ. Partial least squares analysis was used to determine which food groups were important contributors to bone health	(1) Healthy diet: fruits, vegetables, and rice/pasta (2) Processed food diet: processed foods, cakes, and desserts (low intakes of bread and fats/oils (3) Bread and butter diet: bread and fats/oils (low red meat and liquor) (4) Fish and fries diet: fish, fish dishes, potatoes, bread, and fats/oils (5) Nondairy diet: confectionery, chips/nuts, and sauces (low milk intakes)	The healthy diet was associated with decreased bone resorption (urinary pyrridinoline cross-links) ($p<0.001$). The "processed foods" diet and "nondiary" diet were associated with lower hip and spine BMD ($p<0.001$ after adjustment for confounders)

PCA principal components analysis; *FFQ* food frequency questionnaire; *BMD* bone mineral density; *LS* lumbar spine; *BMC* bone mineral content

Fig. 19.2 Example of a variable importance plot generated using partial least squares (PLS) analysis of fruit and vegetable intakes. The *x*-axis, labeled "VAR-ID" shows the individual fruits and vegetables. The *y*-variable labeled "VIP[2]" shows the strength of the relationship between each fruit and vegetable with lumbar spine bone mineral density (BMD); values greater than 1 are considered to be important, whereas those below 0.5 are unimportant. This plot shows that oranges have the strongest relationship with lumbar spine BMD. The *error bars* are 95% confidence intervals

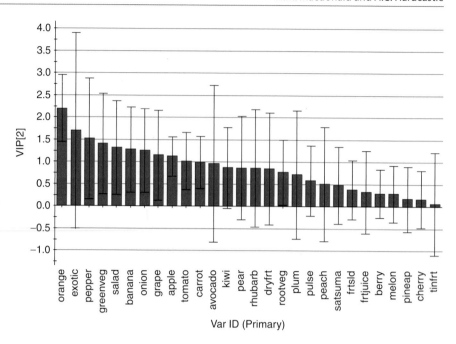

19.8 Conclusions

The study of dietary patterns is useful because it avoids problems that are encountered when studying nutrients only, namely, colinearity of nutrients, database accuracy, and interaction between nutrients which affects their bioavailability. It may also help focus future studies: if we find that a particular dietary pattern is dominated by a particular food group that may be rich in certain nutrients, then studies can be designed to investigate this further. The dietary pattern approach used alone does not help us understand why particular foods may be beneficial for health or assist us in defining the underlying mechanisms.

In conclusion, ietary patterns may be helpful in focusing future research and when used together with a nutrient-based approach, they could help further our knowledge in elucidating the role of nutrition on health and the prevention of chronic diseases.

Acknowledgments The authors wish to thank Lorna Aucott for statistical advice, Jackie Clowes for the opportunity to work on dietary timings, and Marsha Samber for assistance in generating discrete meals from Access databases. We are very grateful to all the women who have taken part in the Aberdeen studies, without whom this work would not have been possible.

References

1. Kant AK, Schatzkin A, Graubard BI, Schairer C. A prospective study of diet quality and mortality in women. *JAMA*. 2000; 283:2109-2115.
2. Willett WC, Howe GR, Kushi LH. Adjustment for total energy intake in epidemiologic studies. *Am J Clin Nutr*. 1997;65:1220S-1228S.
3. Balder HF, Virtanen M, Brants HA, et al. Common and country-specific dietary patterns in four European cohort studies. *J Nutr*. 2003;133:4246-4251.
4. Hoffmann K, Boeing H, Boffetta P, et al. Comparison of two statistical approaches to predict all-cause mortality by dietary patterns in German elderly subjects. *Br J Nutr*. 2005; 93:709-716.
5. Waijers PM, Ocke MC, van Rossum CT, et al. Dietary patterns and survival in older Dutch women. *Am J Clin Nutr*. 2006;83:1170-1176.
6. Kerver JM, Yang EJ, Bianchi L, Song WO. Dietary patterns associated with risk factors for cardiovascular disease in healthy US adults. *Am J Clin Nutr*. 2003;78:1103-1110.
7. Heroux M, Janssen I, Lam M, et al. Dietary patterns and the risk of mortality: impact of cardiorespiratory fitness. *Int J Epidemiol*. 2010;39:197-209.
8. Dauchet L, Kesse-Guyot E, Czernichow S, et al. Dietary patterns and blood pressure change over 5-y follow-up in the SU.VI.MAX cohort. *Am J Clin Nutr*. 2007;85:1650-1656.
9. Nettleton JA, Steffen LM, Ni H, Liu K, Jacobs DR Jr. Dietary patterns and risk of incident type 2 diabetes in the Multi-Ethnic Study of Atherosclerosis (MESA). *Diabetes Care*. 2008;31:1777-1782.

10. Schulze MB, Hoffmann K, Manson JE, et al. Dietary pattern, inflammation, and incidence of type 2 diabetes in women. *Am J Clin Nutr.* 2005;82:675-684; quiz 714-715.

11. Ibiebele TI, van der Pols JC, Hughes MC, Marks GC, Williams GM, Green AC. Dietary pattern in association with squamous cell carcinoma of the skin: a prospective study. *Am J Clin Nutr.* 2007;85:1401-1408.

12. Rouillier P, Senesse P, Cottet V, Valleau A, Faivre J, Boutron-Ruault MC. Dietary patterns and the adenomacarcinoma sequence of colorectal cancer. *Eur J Nutr.* 2005;44:311-318.

13. Kolahdooz F, Ibiebele TI, van der Pols JC, Webb PM. Dietary patterns and ovarian cancer risk. *Am J Clin Nutr.* 2009;89:297-304.

14. Wu AH, Yu MC, Tseng CC, Stanczyk FZ, Pike MC. Dietary patterns and breast cancer risk in Asian American women. *Am J Clin Nutr.* 2009;89:1145-1154.

15. Newby PK, Muller D, Tucker KL. Associations of empirically derived eating patterns with plasma lipid biomarkers: a comparison of factor and cluster analysis methods. *Am J Clin Nutr.* 2004;80:759-767.

16. Nettleton JA, Diez-Roux A, Jenny NS, Fitzpatrick AL, Jacobs DR Jr. Dietary patterns, food groups, and telomere length in the Multi-Ethnic Study of Atherosclerosis (MESA). *Am J Clin Nutr.* 2008;88:1405-1412.

17. Macdonald HM, New SA, Golden MHN, Grubb DA, Reid DM. Food groups affecting perimenopausal and early postmenopausal bone loss in Scottish women. In: Burckhardt P, Dawson-Hughes B, Heaney RP, eds. *Nutritional Aspects of Osteoporosis.* Fourth International Symposium on Nutritional Aspects of Osteoporosis, Switzerland, 2000. New York: Academic Press; 2001:399-407.

18. Tucker KL, Chen H, Hannan MT, et al. Bone mineral density and dietary patterns in older adults: the Framingham Osteoporosis Study. *Am J Clin Nutr.* 2002;76:245-252.

19. Okubo H, Sasaki S, Horiguchi H, et al. Dietary patterns associated with bone mineral density in premenopausal Japanese farmwomen. *Am J Clin Nutr.* 2006;83:1185-1192.

20. Kontogianni MD, Melistas L, Yannakoulia M, Malagaris I, Panagiotakos DB, Yiannakouris N. Association between dietary patterns and indices of bone mass in a sample of Mediterranean women. *Nutrition.* 2009;25:165-171.

21. Cole ZA, Gale CR, Javaid MK, et al. Maternal dietary patterns during pregnancy and childhood bone mass: a longitudinal study. *J Bone Miner Res.* 2009;24:663-668.

22. McTiernan A, Wactawski-Wende J, Wu L, et al. Low-fat, increased fruit, vegetable, and grain dietary pattern, frac-

tures, and bone mineral density: the Women's Health Initiative Dietary Modification Trial. *Am J Clin Nutr.* 2009; 89:1864-1876.

23. Rouillier P, Bertrais S, Daudin JJ, Bacro JN, Hercberg S, Boutron-Ruault MC. Drinking patterns are associated with variations in atherosclerotic risk factors in French men. *Eur J Nutr.* 2006;45:79-87.

24. Tucker KL, Jugdaohsingh R, Powell JJ, et al. Effects of beer, wine, and liquor intakes on bone mineral density in older men and women. *Am J Clin Nutr.* 2009;89:1188-1196.

25. Blumsohn A, Herrington K, Hannon RA, Shao P, Eyre DR, Eastell R. The effect of calcium supplementation on the circadian rhythm of bone resorption. *J Clin Endocrinol Metab.* 1994;79:730-735.

26. Li F, Muhlbauer RC. Food fractionation is a powerful tool to increase bone mass in growing rats and to decrease bone loss in aged rats: modulation of the effect by dietary phosphate. *J Bone Miner Res.* 1999;14:1457-1465.

27. Muhlbauer RC, Li F. Frequency of food intake and natural dietary components are potent modulators of bone resorption and bone mass in rats. *Biomed Pharmacother.* 1997;51: 360-363.

28. Muhlbauer RC, Fleisch H. The diurnal rhythm of bone resorption in the rat. Effect of feeding habits and pharmacological inhibitors. *J Clin Invest.* 1995;95:1933-1940.

29. Muhlbauer RC, Fleisch H. The food-induced stimulation of bone resorption in the rat, assessed by the urinary. *Bone.* 1995;17:449S-453S.

30. Clowes JA, Allen HC, Prentis DM, Eastell R, Blumsohn A. Octreotide abolishes the acute decrease in bone turnover in response to oral glucose. *J Clin Endocrinol Metab.* 2003;88: 4867-4873.

31. de Castro JM. The time of day of food intake influences overall intake in humans. *J Nutr.* 2004;134:104-111.

32. Berteus Forslund H, Lindroos AK, Sjostrom L, Lissner L. Meal patterns and obesity in Swedish women-a simple instrument describing usual meal types, frequency and temporal distribution. *Eur J Clin Nutr.* 2002;56:740-747.

33. Speechly DP, Rogers GG, Buffenstein R. Acute appetite reduction associated with an increased frequency of eating in obese males. *Int J Obes Relat Metab Disord.* 1999;23:1151-1159.

34. de Castro JM. The time of day and the proportions of macronutrients eaten are related to total daily food intake. *Br J Nutr.* 2007;98:1077-1083.

20

Nutritional Factors that Influence Change in Bone Density and Stress Fracture Risk Among Young Female Cross-County Runners

Jeri W. Nieves, Kathryn Melsop, Meredith Curtis, Kristin L. Cobb, Jennifer L. Kelsey, Laura K. Bachrach, Gail Greendale, and MaryFran Sowers

20.1 Introduction

Stress fractures are common among young female competitive athletes, especially among those participating in track and field. There are limited data that suggest that disordered eating, low calcium and dairy product intake, and low dietary fat intake may be related to stress fracture incidence.[1-10] Numerous dietary factors have been hypothesized to relate to BMD including calcium, vitamin D, phosphorous, potassium, vitamin C, fiber, protein, fat, and iron. However, few longitudinal studies have examined the role of diet on skeletal health in female endurance athletes, although this population may have unique nutritional requirements because of their intense physical activity. Potential interactions among foods in the diet may limit the evaluation of single nutrients and bone health. Therefore, it is important to consider the impact of food groups and dietary patterns of the whole diet on bone health. The goal of this study was to identify potential nutritional factors and dietary patterns that predict stress fractures and change in BMD in young female long-distance runners.

20.2 Methods

The population was 150 runners who were recruited from cross-country teams, running clubs, and road race participants. There were 125 (85%) women who provided some follow-up information. The inclusion criteria were that women had to run ≥40 miles per week, compete in races, and should not have used oral contraceptives within the past 6 months. This dietary analysis was within a randomized trial of OC or no intervention for 2 years on BMD and stress fracture. Age, race/ethnicity, and age at menarche were recorded. Based on the number of menstrual cycles, they were classified as normal (>9 cycles/past year), oligomenorrheic (4–9 cycles/past year), or amenorrheic (<4 cycles/past year). A modified version of the 97-item National Cancer Institute Health Habits and History food frequency questionnaire[11] was used, with the inclusion of additional food items[12]. The 97 food items were categorized into 30 food groups and the total intake (g/day) of each food group was calculated by summing the intakes of food items. Body composition, BMC and BMD at the femur, spine, and whole body were measured by Hologic, DXA. Height and weight were measured and body mass index (BMI) (kg/m^2) was calculated. Stress fractures were self-reported and then confirmed by X-ray, bone scan, or magnetic resonance imaging to be counted in this study. Cox proportional hazards models were used to compute adjusted hazard ratios for the rate of a first stress fracture during follow-up as calculated among those with a given nutrient intake divided by the rate among those with a referent nutrient intake. Adjusted annual rates of change of BMD and BMC by

J.W. Nieves (✉)
Clinical Research Center and Columbia University, Helen Hayes Hospital, Route 9W, West Haverstraw, NY 10993, USA
e-mail: jwn5@columbia.edu

P. Burckhardt et al. (eds.), *Nutritional Influences on Bone Health*,
DOI: 10.1007/978-1-84882-978-7_20, © Springer-Verlag London Limited 2010

nutrients and beverages were estimated from linear mixed models, adjusted for clinical site, age, annual menses, and treatment assignment in the randomized trial. Dietary patterns were derived by reduced rank regression, an analysis that determines linear functions of predictors (foods) by maximizing the explained variation in responses (nutrients hypothesized, a priori, including calcium, vitamin D, phosphorous, potassium, vitamin C, fiber, protein, fat, and iron).

20.3 Results

At baseline, the average age was 22 years upon entry and 83% were Whites. The percent body fat was 18% in these runners who ran an average of 34 miles per week. Mean spine BMD z-score was 0.56 and mean hip BMD z-score was 0.31 and one third of the woman reported a history of a stress fracture. An 8% of women had amenorrhea and 26% had oligomenorrhea. The average intake for all nutrients met or exceeded the recommendations except for potassium and phosphorus. Dietary pattern 1 was correlated with the following foods or nutrients: high dairy ($r=0.94$), low fat ($r=-0.36$), and high protein ($r=0.42$) consumption. Dietary pattern 2 was correlated with high fruit and vegetable ($r=0.76$), high fiber ($r=0.61$), high protein ($r=0.24$), and low fat consumption ($r=-0.23$).

There were 18 fractures in 125 women or 14.4% fractured over 2 years. The skeletal sites of the stress fractures were the tibia ($n=10$), foot ($n=5$), femur ($n=2$) and pelvis ($n=1$). We found that higher intakes of calcium, skim milk, milk, and servings of dairy products per day were each related to a reduced rate of stress fracture, although the strongest protection was from higher skim milk consumption. Every additional cup of skim milk consumed per day was associated with a 62% reduced fracture risk. A diet pattern with high dairy and low fat was associated with a 68% reduction in stress fracture risk.

Calcium intake was positively related to the annual gains in BMD of the spine, hip, and total body as well as total body BMC. For every standard deviation increase in calcium intake (approximately 600 mg), women gained an additional 0.0022 g/cm² in hip BMD, 0.0025 g/cm² in total body BMD, and 6.6 g in total body BMC annually. Skim milk, total milk intake, and number of servings of dairy products per day predicted

gains in hip BMD and whole-body BMC. Vitamin D intake predicted gains in spine and hip BMD. Animal protein, a component of milk, predicted gains in whole-body BMD and BMC. There was a positive relationship between increased intake of potassium and significant increases in BMD of the hip and whole-body BMC. For every standard deviation increase in potassium (approximately 900 mg), there was a gain of 6 ± 2.3 g per year in total body BMC. Using the dietary patterns that resulted from the reduced rank regression analysis, we found that individuals with diets high in dairy and low in fat had a greater annual increase in hip BMD, and individuals with diets high in fruits, vegetables, and fiber and low in fat consumption had significantly greater increases in whole-body BMD and BMC. All data were further stratified by menstrual regularity vs. irregularity in order to evaluate the joint effects of menstrual function and diet. Consumption of dairy products predicted positive change in hip BMD in both menstrual groups. Calcium intake predicted positive bone changes in women with both regular and irregular menstrual function, although the magnitudes of the changes were higher in the irregularly menstruating women. The positive effect of animal protein on total body bone was confined to irregularly menstruating women. This suggests that nutritional intake may be more critical in irregularly menstruating women.

20.4 Discussion

The results of our study indicate that in young female runners, higher intakes of calcium, skim milk, and dairy products were associated with lower rates of stress fracture. In fact, a diet pattern with high dairy and low fat consumption was associated with a 68% reduction in stress fracture. In addition, modest increases in total body BMD and BMC were associated with higher intakes of skim milk, dairy foods, calcium, animal protein, and potassium. Small increases in hip BMD were associated with higher intakes of calcium, vitamin D, skim milk, dairy foods, potassium, and a dietary pattern of high dairy and low fat. There were strengths and limitations associated with this analysis. This was a relatively small sample size with a specific population of runners. There is a possibility of uncontrolled or unmeasured confounding. It is possible that menstrual irregularity or OC use may modify the effect of diet, although we have controlled for these variables in the analyses. In fact, stratified analysis showed slightly stronger associations with diet and change in BMD in those individuals with menstrual irregularity. There is a potential for problems in dietary recall and there was limited detail on dietary information (e.g., cola, sodium, caffeine). It is possible that some unmeasured aspects of bone strength may be involved. Several findings of individual nutrients (e.g., potassium) need to be further explored, but are supported in this study by diet pattern analysis, showing the importance of a diet high in fruits and vegetables.

We conclude that, an overall healthy diet, with low fat milk to provide adequate calcium, vitamin D, and sufficient in fruits and vegetables may provide the greatest skeletal benefit to cross-county runners.

Acknowledgments This study was funded by a grant from the U.S. Army Medical Research and Materiel Command, award number DAMD17-98-1-8518.

References

1. Nattiv A. Stress fractures and bone health in track and field athletes. *J Sci Med Sport*. 2000;3(3):268-279.

2. Bennell KL et al. The incidence and distribution of stress fractures in competitive track and field athletes. A twelve-month prospective study. *Am J Sports Med*. 1996;24(2):211-217.

3. Armstrong, D.W., 3rd, et al., *Stress fracture injury in young military men and women*. Bone, 2004. **35**(3): p. 806-16.

4. Bennell KL et al. Risk factors for stress fractures in track and field athletes. A twelve-month prospective study. *Am J Sports Med*. 1996;24(6):810-818.

5. Bennell KL et al. Risk factors for stress fractures in female track-and-field athletes: a retrospective analysis. *Clin J Sport Med*. 1995;5(4):229-235.

6. Myburgh KH et al. Low bone density is an etiologic factor for stress fractures in athletes. *Ann Intern Med*. 1990;113(10): 754-759.

7. Cline AD, Jansen GR, Melby CL. Stress fractures in female army recruits: implications of bone density, calcium intake, and exercise. *J Am Coll Nutr*. 1998;17(2):128-135.

8. Lappe JM, Stegman MR, Recker RR. The impact of lifestyle factors on stress fractures in female Army recruits. *Osteoporos Int*. 2001;12(1):35-42.

9. Schwellnus MP, Jordaan G. Does calcium supplementation prevent bone stress injuries? A clinical trial. *Int J Sport Nutr*. 1992;2(2):165-174.

10. Lappe J et al. Calcium and vitamin d supplementation decreases incidence of stress fractures in female navy recruits. *J Bone Miner Res*. 2008;23(5):741-749.

11. Block GL, et al., Health habits and history questionnaire: diet history and other risk factors. Bethesda, MD: National Cancer Institute; 1989.

12. Nieves JW et al. Teenage and current calcium intake are related to bone mineral density of the hip and forearm in women aged 30-39 years. *Am J Epidemiol*. 1995;141(4):342-351.

A Dietary Pattern That Predicts Physical Performance in an Elderly Population

21

Jeri W. Nieves, Elizabeth Vasquez, Yian Gu, Jose Luchsinger, Yaakov Stern, and Nikolaos Scarmeas

21.1 Introduction

Poor physical performance in the elderly is related to falls and fractures and can easily be measured by lower extremity function tests such as walking speed and chair stands. Dietary intake is a potentially modifiable risk factor for improving physical performance, yet there is limited information regarding the influence of diet on physical performance. In several studies, higher intakes of protein, calcium, magnesium, and vitamin D have been related to improved physical performance in elderly subjects.[1-3] In addition, improved leg strength as measured by either a faster 8-ft. walking speed test or a quicker timed sit-to-stand test was related to higher serum 25(OH)D concentrations in over 4,000 adults over the age of 60.[4] Given that higher lean body mass is related to improved physical performance measures, it is possible that predictors of lean mass may also relate to performance. Increased dietary protein intake based on quintiles of intake between 50 and 90 g/day was associated with greater lean mass over 3 years in the Health ABC participants aged 70–79.[5] In addition, urinary potassium excretion, as a potential marker of fruit and vegetable intake, was significantly and positively related to lean body mass.[6] The objective of this study was to further explore the impact of dietary intake on physical performance in a cohort of 1,155 community dwelling elderly. We were particularly interested in a dietary pattern that would relate to the intake of the following nutrients: protein, calcium, magnesium, potassium, and vitamin D.

21.2 Methods

The study included participants of the Washington Heights-Inwood Columbia Aging Project (WHICAP). Subjects were identified (via ethnicity and age stratification processes) from a probability sample of Medicare beneficiaries residing in an area of three contiguous census tracts within northern Manhattan. Each subject in this study underwent a structured in-person interview including an assessment of health and function as well as a dietary evaluation. Each participant completed chair stands and a 4-m walk speed. The walk speed was measured as a continuous variable (time in seconds) using the average of the times for two walks, at usual pace, over a measured 4-m course. To complete the chair-stand test, participants were asked to rise five times from a seated position as quickly as possible with their hands folded across the chest, and performance was expressed as total time to complete the test.

The following were measured and considered as potential covariates: age (years), education (years), caloric intake (kcal), and body mass index (BMI) were used as continuous variables. Several categorical variables were included in the models including the following: ethnicity, gender, smoking status, alcohol consumption, and the Charlson Index of Comorbidity. The 61-item version of Willett's semiquantitative food frequency questionnaire was administered in English or Spanish. The validity (using two 7-day food records) and reliability (using two 3-month frequency assessments) of this food frequency questionnaire have been previously reported.[7] The 61 food items were categorized into 30 food groups on the basis of similarities in food and nutrient composition, and a total intake (gram/day) of each food group was then calculated by summing the intakes of member food

J.W. Nieves (✉)
Clinical Research Center and Columbia University Helen
Hayes Hospital, Route 9W, West Haverstraw, NY 10993, USA
e-mail: jwn5@columbia.edu

items. We applied reduced rank regression (RRR) to derive a dietary pattern predictive of the five specified nutrients. RRR is a statistical dimension-reduction technique similar to principal component analysis[8] that has been used in nutritional epidemiology to derive dietary patterns. RRR determines linear combinations of a set of predicting variables (30 food groups) by maximizing the explained variation of a set of response variables (five nutrients: protein, calcium, magnesium, potassium, and vitamin D).[9] The first factor explains more response variation than any other linear function of predictors. The response scores were used as independent variables in an ANCOVA model for the two physical performance variables.

21.3 Results

The demographics of the population studied can be found in Table 21.1. The average age of the people in this cohort was 75 years, and 31% were male. The ethnic groups were equally distributed between White, Black, and Hispanic. Almost half of the cohort had less than 12 years of education. Most individuals had at least one additional comorbidity.

The dietary patterns from RRR explained 75% of the total variation in nutrient intakes and 20% of the total variation in food intakes and one primary dietary pattern emerged. High loadings indicate strong associations between the assessed variables and the dietary pattern. This pattern was characterized by elevated consumption of fruits, vegetables, legumes, poultry, and low-fat dairy as evident by the factor loadings noted in Table 21.2. Factor loadings represent the magnitude and direction of each food group's contribution to a specific dietary pattern score. A positive factor loading indicates an increase intake of the food group. A negative loading indicates less intake of the food group. Food groups in the dietary pattern with factor loadings >0.2 or < −0.2 are considered potentially important.

Correlations between the RRR dietary pattern and protein, vitamin D, calcium, magnesium, and potassium were 0.841, 0.343, 0.615, 0.864, and 0.925, respectively. Individuals with greater consumption of food in this dietary pattern, high in fruits and vegetables, legumes, chicken, and low-fat dairy, had a faster walk speed and quicker time to complete five chair stands as compared to those with lower consumption of these food ($p < 0.05$ after controlling for age, gender, BMI, and comorbidity).

Table 21.1 Demographic and descriptive characteristics of the cohort of 1,155 elderly

Variables	
Age (years)	75±5.8
Gender (% male)	31
Ethnicity	
White (%)	30
Black (%)	33
Hispanic (%)	35
BMI (g/cm²)	28±5.6
Education	
Less than 12 years (%)	43
High school graduate (%)	23
Post high school (%)	34
Charlson score	
0	16%
1	29%
2	27%
≥3	28%

Table 21.2 Factor loading of selected dietary pattern with selected food groups

Selected food groups	Factor I
Cruciferous vegetables	0.26
Dark-yellow vegetables	0.28
Green leafy vegetables	0.17
Tomatoes	0.27
Potatoes	0.21
Other vegetables	0.27
Fruits	0.32
Fruit juices	0.22
Legumes	0.22
Nuts	0.16
Fish	0.19
Poultry	0.25
Red meats	0.17
High fat dairy	0.15
Low-fat dairy	0.33

21.4 Discussion

In this elderly cohort, we found that a dietary pattern that is high in fruits and vegetables, legumes, poultry and low-fat dairy explained most of the variations in the five nutrients a priori chosen to be related to physical performance (protein, calcium, magnesium, potassium, and vitamin D). This dietary pattern was found to be related to faster walk speed and time to complete five chair stands, after controlling for age, gender, BMI, and comorbidities. There were several strengths as well as limitations in this analysis. This was a large cohort of community dwelling elderly with extensive data collection. One limitation is that little was known about diet and physical performance so the nutrient selection was based on sparse data. In addition, dietary data collection using a food frequency questionnaire is subject to errors, particularly vitamin D that is confounded by sunlight exposure. The use of RRR allows simultaneous evaluation of correlated nutrients; this allows a combination of all nutrients that are potentially related to physical function to be evaluated all together.

We conclude that a dietary pattern that is high in fruits, vegetables, legumes, poultry, and low-fat dairy is positively related to physical performance. A higher intake of components in this diet resulted in a quicker walk speed and faster time to complete five chair stands. The use of food patterns may lead to an easier public health message regarding the role of diet in physical function as well as overall health.

Acknowledgement Funding from NIA AG07232 and AG028506

References

1. Sharkey JR, Giuliani C, Haines PS, Branch LG, Busby-Whitehead J, Zohoori N. Summary measure of dietary musculoskeletal nutrient (calcium, vitamin D, magnesium, and phosphorus) intakes is associated with lower-extremity physical performance in homebound elderly men and women. *Am J Clin Nutr.* 2003;77(4):847-856.
2. Hitz MF, Jensen JE, Eskildsen PC. Bone mineral density and bone markers in patients with a recent low-energy fracture: effect of 1 y of treatment with calcium and vitamin D. *Am J Clin Nutr.* 2007;86(1):251-259.
3. Swanenburg J, de Bruin ED, Stauffacher M, Mulder T, Uebelhart D. Effects of exercise and nutrition on postural balance and risk of falling in elderly people with decreased bone mineral density: randomized controlled trial pilot study. *Clin Rehabil.* 2007;21(6):523-534.
4. Bischoff-Ferrari HA, Dietrich T, Orav EJ, et al. Higher 25-hydroxyvitamin D concentrations are associated with better lower-extremity function in both active and inactive persons aged > or =60 y. *Am J Clin Nutr.* 2004;80(3):752-758.
5. Houston DK, Nicklas BJ, Ding J, et al. Dietary protein intake is associated with lean mass change in older, community-dwelling adults: the Health, Aging, and Body Composition (Health ABC) Study. *Am J Clin Nutr.* 2008;87(1):150-155.
6. Dawson-Hughes B, Harris SS, Ceglia L. Alkaline diets favor lean tissue mass in older adults. *Am J Clin Nutr.* 2008;87(3): 662-665.
7. Scarmeas N, Stern Y, Mayeux R, Luchsinger JA. Mediterranean diet, Alzheimer disease, and vascular mediation. *Arch Neurol.* 2006;63(12):1709-1717.
8. Hoffmann K, Schulze MB, Schienkiewitz A, Nöthlings U, Boeing H. Application of a new statistical method to derive dietary patterns in nutritional epidemiology. *Am J Epidemiol.* 2004;159(10):935-944.
9. Hu FB. Dietary pattern analysis: a new direction in nutritional epidemiology. *Curr Opin Lipidol.* 2002;13(1):3-9.

Citrus Hesperidin and Bone Health: From Preclinical Studies to Nutritional Intervention Trials

22

Véronique Habauzit, Elizabeth Offord, and Marie-Noëlle Horcajada

22.1 Introduction

Osteoporosis is an age-related systemic condition influenced by the interaction of multiple environmental factors with genetics.[1] Nutrition is one of the most important lifestyle factors that can influence bone mass and strength and ultimately the risk of osteoporosis. Although adequate calcium and vitamin D intakes are essential, other nutrients contained in human diet, especially in plant-derived food such as fruit and vegetables, deserve to be considered.[2] There is a growing accumulation of epidemiological, experimental, and clinical data indicating that higher fruit and vegetables intakes may positively correlate with bone health status in both young and older age groups.[3,4] Beyond their alkaline nature, hypothesized to protect bone from demineralization, fruit and vegetables are an important source of many other nutrients required for the maintenance of skeletal health, including magnesium, zinc, copper, iron, fluoride, and vitamins K, C, and A.[5] Furthermore, the benefits of fruit and vegetables may be associated with the presence of bioactive phytochemical compounds, such as polyphenols. The influence of specific polyphenols belonging to the class of flavonoids (e.g., genistein and daidzein from soy products, quercetin/rutin from onions, resveratrol and kaempferol from grapes and red wine, (+)-catechin and epigallocatechin gallate from green tea, oleuropein from olives, etc.) have been examined primarily in animal models of bone loss and/or bone cell culture systems.[6] Most of these phytonutrients, assessed for their effects on bone, revealed multiple beneficial actions such as promoting osteoblast functions, inhibiting osteoclast activities, and restoring bone mass and bone strength after an induced-bone loss. However safe, pharmacokinetic and bioavailability studies for these phenolic compounds are mostly lacking.[7] As a result, clinical studies with pure phenolic compounds, with the exception of soy isoflavones, assessing bone health parameters (bone mineral density, bone biomarkers, and fractures risk) are not yet available. Because of the large number of molecules, there is a need to focus on the most promising polyphenols to examine end points relative to osteoporosis risk.[8] In this context, hesperidin, a citrus fruit-derived flavonoid, recently appeared to be a natural compound satisfying many of the requirements for development as a dietary active ingredient for the prevention of age-related bone loss.

This chapter will, therefore, summarize the preclinical data obtained with hesperidin prior to clinical testing in nutritional intervention studies in postmenopausal women.

22.2 Dietary Intake, Safety, Bioavailability, and Metabolism of Hesperidin

Hesperidin (hesperetin-7-O-rhamnoglucoside; Fig. 22.1) belongs to the class of flavonoids called flavanones, which occur almost exclusively in citrus fruits and juices. The content of hesperetin (aglycone form of hesperidin) in oranges and orange juices ranges from 31 to 43.2 mg/100 g and from 200 to 700 mg/L, respectively.[9,10] The daily intake of hesperidin has not been precisely evaluated in different populations, but

M.-N. Horcajada (✉)
Nutrition and Health, Nestle, Centre de recherche Nestle,
PO Box 44, Vers chez les blanc, Lausanne 26, Switzerland 1000
e-mail: marienoelle.horcajada@rdls.nestle.com

P. Burckhardt et al. (eds.), *Nutritional Influences on Bone Health*,
DOI: 10.1007/978-1-84882-978-7_22, © Springer-Verlag London Limited 2010

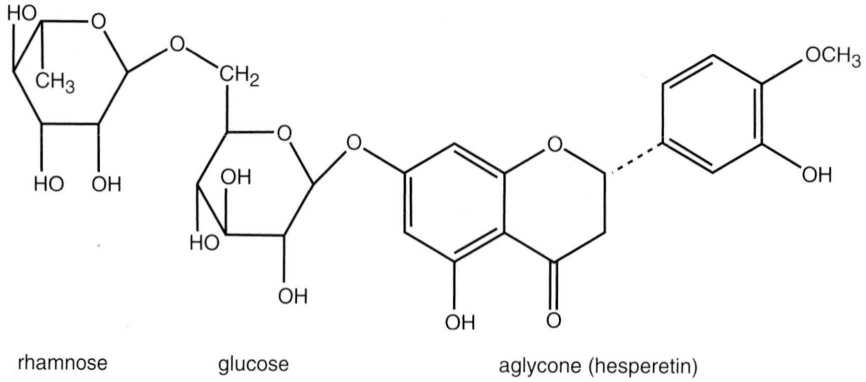

Fig. 22.1 Chemical structure of hesperidin (hesperetin-7-O-rhamno-glucoside)

rhamnose   glucose   aglycone (hesperetin)

it could be quite high in view of the worldwide consumption of citrus products (i.e., in Western countries, intakes of oranges range from 35 to 50 kg per person per year). Thus in Finland, the average daily intake per capita of hesperetin has been estimated to be 28.3 mg, equivalent to 50% of the total flavonoid intake.[11,12] Among naturally occurring flavonoids, hesperidin has been generally accepted to be safe due to the history of safe consumption. Moreover, hesperidin is commonly used as a combination product in traditional medicine for which the administration was found to result in minor side effects compared with placebo.[13]

Over the past few years, understanding of the processes of absorption and metabolism of flavanones has increased. It is now established that hesperidin is present in citrus fruits in the form of glycoside (i.e., a rhamnose-glucoside bound to hesperetin in oranges) that cannot be absorbed in its native form. Similarly to other flavonoids linked to a rhamnose moiety, hesperidin must reach the colon to be hydrolyzed by rhamnosidases of the gut microflora before absorption.[14] Once absorbed, hesperetin enters the circulation as mammalian conjugates (typically glucuronidated, sulfated, and/or methylated metabolites)[15,16] (Fig. 22.2). There are only a few studies on the bioavailability of flavanones in humans. Even if values may fluctuate depending on the source and the dose, maximum measured plasma concentrations of flavanones are in the nM to low μM range.[17] For instance, the maximum concentrations of hesperetin metabolites reached in plasma 5–7 h after the consumption of 130–220 mg given as orange juice were 1.3–2.2 μmol/L.[18,19] A more recent study in humans has demonstrated that daily consumption, for 3 weeks, of 236 mL of orange juice providing close to 230 mg of hesperidin led to an increase of the plasma concentrations of hesperetin from 3.3 up to

22 nmol/L.[20] Thus we can consider that hesperidin has limited bioavailability in humans. However, we have demonstrated that enzymatic removal of the rhamnose sugar from hesperidin to yield hesperetin-7-glucoside (H-7-G) improves its bioavailability by threefold in human subjects.[21] In rodents, the total plasma or serum concentrations detected after oral administration of hesperidin were also in the low μM range.[22-24] In the series of preclinical studies performed in rats (Fig. 22.3), we observed quantitative and qualitative profiles of hesperitin metabolites in accordance with literature cited (Table 22.1).

Despite the moderate bioavailability of citrus flavanones, we can reasonably think that flavanones may reach target cells or organs at sufficiently high concentrations to exert biological and pharmacological effects in both animals and humans. Some of these biological activities have been reported in in vivo experiments to be antioxidant, hypocholesterolemic, veinotonic, anti-inflammatory, and anticarcinogenic.[17,25] In recent years, we and others have shown that hesperidin may have positive activities in promoting bone growth, preventing bone degradation, and modulating bone metabolism in rodent animal models.[26-28]

22.3 Hesperidin and Bone Health: Preclinical Development

22.3.1 Hesperidin and Bone Parameters in Animal Models from Different Age Groups

It has been widely reported that osteoporosis may be prevented by modulating environmental factors

Fig. 22.2 Absorption and metabolism of hesperidin. *H* hesperetin; *Hp* hesperidin; *H-7-G* hesperetin-7-glucoside. Adapted from Scalbert and Williamson[33], Nielsen et al[21]

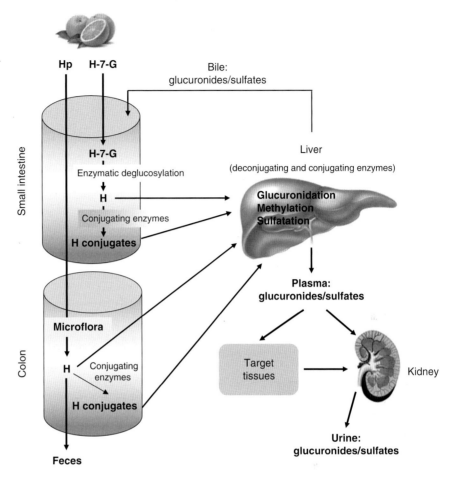

including nutrition throughout life. In our series of preclinical studies, we chose to study the impact of hesperidin on bone parameters (bone mass, bone strength, and biomarkers of bone remodeling) in intact or ovariectomized (OVX) rats (model of postmenopausal osteoporosis) of different ages (3 and 6 months old). Moreover, a rodent model of senile bone loss (21 months old) was used. Finally, the effect of hesperidin on bone mass acquisition and maintenance was evaluated in young growing (3 months old) and adult (6 months old) intact rats (Fig. 22.3). We showed that 0.5% hesperidin in the diet can improve bone mass in intact rats of 3 months, protect against bone loss in 6 months OVX rat,[27] and maintain bone mass in gonad-intact senescent male rats (data not yet published) (Table 22.2). These findings are in agreement with data obtained in OVX mice fed with the same dose of hesperidin[24] or in male orchidectomized rats consuming hesperidin through citrus juice.[29] A further study examining

H-7-G, an intestinal metabolite of hesperidin shown to be more bioavailable, has underlined a greater efficiency of its molecule in inhibiting bone loss due to OVX in 6-month-old rats.[28] In our different studies, the beneficial effect of hesperidin on bone mass has been mainly related to a slowing down of bone resorption (shown by decreased urinary free deoxypyridinoline). However, as first suggested by Chiba et al, hesperidin could not only modulate bone resorption, but also affect bone formation.[24,26]

22.3.2 Hesperidin and Bone Formation in Primary Rat Osteoblasts

Two metabolites of hesperidin (i.e., aglycone form: hesperetin (H), and one of the main conjugated metabolites: hesperetin-7-O-glucuronide (H-7-O-Glu)) have

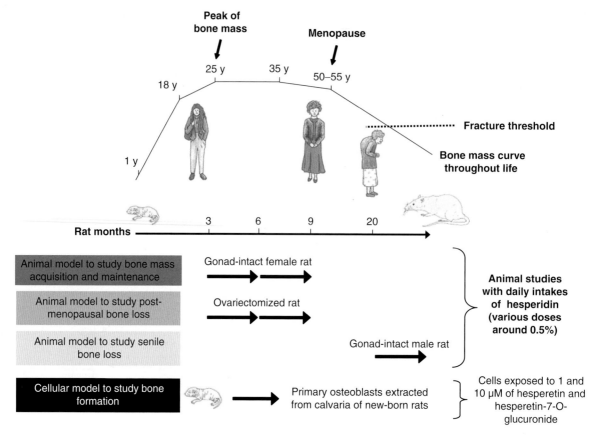

Fig. 22.3 Overview of the preclinical studies performed to test the dietary compound hesperidin as a candidate for the prevention of osteoporosis

been tested at nutritional and physiological concentrations of 1 and 10 µM in primary rat osteoblasts, a cellular model to study bone formation and osteoblastic functions[30, 31] (Fig. 22.3). Both H and H-7-O-Glu were unable to influence proliferation or mineralization, but could stimulate osteoblast differentiation (shown by an increase in alkaline phosphatase (ALP) activity), H-7-O-Glu being apparently more efficient than H at the lower nutritional dose. Both molecules were able to upregulate gene expression of Runx2 and osterix, two transcription factors well known to be implicated in the regulation of osteoblast-related genes. Finally, bone morphogenetic protein (BMP) and mitogen-activated protein kinase (MAPK) could be two of the signaling pathways of the molecular mechanisms of bone formation modulated by both compounds.

22.3.3 Hesperidin and Bone Health: Intervention Studies in Postmenopausal Women

Two randomized placebo-controlled trials are currently ongoing and performed in healthy postmenopausal women not taking an hormone replacement therapy and presenting a normal bone mass (T-score > −1) or a not severe osteopenia (−2 < T-score < −1). The primary objective is to determine the clinical efficacy of hesperidin to protect against postmenopausal bone loss and to influence positively validated biomarkers of bone formation and bone resorption. Secondarily, the safety and tolerability of the daily oral administration of hesperidin are evaluated. More details about these two studies are available at http://clinicaltrials.gov/ct2/home

Table 22.1 Qualitative and quantitative analyses of plasma metabolites of hesperidin assessed in preclinical studies with rats

Reference	Model	Treatment	Study length (months)	Qualitative analysis (percentage of total hesperetin conjugated metabolites)	Plasma concentration of total hesperetin conjugated metabolites (μM)
Horcajada et al[27]	Gonad-intact and OVX female rats, 3 and 6-month old	0.5% Hesperidin in the daily diet	3	ND	*0.5% Hp*: 12.5±2.5
Habauzit et al (data not yet published)	Gonad-intact female rats, 3-month old	0.125; 0.25; 0.5; 1 or 2.5% Hesperidin in the daily diet	3	Depending on the dose, between 6 and 26% aglycone; ~70% glucuronidated metabolites; between 7 and 12% sulfated metabolites	*0.125% Hp*: 1.3±0.5 *0.25% Hp*: 1.8±1.2 *0.5% Hp*: 3.6±0.6 *1% Hp*: 6.7±1.2 *2.5% Hp*: 23.4±4.1
Habauzit et al[28]	OVX female rats, 6-month old	Hesperidin or hesperetin-7-glucoside: 0.25 and 0.5% in the daily diet	3	*0.25% Hp and 0.5% Hp*: <4% aglycone; ~2.5% sulfated metabolites; >90% glucuronidated metabolites *0.25% H-7-G and 0.5% H-7-G*: <3% aglycone; ~34% sulfated metabolites; >60% glucuronidated metabolites	*0.25% Hp*: 1.1±0.3 *0.5% Hp*: 2.1±0.3 *0.25% H-7-G*: 2.3±0.4 *0.5% H-7-G*: 4.9±0.3
Habauzit et al (data not yet published)	Gonad-intact male rats, 20-month old	0.5% Hesperidin in the daily diet	3	*0.5% Hp*: ~5% aglycone; no sulfated forms; >90% glucuronidated metabolites	*0.5% Hp*: 1.4±0.2

ND not determined; *Hp* hesperidin; *H-7-G* hesperetin-7-glucoside; *OVX* ovariectomized

Table 22.2 Impact of hesperidin on bone parameters assessed in preclinical studies with rats

Reference	Model	Treatment	Study length (months)	Main findings
Horcajada et al[27]	Gonad-intact and OVX female rats, 3 and 6-month old	0.5% Hesperidin in the daily diet	3	Whatever the age of animals, ↓ ovariectomy-induced bone loss and ↓ bone resorption (urinary free DPD) No uterotrophic effect In 3-month-old intact rats, ↑ BMD without modulation of femoral bone strength (accelerated bone mass gain) In 6-month-old intact rats, Hp ~ BMD but ↑ femoral bone strength Plasma lipid-lowering effect
Habauzit et al (data not yet published)	Gonad-intact female rats, 3-month old	0.125; 0.25; 0.5; 1; 2.5% Hesperidin in the daily diet	3	↑ Femoral BMD and bone strength ↓ Bone resorption (urinary free DPD) Effective dose: 0.25%
Habauzit et al[28]	OVX female rats, 6-month old	Hesperidin or hesperetin-7-gluco-side: 0.25 and 0.5% in the daily diet	3	↓ Ovariectomy-induced bone loss ↓ Bone resorption (urinary free DPD) No uterotrophic effect Efficiency H-7-G > Hp Higher bioavailability of H-7-glc
Habauzit et al (data not yet published)	Gonad-intact male rats, 20-month old	0.5% Hesperidin in the daily diet	3	Protection of BMD (+ 9% vs. control group) ↓ bone resorption (urinary free DPD) Plasma lipid-lowering effect ↓ Serum IL-6 and ↓ NO production (systemic anti-inflammatory effect)

BMD bone mineral density; *DPD* deoxypyridinoline; *Hp* hesperidin; *H-7-G* hesperetin-7-glucoside; *IL-6* interleukin-6; *NO* nitric oxide; *OVX* ovariectomized

22.4 Conclusions

Dietary measures to maximize bone mass early in life and reduce the loss of bone mass later in life are accepted as one of the best strategies to reduce the risk of osteoporosis. Hence, flavonoids from plant-derived food such as hesperidin may contribute to a positive effect on bone health and thus be part of an integral strategy together with the well-established key-nutrients calcium and vitamin D. Little is known about the mechanisms of action of hesperidin on bone, but we can reasonably think that, similarly to other polyphenols,[8] hesperidin can act at a systemic level by exerting antioxidant and/or anti-inflammatory activities, as well as at a local level by modulating cellular signaling processes regulating both osteoblast[30, 31] and osteoclast functions.[32]

References

1. Duque G, Troen BR. Understanding the mechanisms of senile osteoporosis: new facts for a major geriatric syndrome. *J Am Geriatr Soc.* 2008;56:935-941.
2. Ilich JZ, Kerstetter JE. Nutrition in bone health revisited: a story beyond calcium. *J Am Coll Nutr.* 2000;19:715-737.
3. New SA. Intake of fruit and vegetables: implications for bone health. *Proc Nutr Soc.* 2003;62:889-899.
4. Prynne CJ, Mishra GD, O'Connell MA, et al. Fruit and vegetable intakes and bone mineral status: a cross sectional study in 5 age and sex cohorts. *Am J Clin Nutr.* 2006;83:1420-1428.
5. Prentice A, Schoenmakers I, Laskey MA, de Bono S, Ginty F, Goldberg GR. Nutrition and bone growth and development. *Proc Nutr Soc.* 2006;65:348-360.
6. Habauzit V, Horcajada MN. Phenolic phytochemicals and bone. *Phytochem Rev.* 2008;7:313-344.
7. Sharan K, Siddiqui JA, Swarnkar G, Maurya R, Chattopadhyay N. Role of phytochemicals in the prevention of menopausal bone loss: evidence from in vitro and in vivo, human interventional and pharma-cokinetic studies. *Curr Med Chem.* 2009;16:1138-1157.
8. Williamson G, Holst B. Dietary reference intake (DRI) value for dietary polyphenols: are we heading in the right direction? *Br J Nutr.* 2008;99(suppl 3):S55-S58.
9. Manach C, Scalbert A, Morand C, Rémésy C, Jiménez L. Polyphenols: food sources and bioavailability. *Am J Clin Nutr.* 2004;79:727-747.
10. Kyle JAM, Duthie GG. Flavonoids in foods. In: Andersen OM, Markham KR, eds. *Flavonoids: Chemistry, Biochemistry and Applications.* Boca Raton: CRC Press; 2006.
11. Kumpulainen JT. Intake of flavonoids, phenolic acids and lignans in various populations. In: *Third International Conference on Natural Antioxidants and Anticarcinogens in Food, Health and Disease*, Helsinki; 2001.
12. Knekt P et al. Flavonoid intake and risk of chronic diseases. *Am J Clin Nutr.* 2002;76:560-568.
13. Garg A, Garg S, Zaneveld LJ, Singla AK. Chemistry and pharmacology of the Citrus bioflavonoid hesperidin. *Phytother Res.* 2001;15:655-669.
14. Bokkenheuser VD, Shackleton CH, Winter J. Hydrolysis of dietary flavonoid glycosides by strains of intestinal Bacteroides from humans. *Biochem J.* 1987;248:953-956.
15. Ameer B, Weintraub RA, Johnson JV, Yost RA, Rouseff RL. Flavanone absorption after naringin, hesperidin, and citrus administration. *Clin Pharmacol Ther.* 1996;60:34-40.
16. Matsumoto H, Ikoma Y, Sugiura M, Yano M, Hasegawa Y. Identification and quantification of the conjugated metabolites derived from orally administered hesperidin in rat plasma. *J Agric Food Chem.* 2004;52:6653-6659.
17. Espin JC, Garcia-Conesa MT, Tomas-Barberan FA. Nutraceuticals: facts and fiction. *Phytochemistry.* 2007;68: 2986-3008.
18. Erlund I, Meririnne E, Alfthan G, Aro A. Plasma kinetics and urinary excretion of the flavanones naringenin and hesperetin in humans after ingestion of orange juice and grapefruit juice. *J Nutr.* 2001;131:235-241.
19. Manach C, Morand C, Gil-Izquierdo A, Bouteloup-Demange C, Rémésy C. Bioavailability in humans of the flavanones hesperidin and narirutin after the ingestion of two doses of orange juice. *Eur J Clin Nutr.* 2003;57:235-242.
20. Franke AA, Cooney RV, Henning SM, Custer LJ. Bioavailability and antioxidant effects of orange juice components in humans. *J Agric Food Chem.* 2005;53:5170-5178.
21. Nielsen IL, Chee WS, Poulsen L, et al. Bioavailability is improved by enzymatic modification of the citrus flavonoid hesperidin in humans: a randomized, double-blind, crossover trial. *J Nutr.* 2006;136:404-408.
22. Silberberg M, Gil-Izquierdo A, Combaret L, Remesy C, Scalbert A, Morand C. Flavanone metabolism in healthy and tumor-bearing rats. *Biomed Pharmacother.* 2006;60:529-535.
23. Yamada M, Tanabe F, Arai N, et al. Bioavailability of glucosyl hesperidin in rats. *Biosci Biotechnol Biochem.* 2006;70: 1386-1394.
24. Chiba H, Uehara M, Wu J, et al. Hesperidin, a citrus flavonoid, inhibits bone loss and decreases serum and hepatic lipids in ovariectomized mice. *J Nutr.* 2003;133:1892-1897.
25. Benavente-Garcia O, Castillo J, Marín FR, Ortuño A, Del Río JA. Uses and properties of Citrus flavonoids. *J Agr Food Chem.* 1997;45:4505-4515.
26. Uehara M. Prevention of osteoporosis by foods and dietary supplements. Hesperidin and bone metabolism. *Clin Calcium.* 2006;16:1669-1676.
27. Horcajada MN, Habauzit V, Trzeciakiewicz A, et al. Hesperidin inhibits ovariectomized-induced osteopenia and shows differential effects on bone mass and strength in young and adult intact rats. *J Appl Physiol.* 2008;104:648-654.
28. Habauzit V, Nielsen IL, Gil-Izquierdo A, et al. Increased bioavailability of hesperetin-7-glucoside compared with hesperidin results in more efficient prevention of bone loss

in adult ovariectomised rats. *Br J Nutr.* 2009;102:1-9. doi:10.1017/S0007114509338830.

29. Deyhim F, Garica K, Lopez E, et al. Citrus juice modulates bone strength in male senescent rat model of osteoporosis. *Nutrition.* 2006;22:559-563.

30. Trzeciakiewicz A, Habauzit V, Mercier S, et al. Hesperetin stimulates differentiation of primary rat osteoblasts involving the BMP signalling pathway. *J Nutr Biochem.* 2009;doi: 10.1016/j.jnutbio.2009.01.017.

31. Trzeciakiewicz A, Habauzit V, Mercier S, et al. Molecular mechanism of hesperetin-7-O-glucuronide, the main circulating metabolite of hesperidin, involved in osteoblast differentiation *J Agric Food Chem.* 2010;58:668-675.

32. Kim JY, Jung KJ, Choi JS, Chung HY. Modulation of the age-related nuclear factor-kappaB (NF-kappaB) pathway by hesperetin. *Aging Cell.* 2006;5:401-411.

33. Scalbert A, Williamson G. Dietary intake and bioavailability of polyphenols. *J Nutr.* 2000;130:2073S-2085S.

Acidosis and Bone

23

David A. Bushinsky

23.1 Introduction

Human metabolism leads to the production of ~1 mmol/kg of acid (protons, H^+) per day, which is termed endogenous acid production.[1,2] Additional endogenous acid production occurs during disorders such as diarrhea, diabetic ketoacidosis, and lactic acidosis. This additional acid results in a reduction of systemic pH, which is termed metabolic acidosis. The physiologic response to metabolic acidosis is to rapidly increase extracellular fluid pH toward the physiologic neutral of 7.40 to maintain optimal cellular function.[1] The homeostatic response to metabolic acidosis involves first buffering of the acid, then increasing respiratory rate to lower the partial pressure of carbon dioxide (Pco_2), and finally renal excretion of the additional acid. The initial step, buffering of the additional acid, is critical to the immediate restoration toward neutral pH allowing the preservation of life. The final step, renal excretion of the acid, begins hours after the acid challenge and is complete only days later. Renal acid excretion relies upon normal kidney function; as we age, our ability to excrete acid declines and humans become slightly, but significantly, more acidemic.[3]

Chronic metabolic acidosis, found in patients with chronic kidney disease and renal tubular acidosis, increases urinary Ca excretion secondary to a direct reduction in renal tubular Ca reabsorption.[1] There is little, if any, increase in intestinal Ca absorption resulting in a net loss of body Ca.[1] The source of much of this additional urinary Ca appears to be acid-mediated dissolution and resorption of bone mineral.[1,4] Chronic metabolic acidosis appears to decrease bone mineral content[4] and has been shown to significantly decrease bone density, formation, and growth.[5]

During the sustained metabolic acidosis of severe chronic kidney disease, blood pH remains stable, although substantially reduced, in spite of progressive acid retention, suggesting the availability of large stores of proton buffers.[1,2] During kidney failure, there is ample evidence that acidosis adversely affects bone, which may be corrected by HCO_3^- treatment. Bone carbonate is decreased in acidic uremic patients,[6] which may represent dissolution of bone carbonate or replacement by phosphate, resulting in the incorporation of acid into the mineral. In view of the deleterious effect of metabolic acidosis on bone, the National Kidney Foundation guidelines recommend treatment of metabolic acidosis to help prevent renal osteodystrophy.[7]

The common high protein diet of North Americans, coupled with the known effects of bone to buffer an acid load[1] and the age-related decline in renal function,[3] suggests that excess dietary acid derived from high protein diets may play a role in the etiology of osteoporosis.[1,8] The treatment of postmenopausal women with the base $KHCO_3$, which neutralizes endogenous acid production, leads to improved Ca retention, reduced bone resorption, and increased bone formation.[8,9] Severe, life-threatening metabolic acidosis must be treated; however, the mild metabolic acidosis present in the initial stages of chronic kidney disease and in aging, worsened in the latter case by the common acidogenic high protein diet, is rarely treated.[1]

D.A. Bushinsky
University of Rochester School of Medicine and Dentistry,
601 Elmwood Ave, Box 675, Rochester, NY 14642, USA
e-mail: david_bushinsky@urmc.rochester.edu

P. Burckhardt et al. (eds.), *Nutritional Influences on Bone Health*,
DOI: 10.1007/978-1-84882-978-7_23, © Springer-Verlag London Limited 2010

23.2 Acute Acidosis

23.2.1 Calcium Release

Cultured neonatal mouse calvariae exhibit acid-dependent net Ca efflux (J_{Ca}) during both acute (3 h [10]) and more chronic (>24–99 h) incubations.[2,11–26] The mechanism of acid-mediated Ca efflux from bone during acute incubations is direct physicochemical bone dissolution and is not cell-mediated.[11] This finding was confirmed by demonstrating Ca efflux from synthetic carbonated apatite (CAP) disks, a cell-free model of bone mineral, cultured in physiologically acid medium.[27]

The type of bone mineral in equilibrium with the medium and thus altered by physicochemical forces might be carbonate or phosphate in association with Ca. Bone carbonate is solubilized during an acute reduction in pH, leading to a release of Ca.[28,29] Further support for the role of carbonate in acid-mediated bone mineral dissolution comes from the observation that at a constant pH, whether physiologically neutral or acid, Ca flux from bone is dependent on the medium $[HCO_3^-]$; the lower the $[HCO_3^-]$, the greater the Ca efflux.[30]

23.2.2 Hydrogen Ion Buffering

The in vitro evidence for acid buffering by bone is derived from studies of acidosis-induced proton flux into bone,[2,10,28,31–33] high resolution ion microprobe evidence for a depletion of bone sodium and potassium during acidosis,[16,33–37] and from a depletion of bone carbonate and phosphate during acidosis.[33] When calvariae are cultured in medium acidified by a decrease in $[HCO_3^-]$, there is a net influx of protons into bone, decreasing medium acidity and indicating that the additional acid is being buffered by bone, ultimately leading to an increase in medium pH.[10,28,31–33] During acute acidosis, there appear to be two principal mechanisms by which the acid is buffered: proton for sodium and/or potassium exchange[16,33–37] and consumption of the buffers carbonate and phosphate.[10,28–30,33,38]

23.2.3 Fall in Bone Carbonate and Phosphate

Bone contains ≈80% of the total body carbon dioxide and acute metabolic acidosis decreases bone total carbon dioxide.[39] Bone also contains a substantial amount of the total body phosphate, estimated to be ~90%,[40] largely in the form of hydroxyapatite ($Ca_{10}(PO_4)_6(OH)_2$) and other forms of apatite.[41] During metabolic acidosis, protonation of the phosphate in apatite will consume protons and help restore the pH toward normal.[1,42,43] Using chemical analysis, a model of metabolic acidosis was found to induce the release of bone Ca and carbonate,[28] leading to a progressive loss of bone carbonate.[29]

The high resolution scanning ion microprobe was used to study the bone content of carbonate and phosphate in response to acute metabolic acidosis.[33] There was a marked preferential loss of surface HCO_3^- and of cross-sectional phosphate. When both the in vitro and in vivo studies are considered together, there is clear evidence that bone is a proton buffer capable of maintaining the extracellular fluid pH near the physiologic normal. The loss of bone sodium, potassium, carbonate, and phosphate suggests that in addition to sodium and potassium for proton exchange, bone carbonate and phosphate are lost from the mineral in response to acidosis, each of which helps to restore the pH toward normal.

23.3 Chronic Acidosis

23.3.1 Increased Bone Resorption

Chronic metabolic acidosis causes the release of bone Ca, predominantly by enhanced cell-mediated bone resorption combined with decreased bone formation.[2,12–17,20–24,32,38,44,45] There also continues to be a component of direct physicochemical acid-induced mineral dissolution.[10,11,27–31,33–37,44,46] Osteoblastic collagen synthesis and alkaline phosphatase activity both are decreased after 48 h incubation in a model of metabolic acidosis compared to neutral medium,[13] while RANKL synthesis was increased.[22,26] Release of osteoclastic β-glucuronidase, a lysosomal enzyme whose secretion correlates with osteoclast-mediated bone resorption, is increased during culture in Met. An increase in $[HCO_3^-]$, modeling metabolic alkalosis, decreases Ca efflux from bone through an increase in osteoblastic bone formation and a decrease in osteoclastic bone resorption.[15]

Support for a direct effect of metabolic acidosis to inhibit osteoblastic bone formation was obtained using primary cells isolated from the calvariae. These isolated cells, almost exclusively osteoblasts, synthesize collagen and form nodules of apatitic bone.[44] Compared to cells incubated in neutral medium, cells incubated in a model of metabolic acidosis produced fewer nodules and had decreased Ca influx into the nodules.[44]

23.3.2 Mechanism of Proton Signaling

Bone responds to metabolic acidosis through a coordinated homeostatic response aimed at normalizing systemic pH, often at the cost of decreased mineral content; however, the mechanism by which extracellular pH is sensed was previously not clear. A novel class of G-protein-coupled receptors that respond to both protons and lysosphingolipids has been recently characterized.[47] To test the hypothesis that OGR1 acts as an H^+ sensing receptor in bone cells,[18] we demonstrated that OGR1 was present in cultured neonatal mouse calvariae and then investigated whether an inhibitor of OGR1 ($CuCl_2$) would diminish acidosis-induced Ca efflux from bone, whether metabolic acidosis would increase intracellular calcium in cultured bone cells, and whether transfection of OGR1 into a heterologous cell type would permit cells to mimic the intracellular Ca response to acidosis of primary bone cells.[18] We found that $CuCl_2$ inhibits the acidosis-induced increase in Ca efflux from bone cells and that primary mouse calvarial bone cells respond to a decrease in extracellular pH with an increase in intracellular Ca. We then found that Chinese hamster ovary fibroblasts (CHO cells) increased intracellular Ca in response to a model of metabolic acidosis only after being transfected with murine OGR1 cDNA. Thus OGR1 appears to have a primary role as a proton sensor in bone cells.

23.3.3 Role of PGE_2

PGE_2 levels increase in response to chronic metabolic acidosis, leading to enhanced renal acid excretion. Prostaglandins, especially PGE_2, are potent multifunctional regulators with effects on both bone resorption and formation. Prostaglandins promote new bone formation in vivo and in isolated osteoblasts. However, in bone organ culture, PGE_2 has been shown to directly stimulate bone resorption and to stimulate RANKL expression in calvarial osteoblasts. The relative effects of prostaglandins on bone may be dependent on the timing or magnitude of dose,[48] as has been found for PTH, or dependent on stage of osteoblast differentiation.

Incubation of neonatal mouse calvariae in acidic medium increases medium PGE_2 in parallel with an increase in net Ca efflux.[23] Inhibition of PGE_2 production by indomethacin strongly limited this acidosis-induced bone Ca release as well as acid stimulation of RANKL.[22] Incubation of primary mouse calvarial bone cells, which consist mostly of osteoblasts,[49] in a model of metabolic acidosis led to a marked increase in medium PGE_2 levels, which was again completely suppressed by indomethacin.[23] Cortisol inhibits acid-induced bone resorption through a decrease in osteoblastic PGE_2 production. These results suggest that acid-induced, cell-mediated Ca efflux from bone is regulated, at least in part, by an increase in endogenous PGE_2 production in the osteoblast leading to an increase in RANKL.

Prostaglandin synthesis is regulated by the release of arachidonic acid from membrane phospholipids. The rate-limiting step converting arachidonic acid to specific prostanoids is catalyzed by cyclooxygenase (COX). There are two forms of COX: COX1, which is constitutively expressed, and COX2, which is the inducible form of the enzyme. Both forms of COX are expressed in osteoblasts. COX2 expression is regulated by several bone-resorbing factors. NS-398, a specific COX2 inhibitor, significantly inhibits H^+-induced Ca release from calvariae, which supports the hypothesis that this enzyme is stimulated by acidosis.[23–25] We tested the effects of COX2 knockout using calvariae from the offspring of matings of COX2[+/−] mice and correlating genotype and phenotype. We found COX2 is necessary for acid-induced bone Ca release and it appears that the gene dosage of COX2 sets the level of basal and of H^+-induced bone resorption. Using northern analysis, as well as real-time PCR, initial studies indicate that incubation of primary bone cells in Met causes greater stimulation of COX2 RNA levels than in Ntl, with no change in COX1.

23.3.4 Regulation of Gene Expression

External pH modulates gene expression in several cell types. To determine if metabolic acidosis would specify gene expression in osteoblasts, we examined several immediate early response genes in primary neonatal mouse calvarial cells, including egr-1, junB, c-jun, junD, and c-fos. In response to incubation in acidic medium, only the magnitude of egr-1 stimulation was dependent on medium pH.[19] Osteoblasts express type 1 collagen as the major component of the bone extracellular matrix, which subsequently becomes mineralized. Similarly to egr-1, type I collagen RNA synthesis was decreased by acidosis and increased by alkalosis.[19]

Primary mouse calvarial cells differentiate in culture to form bone nodules. These osteoblastic cells express a number of bone-specific matrix proteins, including bone sialoprotein, osteocalcin, osteonectin (ON), osteopontin (OP), and matrix gla protein (MGP).[50] Since acidic medium decreases bone nodule number, size, and Ca content,[44] we hypothesized that acidosis would alter the pattern of matrix gene expression in these long-term cell cultures. After 3–4 weeks in neutral medium OP RNA levels increased while incubation in acid medium completely inhibited this increase.[20] The RNA levels of two other proteins, ON and transforming growth factor β_1, did not vary with pH. RNA for MGP was also induced by incubation in neutral differentiation medium, while acidic medium almost totally prevented the increase in MGP RNA levels. The inhibition of MGP and OP RNA levels by acidosis was found to be reversible.[20]

We hypothesized that the acidosis-induced bone resorption was a result of alterations in osteoblastic expression of osteoclastogenic factors. Such factors include macrophage colony stimulating factor (M-CSF), a growth factor for osteoclast precursor cells, RANKL and osteoprotegerin (OPG), a decoy receptor for RANKL. Activation of RANK by RANKL

initiates a differentiation cascade that culminates in mature, bone-resorbing osteoclasts, as well as stimulation of mature osteoclast activity. Analysis of RNA extracted from calvariae incubated for 24 or 48 h in neutral or acidic medium by RT-PCR indicated that expression of RANKL RNA was upregulated by acidosis, while expression of M-CSF, OPG, and β-actin were not altered.[22] Analysis of culture supernatants by ELISA demonstrated that calvariae in acidic medium produced greater amounts of soluble RANKL protein than calvariae cultured at neutral pH; production of OPG was not affected.[26]

To examine the role of PGE_2 synthesis in RANKL expression, calvariae were incubated in the absence or presence of indomethacin to inhibit COX activity; Ca flux, as well as RANKL RNA content, was determined. Indomethacin significantly inhibited acid-induced Ca flux and completely suppressed the induction of RANKL RNA by Met.[22] Thus acidosis-induced synthesis of PGE_2 causes an autocrine or paracrine stimulation of osteoblastic prostaglandin receptors. Activation of these receptors consequently induces an increase in RANKL RNA expression, which in turn increases osteoclastogenesis and activation of mature osteoclasts.

23.4 Overview of the Response of Bone to Acid

Thus metabolic acidosis induces changes in the bone mineral, which are consistent with its role as an H^+ buffer.[2] Over the first few hours, buffering of the acidic medium pH[10,31–33] occurs through physicochemical bone mineral dissolution,[28,36] releasing Ca as well as the buffers, carbonate and phosphate.[10,29,30,33,38] There is an exchange of bone Na and K for H^+.[16,33–37] Hours later, cellular mechanisms increase bone resorption and decrease bone formation, both of which normalize systemic pH.[11–17] Increased bone resorption further releases bone carbonate and phosphate,[38,45] and decreased bone formation lessens the amount of acid produced during bone mineralization. In cells, the acidic pH is sensed by the H^+ receptor OGR1[18] and acidosis alters expression of a number of genes in osteoblasts.[19–22] Acidosis increases osteoblastic PGE_2 synthesis,[23–25] leading to an increase in RANKL expression and osteoclastic bone resorption.[22,26]

Acknowledgments Supported by grants RO1 DK 75462 and RO1 AR 46289 from the National Institutes of Health.

References

1. Lemann J Jr, Bushinsky DA, Hamm LL. Bone buffering of acid and base in humans. *Am J Physiol Renal Physiol.* 2003;285:F811-F832.

2. Bushinsky DA. Acidosis and renal bone disease. In: Olgaar, Salusky IB, Silver J, eds. *The Spectrum of Renal Osteodystropy and Calcification in Uremia.* 1st ed. 2009.

3. Frassetto LA, Morris RC Jr, Sebastian A. Effect of age on blood acid-base composition in adult humans: role of age-related renal functional decline. *Am J Physiol (Renal Fluid Electrolyte Physiol 40).* 1996;271:F1114-F1122.

4. Barzel US. The skeleton as an ion exchange system: Implications for the role of acid-base imbalance in the genesis of osteoporosis. *J Bone Min Res.* 1995;10:1431-1436.

5. Domrongkitchaiporn S, Pongsakul C, Stitchantrakul W, et al. Bone mineral density and histology in distal renal tubular acidosis. *Kidney Int.* 2001;59:1086-1093.

6. Pellegrino ED, Blitz RM. The composition of human bone in uremia. *Medicine.* 1965;44:397-418.

7. National Kidney Foundation. K/DOQI clinical practice guidelines for bone metabolism and disease in chronic kidney disease. *Am J Kidney Dis.* 2003;42:S1-S201.

8. Frassetto L, Morris RC Jr, Sebastian A. Long-term persistence of the urine calcium-lowering effect of potassium bicarbonate in postmenopausal women. *J Clin Endocrinol Metab.* 2005;90:831-834.

9. Jehle S, Zanetti A, Muser J, Hulter HN, Krapf R. Partial neutralization of the acidogenic western diet with potassium citrate increases bone mass in postmenopausal women with osteopenia. *J Am Soc Nephrol.* 2006;17:3213-3222.

10. Bushinsky DA, Krieger NS, Geisser DI, Grossman EB, Coe FL. Effects of pH on bone calcium and proton fluxes in vitro. *Am J Physiol (Renal Fluid Electrolyte Physiol 14).* 1983;245: F204-F209.

11. Bushinsky DA, Goldring JM, Coe FL. Cellular contribution to pH-mediated calcium flux in neonatal mouse calvariae. *Am J Physiol (Renal Fluid Electrolyte Physiol 17).* 1985; 248:F785-F789.

12. Bushinsky DA. Net calcium efflux from live bone during chronic metabolic, but not respiratory, acidosis. *Am J Physiol (Renal Fluid Electrolyte Physiol 25).* 1989;256:F836-F842.

13. Krieger NS, Sessler NE, Bushinsky DA. Acidosis inhibits osteoblastic and stimulates osteoclastic activity in vitro. *Am J Physiol (Renal Fluid Electrolyte Physiol 31).* 1992;262: F442-F448.

14. Bushinsky DA. Stimulated osteoclastic and suppressed osteoblastic activity in metabolic but not respiratory acidosis. *Am J Physiol (Cell Physiol 37).* 1995;268:C80-C88.

15. Bushinsky DA. Metabolic alkalosis decreases bone calcium efflux by suppressing osteoclasts and stimulating osteoblasts. *Am J Physiol (Renal Fluid Electrolyte Physiol 40).* 1996;271:F216-F222.

16. Bushinsky DA, Gavrilov K, Stathopoulos VM, Krieger NS, Chabala JM, Levi-Setti R. Effects of osteoclastic resorption on bone surface ion composition. *Am J Physiol (Cell Physiol 40).* 1996;271:C1025-C1031.

17. Bushinsky DA, Nilsson EL. Additive effects of acidosis and parathyroid hormone on mouse osteoblastic and osteoclastic function. *Am J Physiol (Cell Physiol 38).* 1995;269: C1364-C1370.

18. Frick KK, Krieger NS, Nehrke K, Bushinsky DA. Metabolic acidosis increases intracellular calcium in bone cells through activation of the proton receptor OGR1. *J Bone Min Res.* 2009;24:305-313.

19. Frick KK, Jiang L, Bushinsky DA. Acute metabolic acidosis inhibits the induction of osteoblastic *egr*-1 and type 1 collagen. *Am J Physiol (Cell Physiol 41).* 1997;272:C1450-C1456.

20. Frick KK, Bushinsky DA. Chronic metabolic acidosis reversibly inhibits extracellular matrix gene expression in mouse osteoblasts. *Am J Physiol (Renal Physiol 44).* 1998; 275:F840-F847.

21. Frick KK, Bushinsky DA. In vitro metabolic and respiratory acidosis selectively inhibit osteoblastic matrix gene expression. *Am J Physiol (Renal Physiol 46).* 1999;277: F750-F755.

22. Frick KK, Bushinsky DA. Metabolic acidosis stimulates RANK ligand RNA expression in bone through a cyclooxygenase dependent mechanism. *J Bone Miner Res.* 2003;18: 1317-1325.

23. Krieger NS, Parker WR, Alexander KM, Bushinsky DA. Prostaglandins regulate acid-induced cell-mediated bone resorption. *Am J Physiol Renal Physiol.* 2000;279:F1077-F1082.

24. Bushinsky DA, Parker WR, Alexander KM, Krieger NS. Metabolic, but not respiratory, acidosis increases bone PGE_2 levels and calcium release. *Am J Physiol (Renal Fluid Electrolyte Physiol).* 2001;281:F1058-F1066.

25. Krieger NS, Frick KK, LaPlante SK, Michalenka A, Bushinsky DA. Regulation of COX-2 mediates acid-induced bone calcium efflux in vitro. *J Bone Min Res.* 2007;22: 907-917.

26. Frick KK, LaPlante K, Bushinsky DA. RANK ligand and TNF-α mediate acid-induced bone calcium efflux in vitro. *Am J Physiol Renal Physiol.* 2005;289:F1005-F1011.

27. Bushinsky DA, Sessler NE, Glena RE, Featherstone JDB. Proton-induced physicochemical calcium release from ceramic apatite disks. *J Bone Miner Res.* 1994;9:213-220.

28. Bushinsky DA, Lechleider RJ. Mechanism of proton-induced bone calcium release: calcium carbonate-dissolution. *Am J Physiol (Renal Fluid Electrolyte Physiol 22).* 1987;253:F998-F1005.

29. Bushinsky DA, Lam BC, Nespeca R, Sessler NE, Grynpas MD. Decreased bone carbonate content in response to metabolic, but not respiratory, acidosis. *Am J Physiol (Renal Fluid Electrolyte Physiol 34).* 1993;265:F530-F536.

30. Bushinsky DA, Sessler NE. Critical role of bicarbonate in calcium release from bone. *Am J Physiol (Renal Fluid Electrolyte Physiol 32).* 1992;263:F510-F515.

31. Bushinsky DA. Net proton influx into bone during metabolic, but not respiratory, acidosis. *Am J Physiol (Renal Fluid Electrolyte Physiol 23).* 1988;254:F306-F310.

32. Bushinsky DA. Effects of parathyroid hormone on net proton flux from neonatal mouse calvariae. *Am J Physiol (Renal Fluid Electrolyte Physiol 21).* 1987;252:F585-F589.

33. Bushinsky DA, Smith SB, Gavrilov KL, Gavrilov LF, Li J, Levi-Setti R. Acute acidosis-induced alteration in bone

bicarbonate and phosphate. *Am J Physiol Renal Physiol.* 2002;283:F1091-F1097.

34. Chabala JM, Levi-Setti R, Bushinsky DA. Alteration in surface ion composition of cultured bone during metabolic, but not respiratory, acidosis. *Am J Physiol (Renal Fluid Electrolyte Physiol 30).* 1991;261:F76-F84.

35. Bushinsky DA, Levi-Setti R, Coe FL. Ion microprobe determination of bone surface elements: effects of reduced medium pH. *Am J Physiol (Renal Fluid Electrolyte Physiol 19).* 1986;250:F1090-F1097.

36. Bushinsky DA, Wolbach W, Sessler NE, Mogilevsky R, Levi-Setti R. Physicochemical effects of acidosis on bone calcium flux and surface ion composition. *J Bone Miner Res.* 1993;8:93-102.

37. Bushinsky DA, Gavrilov K, Chabala JM, Featherstone JDB, Levi-Setti R. Effect of metabolic acidosis on the potassium content of bone. *J Bone Min Res.* 1997;12:1664-1671.

38. Bushinsky DA, Chabala JM, Gavrilov KL, Levi-Setti R. Effects of in vivo metabolic acidosis on midcortical bone ion composition. *Am J Physiol (Renal Physiol 46).* 1999;277:F813-F819.

39. Bettice JA. Skeletal carbon dioxide stores during metabolic acidosis. *Am J Physiol (Renal Fluid Electrolyte Physiol 16).* 1984;247:F326-F330.

40. Bushinsky DA. Disorders of calcium and phosphorus homeostasis. In: Greenberg A, ed. *Primer on Kidney Diseases.* 4th ed. San Diego: Academic Press; 2005:120-130.

41. Neuman WF, Neuman MW. *The Chemical Dynamics of Bone Mineral.* Chicago: University Chicago Press; 1958.

42. Bushinsky DA. Acid-base imbalance and the skeleton. *Eur J Nutr.* 2001;40:238-244.

43. Krieger NS, Frick KK, Bushinsky DA. Mechanism of acid-induced bone resorption. *Current Opin in Nephrol Hypertens.* 2004;13:423-436.

44. Sprague SM, Krieger NS, Bushinsky DA. Greater inhibition of in vitro bone mineralization with metabolic than respiratory acidosis. *Kidney Int.* 1994;46:1199-1206.

45. Bushinsky DA, Smith SB, Gavrilov KL, Gavrilov LF, Levi-Setti R. Chronic acidosis-induced alteration in bone bicarbonate and phosphate. *Am J Physiol Renal Physiol.* 2003; 285:F532-F539.

46. Bushinsky DA, Sessler NE, Krieger NS. Greater unidirectional calcium efflux from bone during metabolic, compared with respiratory, acidosis. *Am J Physiol (Renal Fluid Electrolyte Physiol 31).* 1992;262:F425-F431.

47. Tomura H, Mogi C, Sato K, Okajima F. Proton-sensing and lysolipid-sensitive G-protein-coupled receptors: a novel type of multi-functional receptors. *Cellular Signal.* 2005;17: 1466-1476.

48. Raisz LG, Fall PM, Petersen DN, Lichtler A, Kream BE. Prostaglandin E_2 inhibits alpha 1(1) procollagen gene transcription and promoter activity in the immortalized rat osteoblastic clonal cell line Py1a. *Mol Endocrin.* 1993;7: 17-22.

49. Krieger NS, Hefley TJ. Differential effects of parathyroid hormone on protein phosphorylation in two osteoblast-like cell populations isolated from neonatal mouse calvaria. *Calc Tiss Int.* 1989;44:192-199.

50. Stein GS, Lian JB, Stein JL, van Wijnen AJ, Montecino M. Transcriptional control of osteoblast growth and differentiation. *Physiol Rev.* 1996;76:593-629.

Acid–Base Homeostasis and the Skeleton: An Update on Current Thinking

24

Susan A. Lanham-New

Abbreviations

BMC   Bone mineral content
BMD   Bone mineral density
IGF-1   Insulin like growth factor 1
NRAE   Net renal acid excretion
PRAL   Potential renal acid load
RDA   Recommended daily allowance

24.1 Introduction

The health benefits of a high consumption of fruit and vegetables and the influence of this food group on a variety of diseases have been gaining increasing prominence in the literature. Of interest to the bone field is the role that bone plays in acid–base balance. Natural, pathological, and experimental states of acid loading/acidosis have been associated with hypercalciuria and negative calcium balance, and more recently, the detrimental effects of "acid" from the diet on bone mineral have been demonstrated. More recently, the possibility of a positive link between a high consumption of fruit and vegetables and indices of bone health has been more fully explored. Further support for a positive link between fruit and vegetable intake and bone health can be found in the results of the DASH and DASH-Sodium intervention trials (dietary approaches to stopping hypertension).

S.A. Lanham-New
Division of Nutritional Sciences, University of Surrey, Guildford, Surrey, GU2 7XH, UK
e-mail: s.lanham-new@surrey.ac.uk

We now urgently require the implementation of (a) fruit and vegetable/alkali administration: bone health intervention trials, including fracture risk as an endpoint; and (b) reanalysis of existing dietary: bone mass/metabolism datasets to look specifically at the impact of dietary "acidity" on the skeleton.

24.2 Background

Our approach to examining the relationship between nutrition and bone health has been to focus on specific (or variety) of nutrients consumed regularly in the human diet. While this has enabled a greater understanding of the influence of the important bone minerals (i.e., calcium, phosphorus, and magnesium) to bone metabolism, there are still considerable gaps in our knowledge. We can also consider the "foods" we consume rather than the nutrients contained within them. It is interesting to note that across Nations and Countries, there is a consensus of agreement as to the proportions with which we should be eating food, even though they are displayed in different formats (e.g., UK and Australia use a plate; USA and Singapore use a pyramid; Finland uses a plate/pyramid combination).

24.3 Acid–Base Balance: Introductory Comments

Acid–base homeostasis is important for health. We know that extracellular fluid pH remains between 7.35 and 7.45, and thus it is a key requirement of our metabolic system to ensure that hydrogen ion concentrations are maintained between 0.035 and 0.045 mEq/L.[1]

P. Burckhardt et al. (eds.), *Nutritional Influences on Bone Health*,
DOI: 10.1007/978-1-84882-978-7_24, © Springer-Verlag London Limited 2010

It is essential to survival that H+ concentrations are kept within these particularly narrow limits, and hence, the body's adaptive response involves three specific mechanisms: (a) buffer systems; (b) exhalation of CO_2; and (c) kidney excretion.

Daily, humans eat substances that both generate and consume protons, and as a net result, adult humans on a normal Western diet generate ~1 mEq per kg body weight of acid per day. The more acid precursors a diet contains, the greater the degree of systemic acidity. As humans become older, their overall renal function declines, which includes their ability to excrete acid.[2]

24.4 Link Between Acid–Base Homeostasis and Bone

There are a number of points that should be considered when examining a link between acid–base maintenance and the skeleton:

First, the theoretical considerations of the role that alkaline bone mineral may play in the defense against acidosis, which date back as far as the late 1880s/ early nineteenth century. The pioneering work of Lemann and Barzel showed extensively the effects of "acid" from the diet on bone mineral in both man and animal.[3,4]

There was much debate on the consideration of the skeleton as a source of buffer, contributing to both the preservation of the body's pH and defense of the system against acid–base disorders at the first-ever Conference on Osteoporosis held in 1969.[5]

Second, the effect of dietary acidity on the skeleton needs only to be relatively small for there to be a large impact over time. Wachman and Bernstein put forward a hypothesis linking the daily diet to the development of osteoporosis based on the role of bone in acid–base balance and noted specifically that 'the increased incidence of osteoporosis with age may represent, in part, the results of a life-long utilization of the buffering capacity of the basic salts of bone for the constant assault against pH.'[6]

Third, there are clear mechanisms for a deleterious effect of acid on bone. Novel work in the 1980s by Arnett and Dempster demonstrated a direct enhancement of osteoclastic activity following a reduction in extracellular pH. This effect was shown to be independent of the influence of parathyroid hormone.[7] Furthermore, osteoclasts and osteoblasts appear to respond independently

to small changes in pH in the culture media in which they are growing.[8]

24.5 Vegetarianism and Bone

The potentially deleterious effect of specific food on the skeleton has been a topic of debate.[9–12] Work by Remer and Manz[13] examining the potential renal acid loads (known as PRAL) of a variety of food has found that many grain products and hard cheese are acidic food.[13] These food, which are likely to be consumed in large quantities in lactoovovegetarians, may provide an explanation for the lack of a positive effect on bone health indices in studies comparing vegetarians vs. omnivores.[14–16]

24.6 Fruit and Vegetables and Skeletal Health

24.6.1 Observational Studies

A variety of population-based studies published in the latter part of the twentieth century and more recently have demonstrated a beneficial effect of fruit and vegetable/potassium intake on indices of bone health in young boys and girls, premenopausal women, perimenopausal women, postmenopausal women, and elderly men and women.[17]

In trying to clarify the size of the effect of fruit and vegetables/potassium intake on bone health, a recent systematic review on over 4,800 subjects suggests a small (~0.9%) but nonetheless significant effect on bone health.[18] Much more detailed analysis is now urgently required with respect to which types of fruit and vegetables have the most direct impact on the skeleton and whether potatoes are included in the calculations for many of these observational studies. Potatoes have a PRAL value of −4.0 mEq/100 g edible portion, but are categorized differently among countries with respect to food groups. For example, in the UK Balance of Health, potatoes are included in the bread, rice, and other starch food group, whereas in Denmark it is included in the fruit and vegetable group. Furthermore, in the UK, potatoes are not included in the five portions a day recommendation, whereas in other European countries potatoes are included.

24.6.2 Dietary Intervention Studies

Further support for a positive link between fruit and vegetable intake and bone health can be found in the results of the DASH and DASH-Sodium intervention trials. In DASH, diets rich in fruit and vegetables were associated with a significant fall in blood pressure compared with baseline measurements. However, of particular interest to the bone field were findings that increasing fruit and vegetable intake from 3.6 to 9.5 daily servings decreased the urinary calcium excretion from 157 mm/day to 110 mg/day.[19] It is key to point out, however, that the authors suggested this was due to the "high fiber content of the diet possibly impeding calcium absorption," but a more likely explanation put forward by Barzel[20] was a reduction in the "acid load" with the fruit and vegetable diet compared to the control diet.[20] This study is the first population-based fruit and vegetable intervention trial showing a positive effect on calcium economy (albeit a secondary finding).

Lin et al. (2003) have reported the findings of the DASH-Sodium trial in which two dietary patterns on indices of bone metabolism were examined.[21] The DASH diet emphasizes fruits, vegetables, and low-fat dairy products and is reduced in red meat, and in this second DASH II trial, three levels of sodium intake were investigated (50, 100 and 150 nmol/L). Subjects consumed the control diet at the 150 mmol sodium intake/d levels for 2 weeks and were then randomly assigned to eat either the DASH diet or the control diet at all three sodium levels for a further 4 weeks in random order. The DASH diet, compared with the control diet, was found to significantly reduce both bone formation (by measurement of the marker osteocalcin) by 8–10% and bone resorption (by measurement of the marker CTx) by 16–18. This is an important intervention study that shows a clear benefit of the high intake of fruit and vegetables on markers of bone metabolism. Research is now required to determine the long-term clinical impact of the DASH diet on bone health and fracture risk, as well as clarification of the exact mechanisms involved with respect to this diet on skeletal protection.

24.7 Dietary Acidity and Bone

Determination of the acid–base content of diets consumed by individuals and populations is a useful way to quantify the link between acid–base balance and skeletal health. On a daily basis, humans eat substances that both generate and consume protons, and as a net result, consumption of a normal Western diet is associated with chronic, low-grade metabolic acidosis. The severity of the associated metabolic acidosis is determined, in part, by the net rate of endogenous noncarbonic acid production (NEAP) that varies with diet. Since 24-h urine collections are impractical for population-based studies, an alternative is to examine the net acid content of the diet. Frassetto et al. have found that the protein-to-potassium ratio predicts net acid excretion, and in turn, NRAE predicts calcium excretion. They propose a simple algorithm to determine the net rate of endogenous NEAP from considerations of the acidifying effect of protein (via sulfate excretion) and the alkalizing effect of potassium (via provision of salts of weak organic acids).[22,23]

24.8 Alkali Supplementation Studies and the Skeleton

24.8.1 Clinical Studies

The clinical application of the effect of normal endogenous acid production on bone is of considerable interest, with extensive work in this area by Lemann (at the subject level) and Bushinsky (at the cellular level).[24,25] Sebastian et al. demonstrated that potassium bicarbonate administration resulted in a decrease in urinary calcium and phosphorus, with overall calcium balance becoming less negative (or more positive).[26] Changes were also seen in markers of bone metabolism, with a reduction in urinary excretion of hydroxyproline (bone resorption) and an increased excretion of serum osteocalcin (bone formation). The study by Sebastian's group is of significant clinical importance and may have valued implications for the prevention and treatment of postmenopausal osteoporosis, but we need more long-term studies of the effect of alkali administration on aging bone loss. Results of the Aberdeen APOSS cohort show that in healthy postmenopausal women, long-term effects of alkali supplementation did not reduce bone loss over a 24-month period,[27] but more research in other population groups and using an alkali food approach rather than a supplementation one would be pertinent.

24.9 Concluding Remarks

It is also important to note that the positive associations found between fruit and vegetable consumption and bone may be due to some other, yet unidentified, "dietary" component rather than alkali-excess effect,[28] and there is good animal evidence to support this. Muhlbauer et al.[29] have shown that vegetables, herbs, and salads commonly consumed in the human diet affect bone resorption in the rat by a mechanism that is not mediated by their base excess,[29] but perhaps through pharmacologically active compounds, which need exploring further.[30]

Future research in this area needs to focus on the following: (a) investigating levels of potassium-rich, bicarbonate-rich food in relation of markers of bone health in a wide range of populations groups, including the young, postmenopausal women, and the elderly long-term, as well as intervention trials centered specifically on potassium-rich, bicarbonate-rich food (e.g., fruit and vegetables) as the supplementation vehicle; and (b) assessing a wide range of bone health indices (including fracture risk). Furthermore, we need more experimental studies to examine the mechanisms under which potassium-rich, bicarbonate-rich food are beneficial to bone metabolism.

References

1. New SA. The role of the skeleton in acid-base homeostasis. The 2001 Nutrition Society Medal. *Proc Nutr Soc.* 2002;61:151-164.
2. Frassetto LA, Sebastian A. Age and systemic acid-base equilibrium: analysis of published data. *J Gerontol.* 1996;51A:B91-B99.
3. Barzel US. The effect of excessive acid feeding on bone. *Calcif Tissue Res.* 1969;4:94-100.
4. JJr L, Litzow JR, Lennon EJ. The effects of chronic acid load in normal man: further evidence for the participation of bone mineral in the defence against chronic metabolic acidosis. *J Clin Invest.* 1966;45:1608-1614.
5. Barzel US. The role of bone in acid-base metabolism. In: Barzel US, ed. *Osteoporosis.* New York: Grune & Stratton; 1970:199-206.
6. Wachman A, Bernstein DS. Diet and osteoporosis. *Lancet.* 1968;I:958-959.
7. Arnett TR, Dempster DW. Effect of pH on bone resorption by rat osteoclasts in vitro. *Endocrinology.* 1986;119:119-124.
8. Bushinsky DA. Acid-base imbalance and the skeleton. In: Burckhardt P, Dawson-Hughes B, Heaney RP, eds. *Nutritional Aspects of Osteoporosis '97. Proceedings of the Third International Symposium on Nutritional Aspects of Osteoporosis, Switzerland: 1997.* Italy: Ares-Serono Symposia; 1998:208-217.
9. New SA, Millward DJ. Calcium, protein and fruit & vegetables as dietary determinants of bone health. *Am J Clin Nutr.* 2003;77:1340-1341 [letter].
10. Plant J, Tidey G. *Understanding, Preventing and Overcoming Osteoporosis.* London: Virgin; 2003.
11. New SA, Francis RF. Book review: understanding, preventing and overcoming osteoporosis by Plant & Tidey. *Sci Parliam.* 2003;85:13-15.
12. New SA. Impact of food clusters on bone. In: Dawson-Hughes B, Burckhardt P, Heaney RP, eds. *Nutritional Aspects of Osteoporosis 2000 (4th International Symposium on Nutritional Aspects of Osteoporosis, Switzerland, 1997). Challenges of Modern Medicine. Ares-Serono Symposia Publications.* San Diego: Academic Press; 2001:379-397.
13. Remer T, Manz F. Potential renal acid load of foods and its influence on urine pH. *J Am Diet Assoc.* 1995;95:791-797.
14. Fox D. Hard cheese. *New Sci.* 2001.
15. New SA, Macdonald HM, Reid DM, Dixon AStJ. Hold the soda. *New Sci.* 2002;2330:54-55.
16. Loveridge N. Lanham-New SA. Healthy ageing: bone health. In: Stanner S, Thompson R, Buttriss JL, eds. *BNF Taskforce on Healthy Ageing – The Role of Nutrition and Lifestyle.* British Nutrition Foundation. Oxford: Wiley-Blackwell; 2009.
17. Lanham-New SA. The balance of bone health: tipping the scales in favour of the potassium case. *J Nutr.* 2008;138:172S-177S.
18. Darling AL, Torgerson DJ, Hewitt C, Millward DJ, Lanham-New SA. Protein intake and bone health: a systematic review and meta-analysis. *Proc Nutr Soc.* 2008;67:E366.
19. Appel LJ, Moore TJ, Obarzanek E, et al. A clinical trial of the effects of dietary patterns on blood pressure. *New Engl J Med.* 1997;336:1117-1124.
20. Barzel US. Dietary patterns and blood pressure. *New Engl J Med.* 1997;337:637 [letter].
21. Lin P, Ginty F, Appel L, et al. Impact of sodium intake and dietary patterns on biochemical markers of bone and calcium metabolism. *J Bone Miner Res.* 2001;16(S1):S511.
22. Frassetto L, Todd K, Morris RC Jr, Sebastian A. Estimation of net endogenous noncarbonic acid production in humans from dietary protein and potassium contents. *Am J Clin Nutr.* 1998;68:576-583.
23. Remer T, Manz F. Estimation of the renal net acid excretion by adults consuming diets containing variable amounts of protein. *Am J Clin Nutr.* 1994;59:1356-1361.
24. Lemann J Jr, Pleuss JA, Gray RW, Hoffmann RG. Potassium administration increases and potassium deprivation reduces urinary calcium excretion in healthy adults. *Kidney Int.* 1991;39:973-983.

25. Bushinsky DA. Decreased potassium stimulates bone resorption. *Am J Physiol* (Renal Fluid Electrolyte Physiol). 1997; 272:F774-F780.

26. Sebastian A, Harris ST, Ottaway JH, Todd KM, Morris RC Jr. Improved mineral balance and skeletal metabolism in postmenopausal women treated with potassium bicarbonate. *New Engl J Med*. 1994;330:1776-1781.

27. Macdonald HM, Black AJ, Aucott L, et al. Effect of potassium citrate supplementation or increased fruit and vegetable intake on bone metabolism in healthy postmenopausal women: a randomized controlled trial. *Am J Clin Nutr*. 2008;88:465-474.

28. Lanham-New SA. Fruit and vegetables: the unexpected natural answer to the question of osteoporosis prevention? *Am J Clin Nutr.* 2006;83(6):1254-1255 (editorial).

29. Muhlbauer RC, Lozano AM, Reinli A. Onion and a mixture of vegetables, salads and herbs affect bone resorption in the rat by a mechanism independent of their base excess. *J Bone Miner Res*. 2002;17:1230-1236.

30. Lanham-New SA. Is "vegetarianism" a serious risk factor for osteoporotic fracture? *Am J Clin Nutr*. 2009;90(4):910-911 (editorial).

Acid–Base Balance, Bone, and Muscle

25

Bess Dawson-Hughes

25.1 Introduction

Muscle weakness and frailty in the elderly lead to falls, fractures, disability, and loss of independence. Preserving muscle mass and strength is an effective way to lower the risk of falling[1] and to maintain physical function and independence. The muscular and skeletal systems are obviously interrelated functionally; however, their connection extends beyond function. Harold Frost was one of the first to recognize the linkage, as he described in his "mechanostat theory".[2] His theory postulates that the link between muscle mass and bone mass results from the bone's ability to adapt to mechanical strain. Subsequently, it has been shown that strain can trigger a cascade of events through mechano-transduction which increase osteoblastic cell activity and the formation of new matrix proteins.[3,4] Recent work demonstrates that in adolescents, the age of peak lean tissue mass accrual precedes several parameters of bone strength accrual by 4–6 months, suggesting that muscle is an important factor affecting bone strength.[5] Bone and muscle are known to be linked genetically. In a twin study, for example, Seeman et al found that genetic factors accounted for 60–80% of the individual variances of femoral neck BMD and lean mass, and for *>50% of their covariance*.[6] Several investigators have demonstrated associations of lean tissue mass with femoral neck bone strength[7] and mass[7,8] in adults.

With aging, there is a gradual increase in the circulating $[H^+]$. In a comprehensive review, Frassetto and Sebastian identified 26 articles that included data on age and circulating $[H^+]$.[9] From the age of 20 to 80 years, they identified a 6–7% rise in blood $[H^+]$ and a 12–16% decline in plasma $[HCO_3^-]$, with most of the age-related change occurring after the age of 50 years. Renal function is known to decline with aging.[10] Renal insufficiency impairs acid–base homeostasis by reducing HCO_3^- conservation and reducing acid excretion. Typically, the glomerular filtration rate declines by 50% from the age of 20 to 80 years.[11,12]

American diets are generally acidogenic or net acid-producing because of their high content of cereal grains and protein and relatively low content of fruits and vegetables.[13] Metabolism of grains and dietary protein of both animal and plant origin produces noncarbonic acids such as sulfuric acid, and the metabolism of fruits and vegetables produces $KHCO_3$ and other alkaline potassium salts. Adults on American diets typically generate 75–100 mEq of acid per day.[14] The daily ingestion of acid-producing diets in combination with a declining capacity to excrete the acid load is thought to account for the mild but progressive metabolic acidosis seen with aging. In this chapter, evidence for the acid–base balance of the diet affecting both bone and muscle is considered.

25.2 Effects of Acid on Bone

25.2.1 Mechanisms

An acidic environment affects both osteoblastic and osteoclastic activity. Building on the earlier findings of Ludwig

B. Dawson-Hughes
Jean Mayer USDA Human Nutrition Research Center on Aging, Tufts University, 711 Washington Street, Boston, MA 02111, USA,
e-mail: bess.dawson-hughes@tufts.edu

P. Burckhardt et al. (eds.), *Nutritional Influences on Bone Health*,
DOI: 10.1007/978-1-84882-978-7_25, © Springer-Verlag London Limited 2010

who identified the OGR1 receptor on osteoblasts,[15] Tomura et al have identified the presence of a family of G protein-coupled hydrogen sensing receptors on rat osteoblasts that are coupled either to increased calcium release or altered adenylate cyclase activity.[16] Frick et al have recently provided evidence that exposure to acid induces a rapid increase in ionized calcium concentration in osteoblasts and in other cells transfected with OGR1 receptors.[17] They postulate that hydrogen ions activate OGR1 receptors on osteoblasts which leads to increases in intracellular ionized calcium, and the latter mediates increases in COX-2 and RANKL expression, with resulting increased resorption.[17] In an in vitro study in rats,[18] a reduction in medium pH from 7.4 to 6.8 was associated with a 14-fold increase in the mean area resorbed per bone slice ($p < 0.01$). In a similar in vitro study, changes in resorption rate were detectable within the physiologic range of pH.[19] Komarova et al have identified a proton receptor on rat osteoclasts.[20] In addition to its effects on osteoblasts and osteoclasts, acid appears to have a direct physico-chemical effect on bone. In a synthetic bone mineral model in which there was no cell-mediated resorption,[21] Bushinsky showed that H^+ ions cause efflux of calcium from the apatite surface. Thus, bone serves as a buffer, and in the process of neutralizing acid arising from American diets, calcium is lost from bone.

25.2.2 Human Studies

25.2.2.1 Bone Turnover

Several short-term (7–18-day) alkali intervention studies in humans have identified significant reductions in biochemical markers of bone turnover. In a crossover study in nine young subjects consuming acid-producing metabolic diets, Maurer et al[22] found that neutralization of endogenous acid with a combination of sodium and potassium bicarbonate over 7 days significantly lowered urinary pyridinoline and NTX, indicators of bone resorption. Over the following 7-day recovery period, during which the alkali was discontinued, pyridinoline and NTX excretion returned to their starting levels.[22] In another crossover study, Sebastian et al examined the effect of 60–120 mmol/day of $KHCO_3$ on serum osteocalcin, a marker of bone formation, over an 18-day period in 18 postmenopausal

women consuming high-protein metabolic diets.[23] The mean osteocalcin level rose from 5.5 ± 2.8 (SD) to 6.1 ± 2.8 ng/mL ($p < 0.001$) with alkalinization. Urine calcium excretion declined in this study from 236 ± 86 (SD) to 172 ± 81 mg/day ($p < 0.001$). In the DASH study, increasing fruit and vegetable intake from 3.6 to 9.5 servings per day significantly reduced the markers of bone turnover.[24]

25.2.2.2 Bone Loss

Jehle et al recently published the first randomized controlled trial that examined the effect of alkali on the rates of bone loss.[25] In 161 postmenopausal women at a mean age of 60 years, treatment with a relatively low dose of 30 mmol/day of potassium citrate significantly reduced bone loss from the spine and hip, but not the radius or total body, over a 1-year period, when compared with the treatment with potassium chloride.[25] On the contrary, a recent randomized, placebo-controlled trial revealed that treatment with potassium citrate in a dose of 55.5 mEq/day for 2 years did not significantly reduce bone loss from the spine or hip in a similar population.[26] Thus the effect of alkali administration on the rates of bone loss is unresolved.

25.3 Acid–Base Balance and Muscle

25.3.1 Muscle Changes with Aging

Atrophy in muscle mass begins around the age of 25 years, accelerates after the age of 50 years, and continues to occur rapidly at least through the age of 80 years, as documented in the analyses of whole vastus lateralis muscles removed at autopsy from cadavers of 42 healthy males, aged 15–83 years.[27] The loss occurred mainly in the total number of fibers, with no predominance in the loss of either Type I (slow-twitch) or II (fast-twitch) fibers.[28] From the age of 55 to 80 years, there was a 50% loss in fiber number and a 30% loss in muscle area.[28] A recent longitudinal study in a small group of healthy elderly volunteers who had biopsies of the vastus lateralis and thigh CT scans at a mean age of 71 years and again 8.9 years later confirmed that the fiber number, but not the fiber size, declined, and that thigh cross-sectional muscle area by CT scan also declined significantly.[29]

The decline in muscle mass that occurs with aging is accompanied by a gradual loss in muscle strength or the capacity to perform work.[30,31] Peak muscle power, defined as the capacity to perform work per unit time (or the product of the force and velocity of muscle shortening), declines earlier and more dramatically than muscle strength.[32] Impairment in peak muscle power is a strong predictor of functional limitation and disability in the elderly.[33-35] Bosco reported that leg extensor power assessed by jumping declined with age from 20.21 $W \times kgBW^{-1}$ at the age of 19–26 years to 10.49 at the age of 41–48 years to 4.98 at the age of 71–73.[30]

25.3.2 Proposed Mechanism for the Link of Acid–Base Balance with Muscle

The following sequence provides a proposed mechanism by which correcting acidosis may reduce the loss of muscle mass in humans. With muscle breakdown, the amino acids released into the blood stream provide the substrate for the hepatic synthesis of glutamine. Glutamine is used by the kidney to synthesize ammonia.[36] With the availability of glutamine, the kidney can increase its production of ammonia. Ammonia molecules spontaneously accept protons and are excreted as ammonium ions; the excretion of ammonium thus removes protons and mitigates the acidosis. The signaling mechanism(s) by which an acidic environment triggers muscle breakdown have not been fully delineated.

There are several clinical states, of which both acidosis and muscle wasting are features, including starvation,[37,38] trauma, sepsis and burns,[36,39-41] chronic renal failure,[42] and individuals on weight loss diets.[43,44] Correction of the acidosis (but not its underlying cause) has been shown to correct the nitrogen (muscle) wasting in several conditions, including chronic renal failure[45] and ketogenic weight-loss diets.[46] Correction of metabolic acidosis has also permitted the resumption of normal growth rates in children with chronic renal failure.[47]

Muscle mass and muscle strength are well known to be correlated. However, in the Health Aging and Body Composition (Health ABC) Study, a carefully conducted 3-year observational study in 1,880 older adults in the U.S., loss in muscle mass, as assessed by thigh muscle cross-sectional area and DXA scans, accounted for only 5% of the observed loss in muscle strength.[48] This study indicates that other as yet undefined mechanisms in addition to the loss of muscle mass are likely to be involved in the loss of muscle strength that occurs with aging.

25.3.3 Human Studies of Alkali Supplementation During Exercise

There are few data describing the impact of dietary alkali on muscle performance in healthy adults. However, several short-term studies are available in adults participating in exercise intervention studies. During exercise, lactic acid efflux across the muscle membrane is an important regulator of intracellular pH.[49] Intracellular acidosis acts directly on the myofibrils and accounts for some of the suppression of muscle contractile force and fatigue during high-intensity exercise of very short duration (e.g., 1–7 min).[50] An increase in extracellular bicarbonate buffering capacity by the ingestion of $NaHCO_3$ facilitates the efflux of lactate and H^+ from muscle cells, thereby delaying the critical decrease in intracellular pH, which negatively affects muscle glycolysis and contributes to fatigue and delayed exercise recovery.[51]

The impact of supplemental HCO_3^- on physical performance has been studied in healthy young subjects. Price et al[52] noted that when compared with control, treatment with $NaHCO_3$ improved exercise tolerance during cycling. $NaHCO_3$, when compared with control, also increased quadriceps torques.[51] Two more recent studies in young men[53] and women[54] have confirmed that preexercise metabolic alkalosis induced by acute ingestion of alkali enhances muscle performance benefits of exercise. This suggests that HCO_3^- improves nonoxidative glycolysis in isometric contraction, resulting in reduced fatigue and enhanced recovery.

Other acute intervention studies have found no impact of HCO_3^- on sprint performance,[55] power output and fatigue,[56] or resistance exercise performance.[57] The relevance of these acute studies to muscle performance in a nonexercise setting is not certain.

25.3.4 Human Studies of Alkali Supplementation Not During Exercise

In 14 healthy postmenopausal women, Frassetto et al found that supplementation with 90 mmol/day of $KHCO_3$ over an 18-day period reduced nitrogen excretion from 14.0 ± 0.63 to 13.2 ± 0.51.[58] In these subjects who were studied on constant protein diets and who had constant exercise levels, the decline in nitrogen excretion was interpreted as conservation of skeletal muscle mass. Frassetto et al calculated that treatment with 90 mmol/day of $KHCO_3$ could theoretically more than offset the chronic losses of muscle mass that occur at an average rate of about 1.0 kg of lean body mass (or 32 g of nitrogen) every 5 years in men and women over the age of 50 years.[58]

25.4 Recent Clinical Trial Results

We recently completed a study designed to determine the effects of potassium bicarbonate and its components on selected changes in bone turnover markers and muscle performance in older men and women. In this double-blind, controlled trial, 171 men and postmenopausal women at the age of 50 years and older were randomized to treatment with placebo or 67.5 mmol of potassium bicarbonate, sodium bicarbonate, or potassium chloride daily for 3 months. These treatments were tested to enable us to determine whether potassium and/or bicarbonate affected the bone outcomes (there was no reason to expect that potassium would affect muscle). All the subjects received 600 mg of calcium as triphosphate daily. The main outcomes, 24-h urinary NTX and calcium excretion, nitrogen excretion, and muscle power and endurance, were measured at entry and after 3 months. Changes in these measures were compared across treatment groups of the 162 participants included in the analyses.

Three-month changes in 24-h urinary NAE/Cr, NTX/Cr, and calcium/Cr excretion by the groups are shown in Fig. 25.1. Bicarbonate significantly reduced each of these measures whereas potassium had no effect. The small increases in calcium excretion in the placebo and potassium chloride groups were expected because all subjects took a calcium supplement throughout the study. Since potassium didn't affect any of our outcomes, the two bicarbonate and the two no bicarbonate (control) groups were combined for further analyses. For the bone related outcomes, men and women were analyzed together, since there was no interaction of bicarbonate with sex in its effects on calcium or NTX excretion.[59] Subjects supplemented with HCO_3^- for 3 months had significantly greater mean changes in calcium/Cr excretion ($p = 0.002$) and urinary NTX/Cr ($p = 0.002$) than subjects in the no HCO_3^- group, after adjustment for sex, baseline value, and changes in sodium/Cr and K/Cr excretion.[59] Moreover, after 3 months on treatment, NAE/Cr was significantly associated with NTX/Cr ($\beta = 0.18$, $p < 0.001$, after the same adjustments).

With respect to the muscle-related findings, there was a significant interaction of sex in the effect of bicarbonate on nitrogen excretion and several measures of lower extremity performance. Bicarbonate significantly reduced nitrogen excretion in the women ($p = 0.004$). Change in NAE/Cr was correlated with the change in nitrogen/Cr excretion in the women ($p = 0.002$) with a similar trend in the men ($p = 0.052$). Bicarbonate also significantly increased peak leg extensor power in the women, but not in the men. These muscle results from this trial are not yet published.

The reason for the attenuated effect of bicarbonate on nitrogen excretion and the absence of an effect on muscle performance in men may be related to their size. In the trial, we gave all the subjects 67.5 mmol/day. The men didn't have as large a decrement in NAE/Cr during treatment as the women; however, on a weight basis, the NAE/Cr decrements in men and women were similar (−0.04 vs. −0.06 mmol/mol). This is important because in men and women, the bone and muscle responses to treatment were proportional to the declines in NAE. Specifically, changes in calcium, NTX, and nitrogen excretion during treatment were proportional to the decrements in NAE. Thus lower dosing per kg of body weight in the men appears to account for their attenuated response to HCO_3^-.

25.5 Future Directions

Much work remains to determine whether HCO_3^- or alkali-producing diets will have persistent and cumulative benefit to the musculoskeletal system. Specific needs follow.

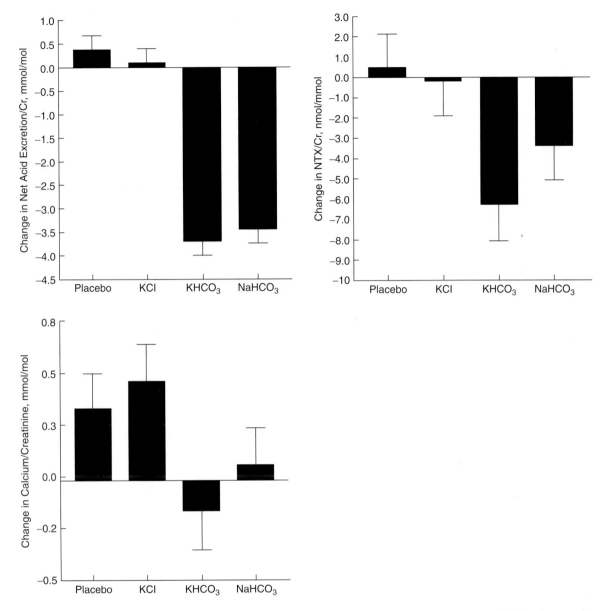

Fig. 25.1 Effect of treatment with placebo, KCl, KHCO$_3$, and NaHCO$_3$ for 3 months on mean (±SEM) change in NAE/Cr, NTX/Cr, and Ca/Cr. Means are adjusted for sex and baseline value. For each variable, the means did not differ significantly between the placebo and KCl groups ($p<0.485$) or between the KHCO$_3$ and NaHCO$_3$ groups ($p>0.243$). In each case, the KCl group did differ significantly from the KHCO$_3$ group ($p<0.018$)

1. The mechanisms by which bicarbonate affects muscle needs to be established. The observed benefits of HCO$_3^-$ to knee extension power output and strength in our 3-months intervention study are not likely to have resulted entirely or even in large part from changes in muscle mass, because only small changes in mass would be expected over the 3-months intervention period. We conclude that other as yet undefined mechanisms are involved. In fact, the mechanisms for much of the age-related loss in muscle strength are currently poorly understood, although several candidate mechanisms (in addition to the loss of muscle mass) have been suggested. These include age-related neurologic

changes, hormonal or metabolic changes, proinflammatory changes, and others.[48] It is important to explore the potential mechanisms further.

2. The optimal dose of alkali for bone and muscle needs to be identified. There are several hints in our study that a higher dose than the 67.5 mmol/day that we used may be optimal. These include the finding that after 3 months of treatment, subjects with the lowest NAE levels had the lowest levels of urinary NTX.[59] The significant positive linear correlations of change in NAE with change in the excretion of NTX, calcium, and nitrogen suggest that further reduction in NAE might be beneficial. Sebastian and colleagues have made the interesting observation that in the preagricultural era, man consumed net alkali-producing diets and excreted on the order of 88 mEq of alkali per day.[13]

3. The current evidence for an effect of bicarbonate on the rates of loss in bone mineral density is mixed and no long-term studies of the effect of alkali on muscle have been done. A large long-term trial needs to be done to evaluate the effects of alkali on change in bone mineral density and to determine whether the short-term benefits to muscle persist over time with ongoing alkali ingestion.

4. Alternatives to potassium bicarbonate pills need to be explored. High-dose bicarbonate requires that many pills be taken. Food fortification may provide an easier and more suitable alternative.

References

1. Campbell AJ, Robertson MC, Gardner MM, Norton RN, Tilyard MW, Buchner DM. Randomised controlled trial of a general practice programme of home based exercise to prevent falls in elderly women. *BMJ*. 1997;315:1065-1069.
2. Frost HM. Bone "mass" and the "mechanostat": a proposal. *Anat Rec*. 1987;219:1-9.
3. Chow JW. Role of nitric oxide and prostaglandins in the bone formation response to mechanical loading. *Exerc Sport Sci Rev*. 2000;28:185-188.
4. Kohrt WM, Bloomfield SA, Little KD, Nelson ME, Yingling VR. American College of Sports Medicine Position Stand: physical activity and bone health. *Med Sci Sports Exerc*. 2004;36:1985-1996.
5. Jackowski SA, Faulkner RA, Farthing JP, Kontulainen SA, Beck TJ, Baxter-Jones AD. Peak lean tissue mass accrual precedes changes in bone strength indices at the proximal femur during the pubertal growth spurt. *Bone*. 2009;44:1186-1190.
6. Seeman E, Hopper JL, Young NR, Formica C, Goss P, Tsalamandris C. Do genetic factors explain associations between muscle strength, lean mass, and bone density? A twin study. *Am J Physiol*. 1996;270:E320-E327.
7. Travison TG, Araujo AB, Esche GR, Beck TJ, McKinlay JB. Lean mass and not fat mass is associated with male proximal femur strength. *J Bone Miner Res*. 2008;23:189-198.
8. Aloia JF, McGowan DM, Vaswani AN, Ross P, Cohn SH. Relationship of menopause to skeletal and muscle mass. *Am J Clin Nutr*. 1991;53:1378-1383.
9. Frassetto LA, Morris RC Jr, Sebastian A. Effect of age on blood acid-base composition in adult humans: role of age-related renal functional decline. *Am J Physiol*. 1996;271:t-22.
10. Lindeman RD, Tobin J, Shock NW. Longitudinal studies on the rate of decline in renal function with age. *J Am Geriatr Soc*. 1985;33:278-285.
11. Davies DF, Shock NW. Age changes in glomerular filtration rate, effective renal plasma flow, and tubular excretory capacity in adult males. *J Clin Invest*. 1950;29:496-507.
12. Rowe JW, Andres R, Tobin JD, Norris AH, Shock NW. The effect of age on creatinine clearance in men: a cross-sectional and longitudinal study. *J Gerontol*. 1976;31:155-163.
13. Sebastian A, Frassetto LA, Sellmeyer DE, Merriam RL, Morris RC Jr. Estimation of the net acid load of the diet of ancestral preagricultural Homo sapiens and their hominid ancestors. *Am J Clin Nutr*. 2002;76:1308-1316.
14. Barzel US. The skeleton as an ion exchange system: implications for the role of acid-base imbalance in the genesis of osteoporosis. *J Bone Miner Res*. 1995;10:1431-1436.
15. Ludwig MG, Vanek M, Guerini D, et al. Proton-sensing G-protein-coupled receptors. *Nature*. 2003;425:93-98.
16. Tomura H, Mogi C, Sato K, Okajima F. Proton-sensing and lysolipid-sensitive G-protein-coupled receptors: a novel type of multi-functional receptors. *Cell Signal*. 2005;17:1466-1476.
17. Frick KK, Krieger NS, Nehrke K, Bushinsky DA. Metabolic acidosis increases intracellular calcium in bone cells through activation of the proton receptor OGR1. *J Bone Miner Res*. 2008;24:305-313.
18. Arnett TR, Dempster DW. Effect of pH on bone resorption by rat osteoclasts in vitro. *Endocrinology*. 1986;119:119-124.
19. Arnett TR, Spowage M. Modulation of the resorptive activity of rat osteoclasts by small changes in extracellular pH near the physiological range. *Bone*. 1996;18:277-279.
20. Komarova SV, Pereverzev A, Shum JW, Sims SM, Dixon SJ. Convergent signaling by acidosis and receptor activator of NF-kappaB ligand (RANKL) on the calcium/calcineurin/NFAT pathway in osteoclasts. *Proc Natl Acad Sci U S A*. 2005;102:2643-2648.
21. Bushinsky DA. Metabolic alkalosis decreases bone calcium efflux by suppressing osteoclasts and stimulating osteoblasts. *Am J Physiol*. 1996;271:F216-F222.
22. Maurer M, Riesen W, Muser J, Hulter HN, Krapf R. Neutralization of Western diet inhibits bone resorption independently of K intake and reduces cortisol secretion in humans. *Am J Physiol Renal Physiol*. 2003;284:F32-F40.
23. Sebastian A, Morris RC Jr. Improved mineral balance and skeletal metabolism in postmenopausal women treated with potassium bicarbonate. *New Engl J Med*. 1994;331:279.
24. Lin P, Ginty F, Appel LJ. Impact of sodium intake and dietary patterns on biochemical markers of bone and calcium metabolism. *J Bone Miner Res*. 2001;16:S511.
25. Jehle S, Zanetti A, Muser J, Hulter HN, Krapf R. Partial neutralization of the acidogenic Western diet with potassium

citrate increases bone mass in postmenopausal women with osteopenia. *J Am Soc Nephrol*. 2006;17:3213-3222.

26. Macdonald HM, Black AJ, Aucott L, et al. Effect of potassium citrate supplementation or increased fruit and vegetable intake on bone metabolism in healthy postmenopausal women: a randomized controlled trial. *Am J Clin Nutr*. 2008; 88:465-474.

27. Lexell J, Taylor CC, Sjostrom M. What is the cause of the ageing atrophy? Total number, size and proportion of different fiber types studied in whole vastus lateralis muscle from 15- to 83-year-old men. *J Neurol Sci*. 1988;84:275-294.

28. Frontera WR, Suh D, Krivickas LS, Hughes VA, Goldstein R, Roubenoff R. Skeletal muscle fiber quality in older men and women. *Am J Physiol Cell Physiol*. 2000;279:C611-C618.

29. Frontera WR, Reid KF, Phillips EM, et al. Muscle fiber size and function in elderly humans: a longitudinal study. *J Appl Physiol*. 2008;105:637-642.

30. Bosco C, Komi PV. Influence of aging on the mechanical behavior of leg extensor muscles. *Eur J Appl Physiol Occup Physiol*. 1980;45:209-219.

31. Hughes VA, Frontera WR, Wood M, et al. Longitudinal muscle strength changes in older adults: influence of muscle mass, physical activity, and health. *J Gerontol A Biol Sci Med Sci*. 2001;56:B209-B217.

32. Metter EJ, Conwit R, Tobin J, Fozard JL. Age-associated loss of power and strength in the upper extremities in women and men. *J Gerontol A Biol Sci Med Sci*. 1997;52: B267-B276.

33. Bassey EJ, Fiatarone MA, O'Neill EF, Kelly M, Evans WJ, Lipsitz LA. Leg extensor power and functional performance in very old men and women. *Clin Sci (Lond)*. 1992;82: 321-327.

34. Foldvari M, Clark M, Laviolette LC, et al. Association of muscle power with functional status in community-dwelling elderly women. *J Gerontol A Biol Sci Med Sci*. 2000; 55:M192-M199.

35. Suzuki T, Bean JF, Fielding RA. Muscle power of the ankle flexors predicts functional performance in community-dwelling older women. *J Am Geriatr Soc*. 2001;49:1161-1167.

36. Souba WW, Smith RJ, Wilmore DW. Glutamine metabolism by the intestinal tract. *J Parent Enter Nutr*. 1985;9:608-617.

37. Owen EE, Robinson RR. Amino acid extraction and ammonia metabolism by the human kidney during the prolonged administration of ammonium chloride. *J Clin Invest*. 1963; 42:263-276.

38. Ruderman NB, Berger M. The formation of glutamine and alanine in skeletal muscle. *J Biol Chem*. 1974;249:5500-5506.

39. Aulick LH, Wilmore DW. Increased peripheral amino acid release following burn injury. *Surgery*. 1979;85:560-565.

40. Askanazi J, Carpentier YA, Michelsen CB, et al. Muscle and plasma amino acids following injury. Influence of intercurrent infection. *Ann Surg*. 1980;192:78-85.

41. Williamson DH. Muscle protein degradation and amino acid metabolism in human injury. *Biochem Soc Trans*. 1980;8: 497.

42. Garibotto G, Russo R, Sofia A, et al. Muscle protein turnover in chronic renal failure patients with metabolic acidosis or normal acid-base balance. *Miner Electrolyte Metab*. 1996;22:58-61.

43. Bell JD, Margen S, Calloway DH. Ketosis, weight loss, uric acid, and nitrogen balance in obese women fed single nutrients at low caloric levels. *Metabolism*. 1969;18:193-208.

44. Vazquez JA, Adibi SA. Protein sparing during treatment of obesity: ketogenic versus nonketogenic very low calorie diet. *Metabolism*. 1992;41:406-414.

45. Papadoyannakis NJ, Stefanidis CJ, McGeown M. The effect of the correction of metabolic acidosis on nitrogen and potassium balance of patients with chronic renal failure. *Am J Clin Nutr*. 1984;40:623-627.

46. Gougeon-Reyburn R, Lariviere F, Marliss EB. Effects of bicarbonate supplementation on urinary mineral excretion during very low energy diets. *Am J Med Sci*. 1991;302:67-74.

47. Gougeon-Reyburn R, Marliss EB. Effects of sodium bicarbonate on nitrogen metabolism and ketone bodies during very low energy protein diets in obese subjects. *Metabolism*. 1989;38:1222-1230.

48. Goodpaster BH, Park SW, Harris TB, et al. The loss of skeletal muscle strength, mass, and quality in older adults: the health, aging and body composition study. *J Gerontol A Biol Sci Med Sci*. 2006;61:1059-1064.

49. Roth DA, Brooks GA. Lactate and pyruvate transport is dominated by a pH gradient-sensitive carrier in rat skeletal muscle sarcolemmal vesicles. *Arch Biochem Biophys*. 1990; 279:386-394.

50. Mainwood GW, Renaud JM. The effect of acid-base balance on fatigue of skeletal muscle. *Can J Physiol Pharmacol*. 1985;63:403-416.

51. Verbitsky O, Mizrahi J, Levin M, Isakov E. Effect of ingested sodium bicarbonate on muscle force, fatigue, and recovery. *J Appl Physiol*. 1997;83:333-337.

52. Price M, Moss P, Rance S. Effects of sodium bicarbonate ingestion on prolonged intermittent exercise. *Med Sci Sports Exerc*. 2003;35:1303-1308.

53. Zoladz JA, Korzeniewski B, Grassi B. Training-induced acceleration of oxygen uptake kinetics in skeletal muscle: the underlying mechanisms. *J Physiol Pharmacol*. 2006;57 (suppl 10):67-84.

54. Edge J, Bishop D, Goodman C. The effects of training intensity on muscle buffer capacity in females. *Eur J Appl Physiol*. 2006;96:97-105.

55. Horswill CA, Costill DL, Fink WJ, et al. Influence of sodium bicarbonate on sprint performance: relationship to dosage. *Med Sci Sports Exerc*. 1988;20:566-569.

56. McCartney N, Heigenhauser GJ, Jones NL. Power output and fatigue of human muscle in maximal cycling exercise. *J Appl Physiol*. 1983;55:t-24.

57. Webster MJ, Webster MN, Crawford RE, Gladden LB. Effect of sodium bicarbonate ingestion on exhaustive resistance exercise performance. *Med Sci Sports Exerc*. 1993;25: 960-965.

58. Frassetto L, Morris RC Jr, Sebastian A. Potassium bicarbonate reduces urinary nitrogen excretion in postmenopausal women. *J Clin Endocrino Metab*. 1997;82:254-259.

59. Dawson-Hughes B, Harris SS, Palermo NJ, Castaneda-Sceppa C, Rasmussen HM, Dallal GE. Treatment with potassium bicarbonate lowers calcium excretion and bone resorption in older men and women. *J Clin Endocrinol Metab*. 2009;94:96-102.

The Effect of Mineral Waters on Bone Metabolism: Alkalinity Over Calcium?

26

Peter Burckhardt

26.1 The Role of Calcium and Bicarbonate

In many countries, the consumption of mineral waters is extremely high, due to fashion and marketing, and in some countries, due to the low quality of tap water. In these countries, the consumption of mineral waters exceeds by far that of milk. But the literature on the bone effects of milk exceeds by far that on mineral waters. Recent studies showed that the positive effect on bone which some mineral waters can have, deserve special attention, especially in respect to their calcium and bicarbonate content.

Mineral waters can decrease bone resorption, bone turnover, PTH secretion, and in a few studies, they have shown to positively influence bone mineral density. One study showed that the consumption of only 0.5 L of a calcium-rich mineral water over 6 months lowered PTH, osteocalcin, and the bone resorption marker CTX in serum and urine.[1] In another study, a calcium-rich water decreased the loss of BMD at the distal radius in postmenopausal women over about 1 year.[2] These effects are explained by the calcium-content of the mineral waters.

On the other hand, bicarbonate, which can also be present in mineral waters, improves calcium balance, and lowers bone resorption and bone turnover. This has been shown with 60–120 mmol K-bicarbonate in postmenopausal women,[3] ±77 mmol K- and Na-bicarbonate in young male volunteers,[4] and 1 mmol/kg in healthy adults,[5] where the effect of K-bicarbonate was slightly stronger

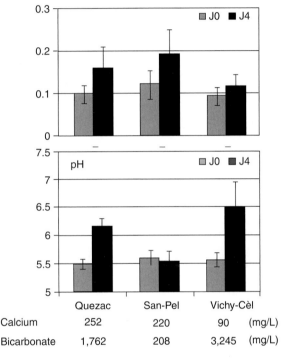

Fig. 26.1 Effect of 3 days on a given mineral water (1 L/day) on the fasting urine of the fourth day in young adult volunteers

than that of Na-bicarbonate. The difference in the nutritional acid load between a supplement of 30 mEq of K-citrate and one of K–Cl significantly improved the changes of BMD over 1 year in postmenopausal osteopenic women.[6] And the consumption of an alkali diet which included a bicarbonate-rich mineral water decreased bone resorption in young volunteers.[7] For these reasons, the effect of mineral waters on bone metabolism might not only be due to calcium, but also an alkali effect.

Before studying this hypothesis, we did a pilot study in four young female volunteers for examining the question of whether 1 L/day of a bicarbonate-rich mineral

P. Burckhardt
Internal Medicine Department Clinique Bois-Cerf/
Hirslanden Avenue d'Ouchy 31, Lausanne 1006,
Switzerland
e-mail: p_burckhardt@bluewin.ch

P. Burckhardt et al. (eds.), *Nutritional Influences on Bone Health*,
DOI: 10.1007/978-1-84882-978-7_26, © Springer-Verlag London Limited 2010

Table 26.1 Composition of the mineral waters given in the EMINOS-studies, 1.5 L/day over 4 weeks

| Mineral water | A | | B | |
Study	Calcium (mg/L)	Bicarbonate (mg/L)	Calcium (mg/L)	Bicarbonate (mg/L)
EMINOS-1	485	403	252	1,762
EMINOS-2	520	291	548	2,172
EMINOS-3	105	391	103	2,989

water would modify the urine pH beyond the 3 days when the water is consumed, i.e., in the fasting urine of the fourth day. For that, we consecutively tested 3 waters during 3 days followed by 4 days wash-out. The results (Fig. 26.1) confirmed that calcium and the pH in the fasting urine are influenced by the characteristics of the mineral waters consumed during the 3 preceding days. Therefore, the question of whether such changes influence bone metabolism has to be answered.

26.1.1 The EMINOS Studies

Three interventional studies were conducted to adress the effects of mineral water composition on bone metabolism. In the first one (EMINOS-1), we compared the effect of two waters over 4 weeks, one rich in calcium, the other moderately rich in calcium, but rich in bicarbonate (Table 26.1). Ten young women consumed 1.5 L of one of the two waters during 4 weeks while being on a self-selected diet, respecting

recommended limits. With the bicarbonate-rich water, urinary telopeptides CTX decreased significantly by 30% in the fasting urine, but not with the calcium-rich water (Fig. 26.2).[8] In the second study, EMINOS-2, we administered to two groups of 15 young women each, on a standardized diet with ± 754 mg/day calcium, 1.5 L/day of one of two calcium-rich waters for 4 weeks. One water also contained a high amount of bicarbonate (Table 26.1). Although these healthy volunteers were on a normal calcium intake even without the mineral water, the water which was rich in both, calcium and bicarbonate, caused not only an increase of the pH in the urine, but also a decrease in serum CTX and PTH, while no change was observed with the water that was only rich in calcium (Fig. 26.3).[9] This showed

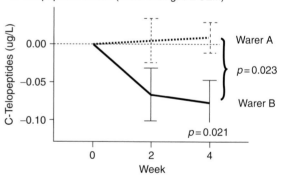

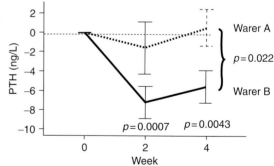

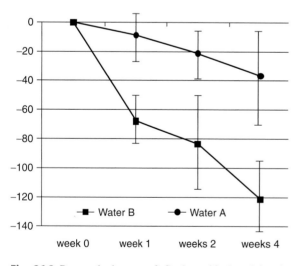

Fig. 26.2 Percental changes of C-telopeptides/creatinine in fasting urine during 4 weeks on a mineral water rich in calcium and bicarbonate (*B*) compared to a calcium-rich water (*A*) in healthy female volunteers (composition of the waters see Table 26.2). At 4 weeks, water B changes significantly compared to week 0 ($p < 0.01$ ANOVA).[8] (EMINOS-1)

Fig. 26.3 Changes in PTH and CTX levels induced by the consumption of two different mineral waters over 4 weeks in healthy female volunteers (composition of the waters see Table 26.2).[9] (EMINOS-2). With permission from *Bone*

Table 26.2 Controlled interventional studies with mineral waters of different PRAL values

References	Mineral water (mg/day)				Calcium intake (mg/day)		PRAL of mineral waters (mEq/day)	Effect on bone metabolism (% changes)		
	Bicarbonate	Sulfate	Calcium	Na	Diet	Total		pl.CTX	pl.PTH	Urine Ca
Meunier[1]	290	1,530	595	7	566	1,162	−10.4	−16.3	−14.2	
	71	8	12	12	546	558	+13.2	+29.6	+3.3	
EMINOS -1.[8]	2,528	215	361	382	1,040	1,401	−20.4	−31		+0
	605	1,781	728	14	1,040	1,768	+13.1	+13		+38
Roux[16]	2,179	4	606	60	400	1,006	−10.4	−30	−11	
	292	1,551	560	7	400	960	+13.2	−7	−7	
EMINOS-2.[9]	3,258	14	822	101	965	1,787	−16.6.	−16	−17	
	437	1,740	780	8	965	1,745	+13.8	+2	+2	
EMINOS-3	4,483	138	155	1,758	±850	±1,000	−40.8	No effect		
	586	20	158	11	±850	±1,000	−1.8	No effect		

that, in calcium-sufficiency, the consumption of a calcium-rich water did not exert a demonstrable effect on bone metabolism, while the mineral water which was also rich in bicarbonate lowered bone resorption significantly. In order to assess the effects of bicarbonate alone, we performed a third study (EMINOS-3), where 30 young female volunteers consumed 1.5 L/day each of two mineral waters with an average-low calcium-content (Table 26.2), one being rich in bicarbonate, in a randomized sequence, for 2 weeks, followed by a wash-out period of 2 weeks. The bicarbonate water increased urinary pH and bicarbonate (fasting urine and 24 h urine) independent of whether it was taken in the first or the second period. But no changes were observed in urinary calcium excretion, the bone resorption marker, or PTH levels. Urinary K-excretion varied inconsistently (n.s.). Therefore, bicarbonate-rich water, which was not rich in calcium, had no effect on bone metabolism.

In order to understand the interrelationship of the minerals found in mineral water, we analyzed them on the basis of the composition of 150 European mineral waters found on the internet, 100 water with calcium-content below 200 mg/L, and 50 waters with a calcium-content above 200 mg/L.[10] American waters could not be included because of their low mineral content. For assessing the conditions that not only lead to high calcium-concentrations, but also to alkalinity, we calculated the PRAL index[11] for each water, using the formula: PRAL (mEq) = (chloride × 0.03 + protein* in g × 0.00049) − (K × 0.021 + Mg × 0.0263 + Ca × 0.013 + Na × 0.04) in mg. Because waters do not contain

proteins, which are the providers of methionin and cystein (sources of SO_4), the formula had to be adapted. In water, SO_4 is in solution. We used the molecular weight of SO_4 (96), and an absorption rate of 70%, which resulted in a conversion factor of 0.0146 for SO_4 (instead of 0.00049 for proteins).

This analysis showed that sulfate and bicarbonate are never found together in the same water in high amounts (Fig. 26.4). In general, calcium is mainly predicted by SO_4. In waters with a positive PRAL value (acid waters), it is predicted mainly by SO_4, i.e., for 83.8% (stepwise regressive analysis, $p < 0.001$). In alkaline waters with a negative PRAL value, calcium was mainly predicted by bicarbonate, but it explained

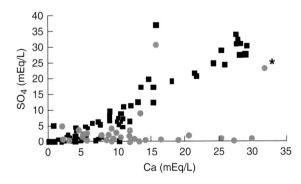

Fig. 26.4 Correlation between calcium (Ca) and Sulfate (SO_4) in 150 European Mineral waters, separated by bicarbonate values: relatively low (*filled square*) or high (*gray circle*) content of bicarbonate (±11.8 mEq/L, respectively 720 mg/L). *Asterisk*: outlier = water from meteoric rocks.[10] With permission from *British Journal of Nutrition*

only 26.5% of the variation ($p < 0.001$). And the PRAL value was mainly predicted by Na, explaining 89.3% of the variation ($p < 0.001$), and not by bicarbonate. This means, that mineral waters with a high calcium content mostly contain relatively high concentrations of SO_4 and are slightly acid, while alkaline mineral waters which are rich in calcium and bicarbonate, suitable for decreasing bone resorption even in calcium sufficiency, are rare.

In this context, is has to be reminded, that SO_4 probably has no effect on urinary calcium excretion.[12,13] One study[14] reported such an effect, but the effect was small (20 mg/24 h), and the calcium intake was about 980 mg/day and uncontrolled.[15] The evidence speaks rather against a calciuric effect of SO_4.

26.2 The Influence of PRAL

As discussed above, the alkali load of a mineral water, especially its bicarbonate-content, seems to provide an additional positive effect on bone metabolism. This led us to examine the importance of the PRAL value of mineral waters, especially the alkali load, on the outcomes of interventional trials. A comparison of the controlled interventional trials,[17] where the PRAL of the mineral waters could be calculated, showed that decreases in bone resorption markers and/or urinary calcium excretion and/or PTH were observed with the

lower PRAL values, independent of the amount of calcium administered in the mineral water (Table 26.2). One study presented an exception, the EMINOS-3 study, where a mineral water with an extremely low PRAL value had no effect on bone metabolism. This water was moderately rich in calcium and contained a significant amount of sodium, 21–250 times more than the other waters with negative PRAL values. Indeed, when the average composition of 150 European mineral waters are considered (Wynn 2009), and the average PRAL value is calculated (-5.9 mE/L), sodium is responsible for 53 % of the PRAL value, while calcium, Mg, and K together predict only 25%. Without Na, the PRAL value of the water used in this study (EMINOS-3) would not be -40.8 mEq/1.5 L, but $+25.5$. Therefore the negative PRAL value of a mineral water which is mainly due to a high Na-content does not exert the same positive effect on bone metabolism as that of a mineral water with a low PRAL value due to calcium.

26.3 Recapitulation

The comparison of all waters used in controlled trials with significant outcomes allows us to understand the various results observed in these studies (Table 26.3). Inhibition of bone resorption could be demonstrated with mineral waters rich in calcium and sulfate in

Table 26.3 Composition of mineral waters, respective intake per day, and effects on bone metabolism in four controlled clinical trials

mg/day	Meunier[1]		Roux[16]		EMINOS-2[9]		EMINOS-3	
	A	B	A	B	A	B	A	B
	0.5 L/day	0.5 L/day	1 L/day	1 L/day	1.5 L/day	1.5 L/day	1.5 L/day	1.5 L/day
HCO3⁻	36	145	292	2,179	436	3,258	587	2,989
SO4⁻	4	765	1,530	4	1,740	14	20	138
Ca⁺⁺	6	298	559	606	780	822	158	103
Na⁺	6	4	7	60	8	101	11	1,172
Mg⁺⁺	4	39	80	27	52	98	29	10
Ca/diet	<700	<700	400	400	965	965	>800	>800
Effect of mineral water	None in Ca-deficiency	Positive in Ca-deficiency	Moderate in Ca-deficiency	Positive in Ca-deficiency	None in Ca-sufficiency	Positive despite Ca-sufficiency	None in Ca-sufficiency	None in Ca-sufficiency

Brand of mineral waters:
EMINOS-2: *A* Adelbodner; *B* Krinisca, EMINOS-3: *A* Henniez; *B* Vichy, Roux: *A* Antica Fonte; *B* Ferrarelle, Meunier: *A* "placebo water"; *B* Antica Fonte
Not indicated: Cl⁻ (below 22 mg/L except Vichy: 235), F⁻ (below 0.5 mg/L), K⁺ (below 12 mg/L, except Vichy: 71)

subjects who were in calcium deficiency, i.e., with a low dietary calcium intake.[1] In fact, for demonstrating such an effect of the calcium in mineral water, subjects with a low calcium intake were chosen for the trial. For an easy comparison, special water with extremely low calcium was chosen, which obviously had no effect. Another trial tried to demonstrate that mineral water rich in bicarbonate, in addition to its calcium content, is more effective at improving bone metabolism.[16] It succeeded by getting significant results in bone metabolism with the bicarbonate-rich water. But the water used as control, which had the same amount of calcium, but a low level of bicarbonate, showed the same profile of actions, mainly antiresorptive one, which however were not significant. This trial was performed in subjects with a relatively low-calcium diet, whose total intake – together with the mineral water – became normal.

The situation is different in calcium sufficiency, i.e., in subjects with a relatively high calcium intake. In this situation, only mineral waters which are also rich in bicarbonate exert an inhibition of bone resorption (EMINOS-2). Bicarbonate-rich waters with a relatively low calcium content have no measurable effect on bone metabolism (EMINOS-3).

References

1. Meunier P, Jenvrin C, Munoz F, de la Gueronnire V, Garnero P, Menz M. Consumption of a high calcium mineral water lowers biochemical indices of bone remodelling in postmenopausal women with low calcium intake. *Osteoporos Int.* 2005;16:1203-1209.
2. Cepollaro C, Orlandi G, Gonnelli S, et al. Effect of calcium supplementation as a high-calcium mineral water on bone loss in early postmenopausal women. *Calcif Tissue Int.* 1996;59:238-239.
3. Sebastian A, Harris S, Ottaway J, Todd K, Morris C. Improved mineral balance and skeletal metabolism in postmenopausal women treated with potassium bicarbonate. *N Engl J Med.* 1994;330:1776-1781.
4. Maurer M, Riesen W, Muser J, Hulter MN, Krapf R. Neutralization of Western diet inhibits bone resorption independently of K intake and reduces cortisol secretion in humans. *Am J Phys Renal Phys.* 2003;284:F32-F40.
5. Morris RC, Schmidlin O, Tanaka M, Forman A, Frassetto L, Sebastian A. Differing effects of supplemental KCl and KHCO3: Pathophysiological and clinical implications. *Semin Nephrol.* 1999;19(5):487-493.
6. Jehle S, Zanetti A, Muser J, Hulter H, Krapf R. Partial neutralization of the acidogenic western diet with potassium citrate increases bone mass in postmenopausal women with osteopenia. *J Am Soc Nephrol.* 2006;17:3213-3222.
7. Buclin T, Cosma M, Appenzeller M, et al. Diet acids and alkalis influence calcium retention in bone. *Osteoporos Int.* 2001;12:493-499.
8. Burckhardt P, Waldvogel S, Aeschlimann J, Arnaud M. Bicarbonate in mineralwater inhibits bone resorption. (EMINOS-1). *J Bone Miner Res.* 2002;17(suppl):M360–S476.
9. Wynn E, Krieg MA, Aeschlimann JM, Burckhardt P. Alkaline mineral water lowers bone resorption even in calcium sufficiency. (EMINOS-2). *Bone.* 2009;44:120-124.
10. Wynn E, Raetz E, Burckhardt P. The composition of mineral waters sourced from Europe and North America in respect to bone health. *Br J Nutr.* 2009;101:1195-1199.
11. Remer T, Manz F. Potential renal acid load of foods and its influence on urine pH. *J Am Diet Assoc.* 1995;95:791-797.
12. Bleich HL, Moore MJ, Lemann J Jr, Adams ND, Gray RW. Urinary calcium excretion in human beings. *N Engl J Med.* 1979;301:535-541.
13. Couzy F, Kastenmayer P, Vigo M, Clough J, Munoz-Box R, Barclay DV. Calcium bioavailability from calcium- and sulfate-rich mineral water, compared with milk, in young adult women. *Am J Clin Nutr.* 1995;62:1239-1244.
14. Brandolini M, Guguen L, Boirie Y, Rousset P, Bertire M, Beaufrre B. Higher calcium urinary loss induced by a calcium sulphate-rich mineral water intake than by milk in young women. *Br J Nutr.* 2005;93(2):225-231.
15. Arnaud M. Nutrition discussion forum. *Br J Nutr.* 2006; 95:650–653 [2008;99:206-209].
16. Roux S, Baudoin C, Boute D, Brazier M, De la Gueronnire V, De Vernejoul M. Biological effects of drinking-water mineral composition on calcium balance and bone remodeling markers. *J Nutr Health Aging.* 2004;8(5):380-384.
17. Burckhardt P. The effects of the alkali load of mineral water on bone metabolism: Interventional studies. *J Nutr.* 2008; 139:435S-437S.

Bone-Anabolic Impact of Dietary High Protein Intake Compared with the Effects of Low Potential Renal Acid Load, Endogenous Steroid Hormones, and Muscularity in Children

27

Thomas Remer and Lars Libuda

Abbreviations

17β-HSD	17β-Hydroxysteroid dehydrogenase
DHEA	Dehydroepiandrosterone
NAE	Net acid excretion
NEAP	Net endogenous acid production
pQCT	Peripheral quantitative computed tomography
PRAL	Potential renal acid load

27.1 Introduction

In addition to genetics, muscle mass and endocrine factors are major determinants of skeletal mineralization, bone mass, and bone strength. Among the modifiable factors which relevantly influence bone parameters, nutrition plays an important role. Until now, almost all corresponding studies on bone have focused on dietary or hormonal influences alone, thereby considering body size-related factors like BMI, fat mass, or lean body mass either as confounders or as additional potential predictors. However, examinations combining all these three determinants (muscularity, specific hormones, and dietary factors) to evaluate their respective possible contributions to bone status are lacking. Therefore, we studied the potential influences on diaphyseal cortical bone of the muscular component as

indexed by muscle area, steroid hormones as quantified in 24-h urine samples, and dietary factors obtained from repeated diet records all combined in healthy children. Regarding nutrition, a special emphasis was placed on dietary alkalinity and protein intake.

27.2 Protein Intake and Dietary Alkalinity in the Ancestral Paleolithic Diet

More than 10,000 years ago, when livestock breeding and cultivation of grain did not exist and our human ancestors primarily lived on wild game, fish, and uncultivated plant foods, nutrient intakes differed considerably from today – not only with respect to fat profile and fiber intake. Especially, protein intake was very high (Table 27.1). This probably supported muscle anabolism, particularly necessary at that time not only for the long walks in search of new food sources, but also, in particular, for a successful hunting.

As a result of the high protein intake and the consequently ingested considerable acid load (in the form of sulfur-containing amino acids and protein-bound phosphorus), an increase in renal calcium losses should have occurred, because renal calcium reabsorption and calcium conservation is clearly negatively affected by the acid loads the kidney has to cope with. Tubular calcium reabsorption at different kidney sites, e.g., in the proximal tubule and the thick ascending limb of Henle's loop is directly reduced by the raising amounts of protons [H+] that have to be renally excreted.[1,2] Additionally, acid-induced reductions in bone mineral content (BMC)

T. Remer (✉)
Department of Nutrition and Health, Research Institute of Child Nutrition/ Forschungsinstitut für Kinderernährung, Heinstück 11, Dortmund 44225, Germany
e-mail: remer@fke-do.de

P. Burckhardt et al. (eds.), *Nutritional Influences on Bone Health*,
DOI: 10.1007/978-1-84882-978-7_27, © Springer-Verlag London Limited 2010

Table 27.1 Dietary PRAL and net acid excretion (NAE) in the Paleolithic Age and today[a]

	Paleolithic diet (3,000 kcal/day)		US diet today (2,500 kcal/day)	
	Intake (g/day)[b]	Urine (mEq/day)	Intake (g/day)[a]	Urine (mEq/day)
Protein	226.0	–	79.0	–
→ Urinary sulfate	–	+110	–	+39
Phosphorus	3.2	+118	1.5	+55
Potassium	10.5	−215	2.5	−51
Calcium	1.6	−20	0.9	−12
Magnesium	1.2	−32	0.3	−8
Dietary PRAL[c]		−39		+23
Organic acids[d]		+45		+45
Urinary NAE[e]		+6		+68

[a]Table adapted from Remer and Manz[5]
[b]Intake data from Eaton and Eaton,[4] with ~30% of energy from protein
[c]Calculated according to Remer and Manz[6] with the only exception that sodium and chloride were not considered
[d]Basal organic acid excretion was calculated as a diet-independent component of net endogenous acid production (NEAP) for an exemplary subject with a body surface area of 1.9 m[2]
[e]Calculated according to Remer and Manz[6,7] and presenting an estimate of overall daily NEAP

are known for decades in a number of pathophysiological conditions. This is consistent with the role of bone as an important proton buffer[3] and it can further explain as to why renal calcium losses increase on diets with a high proton-generating potential.

However, despite a principally acidifying very high animal protein intake, total dietary acid load was probably rather low in ancestral hominids, living as hunter-gatherers. High energy needs and irregular availability of prey forced them to also use all relevant nonanimal food sources available at that time. This, most likely led to regular intakes of "mixed diets" with indeed low-carbohydrate content, but an abundant consumption of tubers, roots, wild fruits, seeds, and wild vegetables.[4] According to the intake estimates published by Eaton and Eaton,[4] the overall diet must have provided a high intake of base-producing minerals (cations) especially potassium and magnesium. If the estimated average amounts of absorbed cationic minerals (which in metabolic steady state largely correspond to the amounts renally excreted) are subtracted from the estimated amounts of absorbed noncombustible anions, a negative potential renal acid load (PRAL) results (Table 27.1) showing that the Paleolithic diet basically yielded a base-forming or alkaline nutrition. Accordingly, a net endogenous acid production (NEAP) – quantifiable in

24-h urine samples as urinary net acid excretion (NAE) – of around 0 mEq/day or slightly above (+6 mEq/day; see calculation in Table 27.1) would have been expected. This is in clear contrast to the acid load which is regularly observed on a typical western diet of today (Table 27.1).

Hence, it can be assumed that urinary calcium losses were rather low in the Paleolithic Age, despite very high protein intakes. In parallel, the overall low PRAL of that diet may have substantially contributed to an improved bone status: Increases in dietary alkalinity (or reductions in nutritional acid load) are positively associated with bone status (Table 27.2) and it is widely assumed that long-term minimization of dietary acidity represents an independent bone-anabolic action.

In addition to that, research in the recent years has provided substantial evidence that dietary protein itself is also bone-anabolic (apart from its acid-forming bone detrimental potential). Subjects ingesting low amounts of protein in the long run, appear to suffer measurable bone losses.[26] The bone-anabolism of higher protein intakes probably operates via increases in circulating and consequently also bone tissue-available IGF-1 levels.[26,27] A recent study of our group in healthy children of the Dortmund Nutritional and Anthropometric Longitudinally Designed (DONALD) Study has

Table 27.2 Literature findings on positive associations of alkaline-based nutrition (high in fruits and vegetables) with bone parameters in observational population studies

Reference	Details	Findings
Eaton-Evans et al[8]	77 females, 46–56 years	Vegetables
Michaelsson et al[9]	175 females, 28–74 years	K intake
New et al[10]	994 females, 45–49 years	K, Mg, fiber, vitamin C
		Past intake: fruit and vegetables
Tucker et al[11]	229 males, 349 females, 75 years	K, Mg, fruit, and vegetables
New et al[12]	62 females, 45–54 years	K, Mg, fiber, vitamin C
		Past intake: fruit and vegetables
Jones et al[13]	215 boys, 115 girls, 8–14 years	K, urinary K
Chen et al[14]	668 females, 48–62 years	Fruit
Miller et al[15]	300 males, 50–91 years	K, Mg
Stone et al[16]	1,075 males, ≥65 years	K, lutein
Tylavsky et al[17]	56 females, Tanner stage 2	Fruits and vegetables
New et al[18]	1,056 females, 45–54 years	Alkali load, K, low protein
McGartland et al[19]	328 boys, 12 years; 369 girls, 15 years	Fruits and vegetables
Macdonald et al[20]	3,226 females, 55 years	K intake
Hirota et al[21]	262 girls, 286 boys, 10–15 years	Fish, fruit, vegetables
Vatanparast et al[22]	85 males, 67 females, 8–20 years	Fruits and vegetables
Chen et al[23]	670 females, 48–63 years	Fruits and vegetables
Prynne et al[24]	132 boys, 125 girls, 16–18 years; females >60 years	Fruits and vegetables
Welch et al[25]	14,563 females and males, 42–82 years	Alkali load

strongly suggested that this dietary protein-related bone anabolism may be, at least partly, abrogated if the protein-associated acidity is not appropriately neutralized by dietary intakes of alkali equivalents.[28] Hence, an alkaline nutrition together with a higher intake of protein, similar to the Paleolithic diet, should have a particular bone-anabolic impact.

27.3 Potential Renal Acid Load, Dietary Methionine and Cysteine, and Diaphyseal Bone Parameters in Children Revisited

The PRAL model for the calculation of the diet-dependent daily acid load in humans is based on the ingested amounts of all those nutrients which after absorption and metabolism or metabolic interactions are

compulsively renally excreted and finally represent the major constituents of the urine ionogram. As shown in Table 27.1, protein (of which the sulfate-containing amino acids are metabolized to organic oxidisable constituents and sulfate), phosphorus, potassium, calcium, and magnesium belong to those nutrients which are considered. The physiologically based acidity calculation model corrects for the average intestinal absorption of the nutrients (PRAL calculation) and in addition – for the estimation of total NEAP of a subject – assumes a rate of urinary excretion of organic acids proportional to body surface area (NEAP = PRAL component + organic acid component). Also sodium and chloride have to be taken into account; however, due to frequently inconsistent data in food composition tables, especially for salted foods, their contribution may be omitted. If the daily intake of cationic sodium and anionic chloride, which are absorbed at almost equal amounts, does not differ, their contribution to overall

NEAP is 0, since it is the anion–cation difference that finally determines daily net acid load. On the other hand, in case of well known sodium and chloride intake amounts, e.g., due to available specific chemical food analyses or particular dietary habits, for example, involving regular intakes of large amounts of sodium bicarbonate-rich mineral waters, both minerals should be taken into account or at least a reasonable estimate of their difference.

The conventional PRAL model assumes constant amounts of methionine and cysteine per 100 g protein intake, irrespective of the protein source, in order to estimate the milliequivalent amounts of H^+ ions and sulfate generated from either daily protein intake or the protein content per 100 g of a certain food.[6,7] However, methionine and cysteine content per 100 g protein markedly varies between different foods. For example, tuna and swordfish have much different methionine and cysteine contents per 100 g edible portion compared to chicken and turkey.[29] Figure 27.1 illustrates these differences for certain food groups each showing an average value for the summed methionine and cysteine amount (in g/100 g of the respective protein) as obtained from several representative food items. It is obvious from these data that (1) animal protein generally yields higher amounts of sulfur

amino acids than vegetable and fruit protein, (2) cereal protein on an average lies in between that of fruit and vegetable and milk, and (3) egg and fish protein have the highest acid generating potential. Accordingly, it has been criticized that estimating sulfuric acid production using a constant value for the sulfur content of protein may present a relevant source of error in the PRAL model, depending on the specific dietary proteins.[30]

For this reason, we reanalyzed our recent findings on the association between long-term dietary PRAL of healthy children and their bone status as determined by peripheral quantitative computed tomography (pQCT)[28] to check whether there may possibly emerge even stronger negative correlations between dietary acidity and bone parameters when food-specific methionine and cysteine content data are considered for PRAL calculation instead of only a single average value[6] for all type of proteins. Calculations and regression analyses were run as described in detail[28] with the only difference that the new PRAL calculation used the mg amounts of methionine and cysteine for individual foods as given in food composition tables[31] or the US Department of Agriculture National Nutrient Database for Standard Reference.[29] Results of reanalyses are shown in Fig. 27.2 along with a graphical

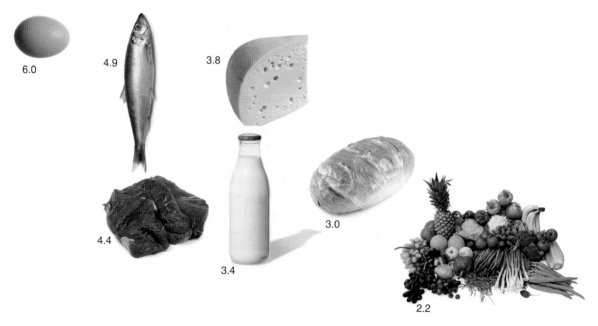

Fig. 27.1 Average methionine and cysteine contents per 100 g protein portion of foods of different food groups (methionine and cysteine summed, g/100 g protein)

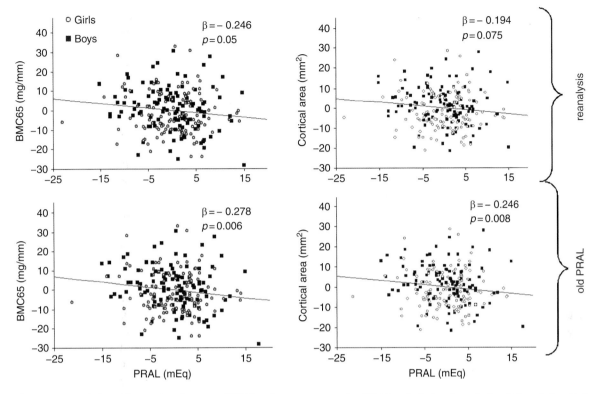

Fig. 27.2 Association of bone mineral content (BMC) and cortical area (CA) with dietary potential renal acid load (PRAL) (1) using food-specific published data on methionine and cysteine content for PRAL calculation (reanalysis of the relationship) and (2) using the conventional PRAL estimate[28]

representation of the original findings ("old PRAL"). It is discernible that use of the more differentiated PRAL model based on the individual sulfate generation potential yielded no substantially different picture for the PRAL association than the previous calculation. Although one might have expected a clearer difference between both the approaches,[30] our observation of similar PRAL-bone relationships are in line with the fact that earlier diet studies using the conventional PRAL method had demonstrated almost accurate estimations of the actually excreted (biochemically analyzed) daily amounts of urinary sulfate in healthy adults on a lactovegetarian, a moderate protein, and a high protein diet.[7] Thus, it can be concluded that food-specific data on methionine and cysteine content possibly allow a more accurate calculation of the diet-induced NEAP for particular diets, for example, based on certain food preferences like fish or eggs. However, for common mixed diets, food-specific sulfur amino acid data appear not to be necessarily required to obtain reasonable PRAL estimates.

Apart from this, it must be kept in mind that the protein-mediated effects on bone become further complicated by the obviously contrasting influences of sulfur amino acid-dependent increases in dietary acid loads on one hand and concurrent bone-anabolic influences via an IGF-1 stimulating protein action on the other.[26,27] In this regard, it is so far not clear which proteins or amino acid combinations actually show the strongest IGF-1-related bone-anabolic impacts (independent of their acidity-related effects) and it cannot be excluded that just those proteins with higher methionine and cysteine contents might be most effective. For example, Larson et al[32] found almost significant trends for an association between either meat or fish intake and circulating IGF-1, but no trends for milk intake, whereas Hoppe et al[33] reported that milk intake, but not meat intake was positively associated with circulating IGF-I in healthy, well-nourished, 2.5-year-old children. A direct positive influence of milk protein on both IGF-1 plasma levels and bone mineral density has been impressively demonstrated by Schurch et al[27] in an intervention trial in elderly patients with osteoporotic hip fractures. These results and further studies[26,28] provide strong evidence that dietary protein exerts an important bone-anabolic influence and is hence a relevant nutritional contributor to bone strength.

27.4 Endogenous Steroid Hormones, Muscularity, and Dietary Influences on Diaphyseal Bone: Reexamination of Existing Measurement Data in Children

27.4.1 Adrenarchal Sex Steroids and Study Inclusion Criteria

Besides genetics, mechanical loads from muscle contraction, metabolic effects, and nutritional influences, also endocrine factors are major determinants of skeletal mineralization, bone mass, and bone strength. Sex hormones play an important role in the regulation of bone formation and bone turn-over. While androgens show an independent influence on bone formation, evidence is now overwhelming that also in males estrogens are responsible for a major part of the bone-anabolic impact of sex steroids.[34] Peripheral aromatase being present in adipose and other tissues in both the sexes

converts a substantial fraction of males' daily secreted testosterone to estradiol. Estrogens inhibit bone remodeling by concurrently suppressing osteoblastogenesis and osteoclastogenesis from marrow precursors.[34]

Sex steroids are also effective in children. Accordingly, positive associations between bone architecture or bone modeling and sex steroids have been observed during growth.[35,36] However, in childhood (i.e., in prepuberty), most of the sex steroid activity is derived from adrenal androgen secretion. During childhood, the adrenal cortex changes in size, cell distribution, and function and begins to secrete steadily increasing amounts of adrenal androgens, even a number of years before the onset of puberty.[37] This phenomenon is termed adrenarche. Adrenal C19 steroid secretion, principally dehydroepiandrosterone (DHEA) and its sulfate ester, continues to rise until the age of 20–30 years. DHEA can be readily converted to more potent sex steroids as estradiol and testosterone. One of DHEA's direct conversion products is androstenediol (Fig. 27.3). The enzymes 17β-hydroxysteroid dehydrogenase (17β-HSD) types 1, 3, and 5 catalyze not only the activation of sex hormone precursors (like androstenedione and Estrone) to testosterone and Estradiol,[38] but also the conversion of DHEA to androstenediol.[38,39] Androstenediol has been shown to exert clear sex steroid effects. Depending on the target tissue, androstenediol's transcriptional regulation of either the androgen or the estrogen receptor preponderates (Fig. 27.3) (for literature, see Remer et al[36]).

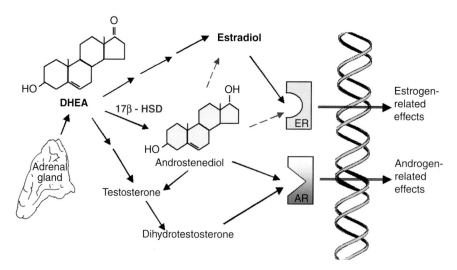

Fig. 27.3 Androstenediol – an androgenic and estrogenic sex steroid and its direct conversion from dehydroepiandrosterone (DHEA)

In healthy children, androstenediol or DHEA have been shown to be associated with bone modeling, independent of the important direct impact of muscularity (i.e., muscle forces) on bone structures. In studies of either dietary or hormonal influences on the proximal radius of children, the local bone-related muscularity – as reflected by pQCT-measured muscle area at the respective bone measurement site – showed the strongest association with most of the analyzed diaphyseal bone outcomes (cortical area (CA), BMC, polar strength strain index (SSI)).[28,35,36]

Until now, sex steroid- and muscularity-related effects on bone as well as dietary influences such as PRAL and protein intake have been studied separately, and a combined examination trying to analyze nutritional and hormonal covariates together is lacking. For this reason, we reanalyzed the existing data on adrenarchal hormone measurements, dietary PRAL, protein and mineral intakes of a group of healthy children for whom parallel data on pQCT measurements at the proximal forearm bone and muscle area were available. All the children included were participants of the DONALD Study. To eliminate potential confounding by increasing puberty-related estrogen levels, which until now could not be reliably and validly quantified in urine samples of children and adolescents, we only included prepubertal children ($n = 107$) (Tanner 1).

27.4.2 Aims and Methods

The aim of the present reexamination was to compare the potential influences of dietary factors with those of adrenarchal steroid hormones including the sex steroid androstenediol after accounting for local bone-related muscularity (Fig. 27.4).

Methodological details regarding steroid profiling, bone analysis, and nutritional examination in the DONALD Study were recently described in detail.[28,35–37,40]

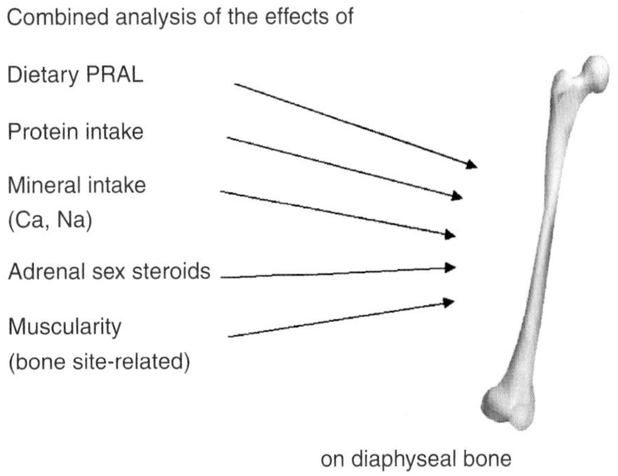

27.4.3 Results

Mean age, body weight, BMI standard deviation scores (BMI-SDS), and energy intake of the 107 prepubertal healthy DONALD participants (57 boys, 50 girls) were

Combined analysis of the effects of

Dietary PRAL

Protein intake

Mineral intake (Ca, Na)

Adrenal sex steroids

Muscularity (bone site-related)

on diaphyseal bone

Fig. 27.4 Study aims

8.6 (SD, 1.9) years, 31.0 (9.8) kg, −0.04 (0.95), and 6.1 (1.0) MJ, respectively. PRAL, protein, calcium, sodium, and soft drink intakes were found to average 9.0 (5.8) mEq/day, 2.0 (0.3) g/kg/day, 714.1 (165.6) mg/day, 1.5 (0.4) g/day, 123.2 (127.6) g/day, respectively. Daily excretion rates of androstenediol (14.0 (14.8) μg/day), total androgens (449.8 (515.6) μg/day), and immediate DHEA metabolites (DHEA&M)[35] (449.8 (515.6) μg/day) lay within the normal ranges as recently published.[37] BMC, CA, and SSI were 43.2 (12.4) mg/mm, 42.8 (10.9) mm^2, and 137.0 (46.3) mm^3, respectively.

In multiple regression analyses, we considered the following potential predictors or covariates in addition to local muscle area, dietary protein intake, and 24-h urinary hormone excretion: age, sex, fat-free mass index, fat mass index, soft drink consumption, intake of sodium, vitamin D, vitamin K, calcium, and PRAL. Variables were included stepwise starting with the block encompassing age, anthropometrics, and muscle area, followed by the nutritional variables and ending with androstenediol, C19, and DHEA&M.

In the final model, of all considered hormones only androstenediol remained significant (log SSI, $p < 0.01$; CA, $p < 0.001$; BMC, $p < 0.001$) with explained variations (R^2) of 2, 5, and 6%, respectively. Only after androstenediol was included, also protein intake, but no other dietary variable showed almost significant trends for CA ($p = 0.06$) and BMC ($p = 0.07$) with explained variations of 1% each. For all bone variables, muscle area explained most of the variation (R^2: 59–66%) ($p < 0.0001$).

To illustrate and compare the magnitude of the association of BMC and CA with daily androstenediol excretion and nutritional factors, log-values of androstenediol excretion, dietary protein density (gram protein intake/ MJ energy intake), and dietary calcium density (gram calcium intake/MJ energy intake) were grouped into three categories respectively: low (<25th percentile), medium (≥25th and ≤75th percentile), and high (>75th percentile). Linear regression models were used, adjusting for potential confounders, identified in the stepwise regression analyses. The adjusted geometric means of geometric means of the bone variables BMC and CA by categories of respective independent variables were predicted by the model when the other variables were held at their mean values. Figure 27.5 shows that the associations of androstenediol and energy-adjusted protein intake, but not energy-adjusted calcium intake, were significant for BMC and CA with almost comparable effect sizes for the hormone and protein intake.

27.4.4 Conclusions

Our results suggest that among the dietary influences on diaphyseal bone in prepubertal children, protein has the strongest impact and this is independent of muscularity and sex steroids. However, in this subgroup of prepubertal children, we did not observe an association between PRAL and bone variables.

As has been recently shown, the association of dietary PRAL with forearm bone is weaker than that of protein intake and it appears from our previous examination in 229 children and adolescents (in which hormones were not accounted for)[28] that the statistical power could have been too small in the current analysis to identify a significant PRAL-bone relationship. Another reason for not finding a significant association between dietary acidity and bone outcomes in our prepubertal DONALD subgroup could have been that overall variation of dietary PRAL in our sample was only moderate (Interquartil range: 5.4–12.2 mEq/day).

The explained variations (R^2) for protein intake (1%) of the bone variables BMC and CA which (among all nutritional factors considered) showed a trend for significance were clearly lower than the R^2 of the sex steroid androstenediol (5–6%). Despite this, our comparison of the bone-related effect sizes of androstenediol with the corresponding effect sizes of the

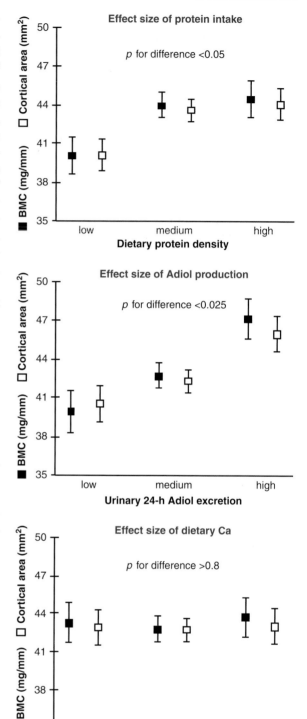

Fig. 27.5 BMC and CA by categories of protein intake, urinary 24-h androstenediol (Adiol) excretion, and Ca intake (means adjusted for muscle area and the respective other variables shown in the figure ± SEM)

bone-anabolic nutrient protein, give us an idea of the relative importance that diet has in comparison to endocrine factors both of which (diet and hormones) are relatively moderate in magnitude as compared to muscularity (data not shown).

Low explained variations of only a few percent are what researchers in nutritional science are frequently confronted with and they should be aware of it. However, nutritional behavior and diet affect bone health and other physiologically and pathophysiologically relevant outcomes in a sustained way in the long run. The importance of preventive long-term effects can best be assessed by examining the respective effect sizes of the dietary intakes of interest and not by their contributions to explained variation. The magnitude of the association (effect size) of diaphyseal bone parameters with protein intake is not that much less than the magnitude discernible for the sex steroid androstenediol. Therefore, minor explained variations of bone outcomes by dietary factors like protein intake (or PRAL[28]) must not be misinterpreted as clinically irrelevant in the long run. Nutritional prevention of reduced bone accretion and bone loss, although somewhat lower in magnitude than bone-anabolic hormonal influences, remains an important challenge.

References

1. Houillier P, Normand M, Froissart M, et al. Calciuric response to an acute acid load in healthy subjects and hypercalciuric calcium stone formers. *Kidney Int.* 1996;50:987-997.
2. Moe OW, Huang CL. Hypercalciuria from acid load: renal mechanisms. *J Nephrol.* 2006;19(suppl 9):S53-S61.
3. Krieger NS, Frick KK, Bushinsky DA. Mechanism of acid-induced bone resorption. *Curr Opin Nephrol Hypertens.* 2004;13:423-436.
4. Eaton SB, Eaton SB III. Paleolithic vs. modern diets–selected pathophysiological implications. *Eur J Nutr.* 2000;39:67-70.
5. Remer T, Manz F. Paleolithic diet, sweet potato eaters, and potential renal acid load. *Am J Clin Nutr.* 2003;78:802-803; author reply 803-804.
6. Remer T, Manz F. Potential renal acid load of foods and its influence on urine pH. *J Am Diet Assoc.* 1995;95:791-797.
7. Remer T, Manz F. Estimation of the renal net acid excretion by adults consuming diets containing variable amounts of protein. *Am J Clin Nutr.* 1994;59:1356-1361.
8. Eaton-Evans J, McIlrath EM, Jackson WE, et al. Dietary factors and vertebral bone density in perimenopausal women from a general medical practice in Northern Ireland. *Proc Nutr Soc.* 1993;52:44A.
9. Michaelsson K, Holmberg L, Mallmin H, et al. Diet, bone mass, and osteocalcin: a cross-sectional study. *Calcif Tissue Int.* 1995;57:86-93.
10. New SA, Bolton-Smith C, Grubb DA, et al. Nutritional influences on bone mineral density: a cross-sectional study in premenopausal women. *Am J Clin Nutr.* 1997;65:1831-1839.
11. Tucker KL, Hannan MT, Chen H, et al. Potassium, magnesium, and fruit and vegetable intakes are associated with greater bone mineral density in elderly men and women. *Am J Clin Nutr.* 1999;69:727-736.
12. New SA, Robins SP, Campbell MK, et al. Dietary influences on bone mass and bone metabolism: further evidence of a positive link between fruit and vegetable consumption and bone health? *Am J Clin Nutr.* 2000;71:142-151.
13. Jones G, Riley MD, Whiting S. Association between urinary potassium, urinary sodium, current diet, and bone density in prepubertal children. *Am J Clin Nutr.* 2001;73:839-844.
14. Chen Y, Ho SC, Lee R, et al. Fruit intake is associated with better bone mass among Hong Kong Chinese early postmenopausal women. *J Bone Miner Res.* 2001;16(suppl 1):S386.
15. Miller DR, Krall EA, Anderson JJ, et al. Dietary mineral intake and low bone mass in men: The VALOR Study. *J Bone Miner Res.* 2001;16(suppl 1):S395.
16. Stone KL, Blackwell T, Orwoll ES, et al. The relationship between diet and bone mineral density in older men. *J Bone Miner Res.* 2001;16(suppl 1):S388.
17. Tylavsky FA, Holliday K, Danish R, et al. Fruit and vegetable intakes are an independent predictor of bone size in early pubertal children. *Am J Clin Nutr.* 2004;79:311-317.
18. New SA, MacDonald HM, Campbell MK, et al. Lower estimates of net endogenous non-carbonic acid production are positively associated with indexes of bone health in premenopausal and perimenopausal women. *Am J Clin Nutr.* 2004;79:131-138.
19. McGartland CP, Robson PJ, Murray LJ, et al. Fruit and vegetable consumption and bone mineral density: the Northern Ireland Young Hearts Project. *Am J Clin Nutr.* 2004;80:1019-1023.
20. Macdonald HM, New SA, Fraser WD, et al. Low dietary potassium intakes and high dietary estimates of net endogenous acid production are associated with low bone mineral density in premenopausal women and increased markers of bone resorption in postmenopausal women. *Am J Clin Nutr.* 2005;81:923-933.
21. Hirota T, Kusu T, Hirota K. Improvement of nutrition stimulates bone mineral gain in Japanese school children and adolescents. *Osteoporos Int.* 2005;16:1057-1064.
22. Vatanparast H, Baxter-Jones A, Faulkner RA, et al. Positive effects of vegetable and fruit consumption and calcium intake on bone mineral accrual in boys during growth from childhood to adolescence: the University of Saskatchewan Pediatric Bone Mineral Accrual Study. *Am J Clin Nutr.* 2005;82:700-706.
23. Chen YM, Ho SC, Woo JL. Greater fruit and vegetable intake is associated with increased bone mass among postmenopausal Chinese women. *Br J Nutr.* 2006;96:745-751.
24. Prynne CJ, Mishra GD, O'Connell MA, et al. Fruit and vegetable intakes and bone mineral status: a cross sectional study in 5 age and sex cohorts. *Am J Clin Nutr.* 2006;83:1420-1428.

25. Welch AA, Bingham SA, Reeve J, et al. More acidic dietary acid-base load is associated with reduced calcaneal broadband ultrasound attenuation in women but not in men: results from the EPIC-Norfolk cohort study. *Am J Clin Nutr.* 2007;85:1134-1141.

26. Heaney RP, Layman DK. Amount and type of protein influences bone health. *Am J Clin Nutr.* 2008;87:1567S-1570S.

27. Schurch MA, Rizzoli R, Slosman D, et al. Protein supplements increase serum insulin-like growth factor-I levels and attenuate proximal femur bone loss in patients with recent hip fracture. A randomized, double-blind, placebo-controlled trial. *Ann Intern Med.* 1998;128:801-809.

28. Alexy U, Remer T, Manz F, et al. Long-term protein intake and dietary potential renal acid load are associated with bone modeling and remodeling at the proximal radius in healthy children. *Am J Clin Nutr.* 2005;82:1107-1114.

29. U.S. Department of Agriculture. National Nutrient Database for Standard Reference; 2009. Available at: http://www.nal.usda.gov/fnic/foodcomp/search/. Accessed June 19, 2009.

30. Frassetto LA, Morris RC Jr, Sebastian A. A practical approach to the balance between acid production and renal acid excretion in humans. *J Nephrol.* 2006;19(suppl 9):S33-S40.

31. Souci SW, Fachmann W, Kraut H. *Die Zusammensetzung der Lebensmittel. Nährwert-Tabellen.* Stuttgart: Medpharm Scientific Publishers; 1994.

32. Larsson SC, Wolk K, Brismar K, et al. Association of diet with serum insulin-like growth factor I in middle-aged and elderly men. *Am J Clin Nutr.* 2005;81:1163-1167.

33. Hoppe C, Udam TR, Lauritzen L, et al. Animal protein intake, serum insulin-like growth factor I, and growth in healthy 2.5-y-old Danish children. *Am J Clin Nutr.* 2004;80:447-452.

34. Syed F, Khosla S. Mechanisms of sex steroid effects on bone. *Biochem Biophys Res Commun.* 2005;328:688-696.

35. Remer T, Boye KR, Hartmann M, et al. Adrenarche and bone modeling and remodeling at the proximal radius: weak androgens make stronger cortical bone in healthy children. *J Bone Miner Res.* 2003;18:1539-1546.

36. Remer T, Manz F, Hartmann MF, et al. Prepubertal healthy children's urinary androstenediol predicts diaphyseal bone strength in late puberty. *J Clin Endocrinol Metab.* 2009;94:575-578.

37. Remer T, Boye KR, Hartmann MF, et al. Urinary markers of adrenarche: reference values in healthy subjects aged 3–18 years. *J Clin Endocrinol Metab.* 2005;90:2015-2021.

38. Luu-The V. Analysis and characteristics of multiple types of human 17 beta-hydroxysteroid dehydrogenase. *J Steroid Biochem Mol Biol.* 2001;76:143-151.

39. Labrie F, Luu-The V, Lin SX, et al. Role of 17 beta-hydroxysteroid dehydrogenases in sex steroid formation in peripheral intracrine tissues. *Trends Endocrinol Metab.* 2000;11:421-427.

40. Libuda L, Alexy U, Remer T, et al. Association between long-term consumption of soft drinks and variables of bone modeling and remodeling in a sample of healthy German children and adolescents. *Am J Clin Nutr.* 2008;88:1670-1677.

Salt Sensitivity, Metabolic Acidosis, and Bone Health

28

Lynda A. Frassetto, Olga Schmidlin, and Anthony Sebastian

28.1 Introduction

The potential link between dietary sodium chloride (NaCl), hypertension, and osteoporosis has been speculated upon for years. Increased NaCl intake is associated with increases in blood pressure both in metabolic balance studies and in population studies.

Acute NaCl infusions and increased diet NaCl induce a hyperchloremic metabolic acidosis. Accumulating clinical and epidemiologic data suggest that chronic low-grade diet and age-related metabolic acidosis increase bone resorption and loss of bone mass.

Acute NaCl loading inhibits endothelial nitric oxide synthase (NOS) in a dose-dependent manner in cell systems and transfected cell lines. Asymmetric dimethylarginine (ADMA) also inhibits the conversion of L-arginine to nitric oxide (NO). NO is a direct vasodilator, and decreases in NO production are associated with higher blood pressures.

Persons, who are particularly sensitive to salt, generally defined as an increase in mean arterial pressure of three to five mmHg after an increase in dietary salt intake, have increased levels of ADMA (resulting in less NO production) and increased urinary calcium excretion compared to salt resistant subjects. In cohort studies, subjects at risk for salt sensitivity, such as those with metabolic syndrome, are more likely to have lower bone mineral density (BMD) and a higher incidence of osteoporotic fractures.

Those considerations raise the possibility that salt sensitivity is the key to predicting who, on a high NaCl diet, would be particularly prone to developing not only high blood pressure, but increased bone breakdown, which can predispose to osteoporosis.

28.2 NaCl, Metabolic Acidosis, and Bone

In in vitro studies, metabolic acidosis activates osteoclasts and bone resorption, deactivates osteoblasts and bone mineralization, and increases calcium loss from bone as the systemic pH decreases.[1,2] Bushinsky et al elegantly demonstrated in mouse calvarie that calcium efflux from bone dose-dependently increases as the systemic pH and plasma bicarbonate concentration decrease, whether the bone cells are alive, dead, or stimulated with PTH or vitamin D. This group has also recently shown that OGR-1 is the proton-sensing receptor on the *osteoblasts* that induces activation of the *osteoclasts* in a high acid environment.[3]

Cross-sectional analyses of human metabolic balance studies demonstrate that increased ingestion of dietary NaCl is independently associated with lower steady-state blood pH (increased acid levels) and lower steady-state plasma bicarbonate levels within the range considered to be clinically normal, (viz. a low-grade chronic metabolic acidosis) compared with the ingestion of a lower dietary NaCl intake.[4] This effect is independent of the diet, net acid load, renal function, and the partial pressure of carbon dioxide, the three other variables that have been shown to regulate systemic pH and bicarbonate.

The dose-dependent acid–base effects of NaCl are even more pronounced in salt-sensitive rats.[5] Batlle et al demonstrated in Dahl/Rapp salt-sensitive and salt-resistant rats that not only urine net acid excretion (NAE) increased

L.A. Frassetto (✉)
UCSF campus box 0126,
505 Parnassus Ave,rm M1202, San Francisco,
CA 94143, USA
e-mail: frassett@gcrc.ucsf.edu

P. Burckhardt et al. (eds.), *Nutritional Influences on Bone Health*,
DOI: 10.1007/978-1-84882-978-7_28, © Springer-Verlag London Limited 2010

as NaCl intake increased, but also the NAE increases in the salt-sensitive rats was significantly greater than in the salt-resistant rats *at all levels of salt intake.* In other words, the salt-sensitive rats had more of a metabolic acidosis with any salt intake than the salt-resistant rats.

More recently, a small prospective study in young healthy subjects has demonstrated that dietary NaCl increases this low-grade chronic metabolic acidosis in a dose-dependent fashion and this is associated with significant dose-dependent increases in urinary excretion of calcium and bone resorption markers such as C-telopeptide.[6] Sharma et al has also shown that salt-sensitive humans had significantly lower blood pH and plasma bicarbonate levels on high salt diets compared to salt-resistant subjects.[7] Whether salt-sensitive subjects have a higher incidence of osteoporosis and fractures would be predicted, but has not been prospectively demonstrated.

28.3 NaCl and Nitric Oxide Synthesis

NO is generated from L-arginine by the enzyme NOS. Vascular endothelial cell-produced NO is a direct vasodilator, leading to decreased blood pressure. Recently, NaCl has also been shown to dose-dependently decrease endogenous nitric oxide synthase (eNOS) activity in both bovine aortic endothelial cells (BAEC) as well as transfected Chinese hamster ovarian cells (CHO-eNOS).[8] The phosphate salt of sodium also dose-dependently decreased eNOS activity.

ADMA, which derives from the methylation of arginine residues in proteins, is a competitive inhibitor of eNOS; increases in ADMA inhibit NO-related vasodilation, leading to increased blood pressure. In 13 salt-sensitive normotensive subjects, Fang el al. demonstrated significantly higher mean blood pressures and ADMA levels on a high salt diet, compared to a low salt diet and compared to 47 salt-resistant subjects on either salt diet.[9]

28.4 Nitric Oxide and Bone

Nitrates are metabolized to NO by multiple factors, including thiol compounds, deoxyhemoglobin in erythrocytes, and enzymes in the cytochrome P450 system.

More recently, the mitochondrial isoform of aldolase dehydrogenase, ALDH-2, has been shown to be a high affinity metabolic pathway for nitrate precursors of NO.[10] Interestingly, several recent clinical studies have suggested that giving nitrates will improve BMD.[11,12] A recent comparison study by Nabhan and Rabie demonstrated in 60 postmenopausal women with osteoporosis that 12 months treatment with isosorbide dinitrate 20 mg three times a day was as effective as alendronate 70 mg weekly in improving BMD and DEXA *T*-score (10.8 vs. 12.1% respectively; $p<0.05$ for each within group increase, $p=0.7$ for between group differences).[11]

NOS have been demonstrated in both osteoclasts and osteoblasts.[13,14] Rats that are deficient in the eNOS gene have significant reduction in bone formation.[15] NO produced by bone cells may play an important role in mechanical strain-induced bone remodeling.[16]

NO may also be the mediator by which estrogen or androgen therapy improves BMD. Studies in castrated or oophorectomized rats with decreases in BMD after surgery had equivalent improvements in BMD when either nitrates or hormone replacement therapy was given.[12,17] Preoperatively treating the rats with the NOS blocker L-NAME prevented the loss of BMD seen in the sex-steroid-deficient rats not given L-NAME.[17]

28.5 Salt Sensitivity and Bone Metabolism

From the previous paragraphs, dietary NaCl might be expected to adversely affect bone metabolism through two pathogenetic pathways: by inducing a low-grade metabolic acidosis and by inhibiting NO production. The data also suggest that these effects will be seen especially in those subjects who are salt sensitive. Schmidlin et al studied the effects of NaCl intake in 25 salt-sensitive (SS) and salt-resistant (SR) normotensive subjects on ADMA production and urine calcium excretion on both a low (30 mmol/day) salt and a high (250 mmol/day) diet in a 2 week crossover metabolic balance study. NaCl loading significantly increased ADMA only in the SS group, $p=0.007$. ADMA levels were significantly correlated with urine calcium excretion only in the salt-sensitive group ($R^2=0.47, p=0.02$), with no correlation in the SR group ($R^2=0.03, p=0.57$).[18]

Studies suggest that subjects with risk factors for the metabolic syndrome are also more likely to be salt sensitive. Chen et al studied 1,881 subjects in northern China and evaluated them for salt sensitivity as well as the presence of markers for the metabolic syndrome; dyslipidemia, abdominal obesity, hyperglycemia, and elevated blood pressure. After adjustment for age, sex, education, physical activity, cigarette smoking, body mass index, and 24-h urinary sodium and potassium excretion, there was a progressive increase in the relative risk for salt sensitivity as the number of risk factors for metabolic syndrome increased (four or five factors; OR 3.54, CI 2.05–6.11).[19] Metabolic syndrome has been associated with lower urine pH values[20] and lower NO levels.[21] Analyses from several large cohort studies have demonstrated in both older men and women an association between metabolic syndrome, lower BMD, and an increased risk of nonvertebral fractures,[22] and between lower BMD and type 2 diabetes.[23,24]

Conversely, subjects who are insensitive to salt, such as those with mutations leading to renal salt wasting, might be expected to have less salt-induced bone resorption. Cruz et al have shown that subjects who are homozygous for the NCCT mutation (of the thiazide sensitive Na–Cl transporter in the distal tubule in the kidney) have significantly higher serum bicarbonate levels, lower urine calcium excretion associated with higher urine Na excretion, and higher BMDs than subjects who are heterozygous for the mutation, and both the groups are higher than the subjects who are homozygous for the wild-type alleles.[25]

28.6 Common Final Pathway?

Are the two pathogenetic pathways interrelated? Is there a relationship between metabolic acidosis and NO synthesis? Studies by Mitch et al over the last decade have demonstrated that in muscle cells metabolic acidosis inhibits the signaling pathway for insulin and IGF-1, leading to decreased intracellular phosphoinositol-3-kinase (PI3K) activity, which in turn leads to activation of nuclear factors, caspase-3 activity, and increased protein degradation.[26] In endothelial cells, IGF-1 is the receptor that activates PI3K leading to increased NO synthesis.[27]

NaCl, then, might in fact have a "double whammy" effect on bone; (1) by inducing a metabolic acidosis and (2) by inhibiting NO production, the latter resulting perhaps separately from metabolic acidosis (inhibiting IGF-1 signaling) and salt loading (enhancing ADMA levels). Those subjects who are particularly sensitive to the effects of NaCl would be those most likely to demonstrate increased bone break down and decreased BMD. This formulation would help strengthen the previously speculated upon but unproven positive association of hypertension and osteoporosis, and perhaps other metabolic diseases, such as diabetes and metabolic syndrome, and osteoporosis.

28.7 Conclusions

Osteoporosis is a disease of multifactoral origin significantly affected by dietary intake. Whether table salt (NaCl) is a factor has been difficult to extrapolate; some studies suggest that it is, while others do not.[28]

In this manuscript, we have reviewed how metabolic acidosis increases bone breakdown, increasing dietary NaCl intake induces a low-grade metabolic acidosis, and rats and humans who are salt-sensitive have a significantly increased metabolic acidosis compared to those who are not salt sensitive.

In addition, we have reviewed how increasing NaCl intake dose-dependently inhibits endothelial NOS, increases ADMA production, and increases urinary calcium excretion, a potential marker of bone breakdown. Exogenous replacement of NO has been shown to improve BMD in surgically castrated rats and postmenopausal women.

Finally, we suggest that subjects with metabolic syndrome may be prone to salt sensitivity. Subjects with metabolic syndrome tend to have lower urine pH levels, and metabolic syndrome is associated in multiple cohort studies with increased risk for lower BMD and osteoporotic fractures.

In conclusion, salt sensitivity imposes a "double jeopardy" on bone by exaggerating the dose-dependent NaCl-induced metabolic acidosis and reducing NO levels, possibly mediated in part through the effects of metabolic acidosis on IGF-1 receptors.

References

1. Arnett TR, Dempster DW. Effect of pH on bone resorption by rat osteoclasts in vitro. *Endocrinology*. 1986;119(1):119-124.

2. Frick KK, Bushinsky DA. Chronic metabolic acidosis reversibly inhibits extracellular matrix gene expression in mouse osteoblasts. *Am J Physiol*. 1998;275(5 pt 2):F840-F847.

3. Frick KK, Krieger NS, Nehrke K, Bushinsky DA. Metabolic acidosis increases intracellular calcium in bone cells through activation of the proton receptor OGR1. *J Bone Miner Res*. 2009;24(2):305-313.

4. Frassetto LA, Morris RC Jr, Sebastian A. Dietary sodium chloride intake independently predicts the degree of hyperchloremic metabolic acidosis in healthy humans consuming a net acid-producing diet. *Am J Physiol Renal Physiol*. 2007; 293(2):F521-F525.

5. Batlle DC, Sharma AM, Alsheikha MW, Sobrero M, Saleh A, Gutterman C. Renal acid excretion and intracellular pH in salt-sensitive genetic hypertension. *J Clin Invest*. 1993;91(5): 2178-2184.

6. Frings-Meuthen P, Baecker N, Heer M. Low-grade metabolic acidosis may be the cause of sodium chloride-induced exaggerated bone resorption. *J Bone Miner Res*. 2008;23(4): 517-524.

7. Sharma AM, Kribben A, Schattenfroh S, Cetto C, Distler A. Salt sensitivity in humans is associated with abnormal acid-base regulation. *Hypertension*. 1990;16(4):407-413.

8. Li J, White J, Guo L, et al. Salt inactivates endothelial nitric oxide synthase in endothelial cells. *J Nutr*. 2009;139(3): 447-451.

9. Fang Y, Mu JJ, He LC, Wang SC, Liu ZQ. Salt loading on plasma asymmetrical dimethylarginine and the protective role of potassium supplement in normotensive salt-sensitive Asians. *Hypertension*. 2006;48(4):724-729.

10. Daiber A, Wenzel P, Oelze M, Münzel T. New insights into bioactivation of organic nitrates, nitrate tolerance and cross-tolerance. *Clin Res Cardiol*. 2008;97(1):12-20.

11. Nabhan AF, Rabie NH. Isosorbide mononitrate versus alendronate for postmenopausal osteoporosis. *Int J Gynaecol Obstet*. 2008;103(3):213-216.

12. Wimalawansa SJ. Rationale for using nitric oxide donor therapy for prevention of bone loss and treatment of osteoporosis in humans. *Ann N Y Acad Sci*. 2007;1117:283-297.

13. Kasten TP, Collin-Osdoby P, Patel N, et al. Potentiation of osteoclast bone-resorption activity by inhibition of nitric oxide synthase. *Proc Natl Acad Sci USA*. 1994;91(9): 3569-3573.

14. Löwik CW, Nibbering PH, van de Ruit M, Papapoulos SE. Inducible production of nitric oxide in osteoblast-like cells and in fetal mouse bone explants is associated with suppression of osteoclastic bone resorption. *J Clin Invest*. 1994; 93(4):1465-1472.

15. Aguirre J, Buttery L, O'Shaughnessy M, et al. Endothelial nitric oxide synthase gene-deficient mice demonstrate marked retardation in postnatal bone formation, reduced bone volume, and defects in osteoblast maturation and activity. *Am J Pathol*. 2001;158(1):247-257.

16. Pitsillides AA, Rawlinson SC, Suswillo RF, Bourrin S, Zaman G, Lanyon LE. Mechanical strain-induced NO production by bone cells: a possible role in adaptive bone (re) modeling? *FASEB J*. 1995;9(15):1614-1622.

17. Wimalawansa SJ. Restoration of ovariectomy-induced osteopenia by nitroglycerin. *Calcif Tissue Int*. 2000;66(1): 56-60.

18. Frassetto L, Schmidlin O, Sebastian A. Is salt sensitivity the link between hypertension and osteoporosis? In: *Seventh ISNAO conference*, Lausanne/Switzerland; 2009:abstract.

19. Chen J, Gu D, Huang J, et al. GenSalt Collaborative Research Group. Metabolic syndrome and salt sensitivity of blood pressure in non-diabetic people in China: a dietary intervention study. *Lancet*. 2009;373:829-835.

20. Maalouf NM, Cameron MA, Moe OW, Adams-Huet B, Sakhaee K. Low urine pH: a novel feature of the metabolic syndrome. *Clin J Am Soc Nephrol*. 2007;2(5):883-888.

21. Barylski M, Kowalczyk E, Banach M, Ciecwierz J, Pawlicki L, Kowalski J. Plasma total antioxidant activity in comparison with plasma NO and VEGF levels in patients with metabolic syndrome. *Angiology*. 2009;60(1):87-92.

22. von Muhlen D, Safii S, Jassal SK, Svartberg J, Barrett-Connor E. Associations between the metabolic syndrome and bone health in older men and women: the Rancho Bernardo Study. *Osteoporos Int*. 2007;18(10):1337-1344.

23. Yaturu S, Humphrey S, Landry C, Jain SK. Decreased bone mineral density in men with metabolic syndrome alone and with type 2 diabetes. *Med Sci Monit*. 2009;15(1):CR5-CR9.

24. de Liefde II, van der Klift M, de Laet CE, van Daele PL, Hofman A, Pols HA. Bone mineral density and fracture risk in type-2 diabetes mellitus: the Rotterdam Study. *Osteoporos Int*. 2005;16(12):1713-1720.

25. Cruz DN. The renal tubular Na-Cl co-transporter (NCCT): a potential genetic link between blood pressure and bone density? *Nephrol Dial Transplant*. 2001;16(4):691-694.

26. Rajan VR, Mitch WE. Muscle wasting in chronic kidney disease: the role of the ubiquitin proteasome system and its clinical impact. *Pediatr Nephrol*. 2008;23(4):527-535.

27. Symons JD, McMillin SL, Riehle C, et al. Contribution of insulin and Akt1 signaling to endothelial nitric oxide synthase in the regulation of endothelial function and blood pressure. *Circ Res*. 2009;104(9):1085-1094.

28. Teucher B, Fairweather-Tait S. Dietary sodium as a risk factor for osteoporosis: where is the evidence? *Proc Nutr Soc*. 2003;62(4):859-866.

Index